During the time of writing this book, I have had the great pleasure of serving on the Executive Board of the American Veterinary Medical Association, including one year as Chair. This experience has truly been a highlight. Many people and organizations have supported me in this experience. These included friends who encouraged me to run, voted for me, supported my efforts in several ways, presented me with opinions and challenges, cared for my animals, and helped me survive the work that never ceased to pile up. They also included colleagues and staff members at Texas A&M, AVMA, Texas VMA, Arkansas VMA, Louisiana VMA, and others. To all of you I dedicate this book.

Feline Behavior

A Guide for Veterinarians

Second Edition

Bonnie V. Beaver, DVM, MS, Dipl. ACVB
Department of Small Animal Medicine and Surgery
College of Veterinary Medicine
Texas A&M University
College Station, Texas

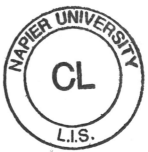

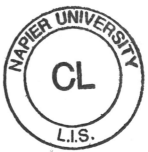
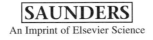
SAUNDERS
An Imprint of Elsevier Science

SAUNDERS

An Imprint of Elsevier Science

11830 Westline Industrial Drive
St. Louis, Missouri 63146

FELINE BEHAVIOR: A GUIDE
FOR VETERINARIANS, SECOND EDITION

ISBN   0-7216-9498-5

NOTICE

Veterinary Medicine is an ever-changing field. Standard safety precautions must be followed, but as new research and clinical experience broaden our knowledge, changes in treatment and drug therapy may become necessary or appropriate. Readers are advised to check the most current product information provided by the manufacturer of each drug to be administered to verify the recommended dose, the method and duration of administration, and contraindications. It is the responsibility of the licensed prescriber, relying on experience and knowledge of the patient, to determine dosages and the best treatment for each individual patient. Neither the publisher nor the author assumes any liability for any injury and/or damage to persons or property arising from this publication.

Previous edition copyrighted 1992.

Some material previously published in *Veterinary Aspects of Feline Behavior.*
© 1980, Mosby, Inc. All Rights Reserved.

International Standard Book Number 0-7216-9498-5

Acquisitions Editor: Ray Kersey
Developmental Editor: Denise LeMelledo
Project Manager: Joy Moore
Designer: Julia Dummitt
Cover Design: Paula Ruckenbrod

Printed in the United States of America.

Last digit is the print number: 9   8   7   6   5   4   3   2   1

Preface

Cats have long been a creature of mystery and fascination. People tend to either love them or hate them. Until recently, little was written about the cat's general behaviors because the animal was simply considered to be a farm-variety mobile mousetrap. Now that they have purred their way into our hearts, they have remained less understood than perhaps they should. The partnership between humans and cats is now resulting in our clients asking "why" about a number of different observations. The uniqueness of this species makes the cat somewhat difficult to really understand. In the past cats have served as models for neurologic research, to learn more about humans. Finally we are studying cats to learn more about cats.

Veterinary practices are changing, with behavior problems becoming an important aspect of client and patient service. Owners expect to have their furry friends around for a long time and demand the best in nutrition, health care, and behavioral medicine. The latter is not just drug therapy; it includes preventive measures, diagnostic procedures, and behavioral modification, too. The importance of providing behavioral health care for patients is a win-win-win opportunity for a veterinarian, his or her client, and the cat.

For veterinarians and cat enthusiasts with a special interest in feline behavior, information has been particularly hard to find, as it is widely scattered and difficult to locate, even with access to a large library. In addition, the internet has provided as much bad advice as it has good. How can one determine which information is based on science and which is not worth reading? Researchers have also had a difficult time determining exactly what work has been done.

Working with feline behavior problems remains both an art and science, but the importance of it and the resources to accomplish it have grown tremendously since the first edition of this book was published in 1980. Interestingly, however, the curriculum of most veterinary colleges does not include behavior to any significant extent, so new graduates must seek continuing education opportunities and reliable publications in order to serve their patients.

The original version of this book, *Veterinary Aspects of Feline Behavior*, was written for several reasons: (1) to describe the cat's behavior and its changing role for humans, (2) to provide the practicing veterinarian with important information on how to treat feline behavior problems, (3) to collect a bibliography for those interested in pursuing specific areas of interest, (4) to bring together diffuse information to portray the complete felid, and (5) to provide a reference of origin from which feline behaviorists may build. Additional information has been learned about cat behavior, and new treatments continue to be developed for feline behavior problems. The discipline has evolved to the point that several veterinarians are now board certified in the American College of Veterinary Behaviorists. These changes and challenges keep veterinary medicine fun.

I would like to thank Drs. Richard Adams and David Williams for their encouragement and support. It takes good people in the right places to help a new discipline develop. Support from my colleagues Drs. Deb Zoran, Lore Haug, and Amanda Florsheim; Ms. Nini Binkley-Hodges, Patty Hug, Linda Knight, Liz Kelley, and other members of the Department of Small Animal Medicine and Surgery has been really appreciated. I am especially appreciative of the veterinarians and their dedicated cat-owning clients throughout the country for their referrals and valuable input. Thanks, too, goes to Ray Kersey at W.B. Saunders.

Bonnie V. Beaver

Contents

1

Introduction to Feline Behavior

HISTORY OF FELINE DEVELOPMENT

Earliest Origins of the Cat

The earliest known ancestors of the Felidae date back 45,000,000 years. Carnivores are believed to have shared at that time a common forest-dwelling ancestor: the Miacidae. The cat was derived from a later subdivision, the *Dinictis*. Approximately 8,000,000 to 10,000,000 years ago, the feline branch with the cat's closest relatives separated from that which gave rise to the modern large cats.[34,150,240] Today it is generally accepted that the modern cat, *Felis catus,* is derived from *Felis libyca,* the Kaffir cat (also known as the *small African bush cat, African wildcat,* and *Caffre cat*), which was numerous in Egypt at that time. The role played by the European wildcat *Felis silvestris* in the development of the modern cat is uncertain, although it is known to have separated from the other small cat branch before *F. libyca.*[240] Some contend that *F. silvestris* (formerly called *F. catus*) was crossed with the Egyptian cat to produce the modern *F. catus* (formerly called *Felis domestica*), whereas others give behavioral, cultural, and physical reasons to refute this theory. Another theory is that the two wild types are actually subspecies (*F. silvestris silvestris* and *F. silvestris libyca*), because the domestic and wild variations have identical karyotypes.[33,186] Molecular studies show a close lineage between the domestic cat and five wildcats, including *F. libyca.*[34,150,240]

Through the ages the human's relationship with the cat has been a curious one. This relation, more inconsistent than that between humans and any other domestic animal, has nurtured the behavior of the modern cat. It is not known when the cat was first considered domesticated. What is recorded is that by 1600 BC cats were domesticated in Egypt.

Spread of the Cat from Ancient Egypt

In ancient Egypt the cat was originally kept to control rodents on farms and in granaries. Later, cats were also used to fish and to hunt and retrieve wild birds. The Egyptian word for cat, *mau,* means "to see." As time passed, the cat came to be associated with religion.

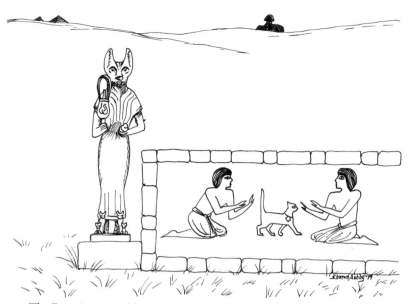

Figure 1-1 The Egyptian cat goddess Bastet.

The belief that a cat could see into the soul is tied to the fascination with cat eyes.[138] Bastet (also called Bast, Bassett), the cat goddess, daughter of the sun god Re, represented the fertility of plants and women, as well as good health (Figure 1-1). As Bastet became the primary goddess, the cat became a prized animal—legally protected, mourned over at death by the owner shaving his eyebrows, and mummified for burial in special cemeteries.

Spread of the domesticated cat occurred slowly, possibly because of tight export restrictions, which limited emigration to the individual cat's own travels.[10,186,213,248] Eventually merchants and soldiers introduced *F. catus* to Asia and Europe, so between 300 and 500 AD the cat is known to have reached Britain. Evaluation of water trade routes and feline populations shows that water posed no problem to migration. The orange genetic allele, which originated in Southeast Asia and India, can be traced as it moved westward.[138] Therefore, the cats probably traveled by ship, coming and going as they pleased.[225] In the Orient, cats were revered for their ability to foresee storms at sea and Mi-Ke (calico) cats ensured a safe voyage as symbols of good luck.[138]

Because Mohammed's favorite animal was the cat, it has always enjoyed favor in Islamic countries. Islamic teachings include specific references to punishment for the harsh treatment of cats and other animals.[54] However, Christianity's treatment of this animal has had a more profound effect on its course of behavioral development. When first introduced into Europe, the cat was believed to have protected the Christ child in the stable from the Devil's mouse.[10] As time passed, the independent nature of the cat and its prominent eyes led to its association with Diana, the moon goddess (Figure 1-2).[96] Legend says she created the cat to mock the sun god Apollo.[10] This association of cats with the moon led to the connection of the cat with the Devil and witchcraft.[62,207] During the Middle Ages, not only were vast numbers of cats exterminated,

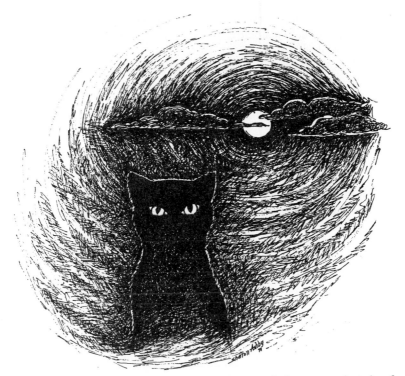

Figure 1-2 Prominent eyes led to the association of the cat with the moon and witchcraft.

but the same fate was met by individuals showing compassion for them. As the European Crusaders returned around 1600 AD, they brought with them an invasion of the brown rat, the plague, and a gradual reacceptance of the only effective rat-control method—the cat. They lived in monasteries to protect manuscripts from rodents. As a result of monk preferences in type, color, and coat, certain breeds were established, including the Korat and Chartreux.[138] Introduction into North America came in the seventeenth century, probably because the cat served as the principal method of rodent control on British vessels bound for the New World. Along with the cat, however, came the witchcraft cult.[62]

When Pasteur discovered microbes in the 1800s, people became extremely conscious of cleanliness. By another twist of fate, the cat came to be considered the only clean animal and was allowed in food markets, acquiring a position of favor by merchants.[62,178]

Domestication of the Cat

Domestication is a process requiring several generations of selective breeding to produce physiologic, morphologic, and/or behavioral changes.[66,109] It is not known how long this process might take. In foxes dramatic changes occurred in 20 generations[135,142]; however, 24 generations in cats did not result in significant differences in the reverse process.[231] For *F. catus* the domestication process has been unique. There has been recent discussion about whether cats may have undergone "self-domestication." This is, humans played little or no role in the changes except allowing cats near them for a better chance for survival and reproductive success. It is more likely humans did play a role that gradually became more significant. Except for the cat, breeding during domestication of most animals had been done by selection of behavioral characteristics, which are more quantitative than qualitative.[179] Response thresholds are heightened, and the resulting behavior is generally an increase in gentleness or ease in training. The cat, however, was first brought into the home for religious reasons, not utilitarian ones.[120,241] Cats followed the urbanization of human populations, so mating was a matter of proximity rather than human selection.[207,226] Not only was it difficult to control mating in cats, but the religious connotation prohibited selective breeding. The date given of domestication varies from 100 BC to as early as 7000 BC, but several infer that even now the cat is not fully domesticated because it can revert to total self-sufficiency.[138,186] The time from ancient Egypt to the present may represent as few as 4000 generations with a constant infusion of genes from uncontrolled populations. Only the small group of purebred cats had true selective breeding,[20] and these are mainly for physical features.[93] The first recorded planned feline breeding did not occur until 999 AD at the Japanese Imperial Palace. It soon became fashionable in that country to control cat matings and environments. With cats under tight control mice devastated the silkworm industry, so by 1602 Japanese cats were again released from these controls.[178]

Although the cat fell from favor and met with mass extermination in Europe, selective breeding was of course not practiced. Even with the Crusaders helping its return to favor, the atmosphere was one of tolerance rather than full acceptance. Historically, then, it took many years before the cat achieved a position in which selective breeding could help develop the behavioral characteristics desired in a domesticated animal.

CURRENT STATUS OF THE FELID

Cat Population Statistics

In recent years there has been a dramatic increase in the number of cats, especially registered cats, in the United States, partly because of their adaptability to apartments and small homes. Exact population figures vary greatly and are inaccurate because of the wild population, but it has been estimated that the cat population numbers from 23,100,000 to 61,000,000.* In the United States 23% of households have at least one cat.[220] Sixty-six percent of cat owners have only one cat,[222] but associated figures estimate 1.4 to 2.2 cats for each house having cats, or 1 cat in every 3.2 single-family dwelling units.† Of this cat population less than 80% are seen annually by veterinarians.‡

The modern cat's lifestyle tends to fall into one of four categories: (1) feral, independent "wildlife," totally ignored by people; (2) feral and interdependent free-roaming or unowned with dependence to humans limited to food; (3) domesticated, interdependent, and free-roaming or loosely owned, such as abandoned pets; and (4) domesticated

---

*References 1, 5, 6, 50, 74, 145, 173, 175, 232, 242.
†References 5, 6, 50, 51, 68, 117, 125, 129, 147, 175, 206, 222, 232, 233, 242.
‡References 5, 6, 74, 102, 145, 174, 220, 232.

household pets.[138] Of this owned group, only 14% of the cats are purebred,[197] compared with 61% of owned dogs.[222] The population is also relatively young, with 11% younger than 1 year, 49% being 1 to 6 years, 27% being 7 to 12 years, and 10% older than 12 years.[197,222]

The number of stray cats has been estimated at between 2% and 28% of the known population.[72,133,147] Whereas 415 humans are born every hour in the United States, 100 to 2000 kittens are born per hour.[55] The significance of this is that at least 30,000 cats must die per day just to maintain a stable population. At the end of a 1-year period 18% to 30% of cats are no longer in their original home.[125,169,196] After 3 years two thirds are no longer in their first home.

An excess population comprises those animals that are available and adoptable but for which no home can be found.[224] Each year as many as 20% of a city's pet population may pass through its animal shelter.[173] An estimated 4 to 9 million cats die each year in these shelters.[7,94,127,151,170] Of all cats euthanized in shelters, 18% to 33% die because of behavior problems.[71,125,137,193,227] At least 28% of cats relinquished to animal shelters are there because of behavior problems.[192] The top four problems cited include housesoiling, problems between pets, aggression toward humans, and destructive behaviors.[192] Interestingly, the presence of at least one other pet in the home dramatically increases the likelihood of relinquishment for behavior problems to approximately 70%, a trend that has been especially true if a new pet was added during the preceding year.[192]

The surplus cat population is related to the cat's reproductive efficiency and cat owners' attitudes. Although most of the U.S. population believes that something should be done about pet overpopulation, most cat owners claim their own litters "just happen."[94] Half believe controlling reproduction is the pet owner's responsibility, but a lot of ignorance remains about the necessity of neutering. People who relinquish cats to animal shelters are significantly more likely to believe a female should have a litter before being neutered and to be ignorant about the estrous cycle compared with cat owners who keep their cat.[148] They also are more likely to believe that cats exhibit behaviors for "spite," to not understand normal play behaviors, and to feel the number of cats in a home does not relate to the incidence of problems.[148]

In 7 years one female cat can be responsible for the birth of up to 781,250 kittens.[127,151,224] In 7.9% of cat-owning households at least one litter of kittens is born during the year and most of those are unplanned.[169] By the time a queen is 3 years old, 74.4% will have had at least one litter,[125,129,196] and many of the females that do have an ovariohysterectomy have already had kittens.[184] The highest cat densities are found in the same areas that have the highest densities of people—a source of food.[184] The presence of these cats indicates that there is a niche that will support that approximate number of cats, so migration and reproduction help replace any permanent losses. Removal of individual cats increases population turnover but does not significantly alter the total number of cats.[247] The large stray feline population may be reflected in another statistic: Only 38% of male cats are castrated and 31% of females are spayed,[242] although local differences are reported.[146]

Worldwide cat ownership is increasing, often in parallel to trends in the United States. In several European countries, the numbers for cats increased so much that they now outnumber dogs, as did the percentage of homes owning cats.[130]

Cat Owner Categorization

In addition to surviving a varied history, the cat has survived many types of owners. Cat owners have been classified in several ways by different researchers, but they tend to be categories for those who have a weak attachment and those who have a strong one.[102,242] The classification "low involvement owner" is applied to 59% of the 14,645,000 cat-owning households in one study of pet owners.[242] Another study called this group "pet dispassionates" and suggested it comprised 41% of pet owners.[117] These individuals devote little time to the care or company of the cat and seem to enjoy having a cat around more than really interacting with it. The animal may be a companion for someone else in the household. This lack of involvement with the pet is reflected in trauma statistics. Of 126 cats (89 males, 37 females) reported injured over slightly more than a year's period, 16.3% were hit by a car, 14.7% were involved in animal interaction, and 39.5% received injuries from causes unknown to the owner.[108] Although the average age for the general population is 3 years, that of the neutered cat is 3 to 5 years longer, and that of the traumatized cat is only 1.3 years.[22,108,242] This is despite the average life span for a cat being 12 years, with ages of 20 years or older not uncommon.[35,218] The current longevity record is 36 years.[243] One study of roadkills indicated that most were kittens or young adults.[31] Because of these low involvement owners, cat populations for the most part still fulfill the criteria of random mating.[203]

A subcategory of the low-involvement group might include owners described as the "pet-for-child people."[117] This group consists of 29% of owners. Here the pet is considered to belong to a child; the adult is not highly committed to the animal but usually ends up being the primary caregiver.

The second classification of cat owners, those with a strong attachment, has been subdivided. "Quality or status conscious owners" represent 21% of all cat owners. The pet is an expression of how this owner views himself or herself and reflects his or her good taste, as would other material possessions. These owners feel that the cat depends on them for love, affection, and care, and as a result, the animal is well groomed and only reluctantly left alone.[58,242]

"High involvement owners" compose the second subdivision of the strong-attachment category.[242] These owners have also been called "pet lovers" and make up 20% to 30% of pet owners.[117,242] Unlike owners in the other two categories, these individuals rely on the cat to supply love and affection or to serve as an emotional crutch, such as a child substitute. Attachments to the cat are frequently described as those to a human family member, friend, or child.[1,67] These people feel the cat enjoys humans, feed it specially prepared foods, have photographs of the pet, take it on vacation, and may celebrate the cat's birthday.[67,222] They estimate spending more than 3 hours a day with the animal, particularly on the weekend.[177] Owners from this group are most likely to bury a deceased pet in a pet cemetery or mausoleum or to leave an estate to their cats. Just this kind of owner made two cats worth $415,000 in 1965 the richest cats in history.[58,242]

Cat owners with a strong attachment to their pets are often in the middle and upper socioeconomic levels and will spend billions of dollars each year on their pets. These individuals have a higher percentage of neutered cats and a preference for lighter-colored cats.[32]

Modern Roles for the Cat

Pets take on many roles in society, and these roles change as the needs of civilization change. Although individual animals can be shown to be unique, all cats are a product of species-specific characteristics.[56] Reasons people have cats vary, but most people indicate that personality and appearance are important features.[176] The cat still controls rodents, but closer contact with humans is now adding new dimensions of purpose. As a research animal, the cat has become invaluable for studies of aggression, neurology, anatomy, ecology, and aging.

Developing children derive significant benefits from having a pet, and the cat has long been important in this regard. The animal can assume different roles during a child's maturation. A child may relate better to pets than to adults and with this friend may be better able to work out many of the normal problems of childhood. Caring for a cat teaches a sense of responsibility to the child, and watching the cat's normal body functions results in self-understanding and a respect for life. The cat also provides companionship. Motivation for learning and creativity is also stimulated by a cat's presence.[58,121,123,219] Even the painful process of the death of a beloved pet can help prepare a child for the future loss of loved ones. It has been shown that especially in boys, and to a lesser extent in girls, interest in pets tends to decrease sharply when adolescence is reached.[116,120,121]

Cats and other pets are assuming an increasingly important role in maintaining the mental health of our society. The fast pace of modern civilization tends to isolate humans from each other, and the animal may be the only constant factor in a person's environment to help maintain psychologic equilibrium. For most owners, a cat provides companionship, something to care for, motivation to exercise, and a feeling of being needed and safety.[69,222,246] The role a pet plays within a family often varies with individuals. For a wife, petting the cat may represent affection for a child substitute or a safe expression of desire for sexual sensations, whereas the pet may represent an object of ego expression for the husband.[63,121] The important role of emotional support has been documented for widows during the first year after the loss of their husbands and in cat owners in general.[229]

Serving as a catalyst and facilitator of human relationships, the cat has been especially helpful to the elderly and the young. The role of a dependent may be difficult to accept by an individual in either age-group, and the cat, as a subordinate, can boost the person's self-esteem.[40,118,122] The psychologic health of cat owners is significantly better than that of nonowners in terms of general responsiveness and being in touch with reality.[246] To the elderly, cat adoption increases life satisfaction and occasionally has health benefits too.[246] To an individual, a pet may serve as a living memory of a deceased spouse. Widows tend to preserve this memory at all costs, whereas widowers often destroy guilt-laden reminders of the past.[120,122] Although it is generally believed that relationships like loving a cat promote good mental health, a minority opinion has been expressed that attachment to a pet is a symptom of alienation toward other humans.[27] This is probably true in cases in which the attachment is pathologic.

Use of the cat has increased in psychotherapy sessions to stimulate communication, provide an object for affection, and allow the patient's mastery of a situation. Cats have also been prescribed for home therapy, working 24 hours a day to draw individuals into an awareness of their surroundings or provide affection and emotional security where it might be lacking. Therapy in institutional settings for the emotionally disturbed and mentally retarded has also received a big boost when cats are part of the settings, because the animals increase the effect of the professional staff and provide continuity during staff turnovers.[119]

Pets often reflect the psychologic state of their families, even to the point of taking on the same neuroses as the family.[215] The animal may receive the abuse that a parent would have otherwise directed toward the child or the abuse from a child mimicking his or her parents.[77,87] The relationship between criminals convicted of having committed violent crimes and a childhood history of animal abuse is well documented. Even the cat's name may indicate its role to the family. "Ugly" or "Shorty" may represent the low regard the owner has for the animal, whereas human names may be indicative of a peer ranking. In a study of cat owners who used veterinary services, 52% of the owners gave their cat a human name and another 26% had chosen a pet-related name.[4] Nicknames were used by 56% of the owners.[3]

The veterinarian is in a unique position in the owner-pet relationship. He or she is privileged to be trusted with helping keep the cat healthy and to be sought out by 71% of cat owners for feline-related information.[222] The increasing use of the cat as a mental health tool forces such patients into an increased dependency on the veterinarian, which necessitates the veterinarian's awareness of human behavior, including methods of communication with affected individuals. In this regard, a special facility has already been established to study the human-animal interrelationship.[128] There will also be the added role for the veterinarian of helping in the selection of pets, so he or she must be aware of characteristics that make each animal desirable or undesirable for a particular emotional or physical need.[11,12,111,118] There are risk factors for cat relinquishment that can be changed through veterinary interactions with clients. Included in these are (1) owners who have specific expectations, (2) cats that can go outdoors, (3) sexually intact cats, (4) owners who never read a book on cat behavior, (5) daily or weekly bouts of housesoiling, and (6) inappropriate care expectations.[170]

If the trend toward pet dependence continues, if civilization continues to gather in suburban areas, and if pets take on neuroses from family members, then the veterinarian will have to be able to treat more and more abnormal behaviors in their feline patients. Although almost two thirds of pet owners believe their pet is well behaved, as many as 82% of cat owners will mention a specific behavior problem if asked.[174] Problems most commonly cited are anxiety, clawing furniture (15% to 20%), climbing on furniture (16%), housesoiling (10% to 13%), bringing birds or mice into the house (8%), fighting (6%), biting people (6%), and destroying items (5%).[86,174,222] As significant as the numbers and types of problems is the report that 24% of cat owners have not tried anything to stop the behavior and 68% have not resolved the problem.[174]

Each animal species has certain behavior patterns that are genetically programmed into all individuals of that species. These are the behaviors that are discussed throughout this book—behaviors that have resulted in *F. catus* through years of evolution. Individual variations resulting from environmental alterations are so inconsistent that they are essentially meaningless. To evaluate any behavioral problem, the veterinarian should decide whether the behavior pattern is objectionable to the owner but normal to the cat or whether it is both objectionable to the owner and abnormal for the cat.[76] Fortunately, euthanasia is no longer the only alternative for a cat showing abnormal behavior.

INTRODUCTION TO EVALUATING BEHAVIOR PROBLEMS

There is a serious lack of knowledge about animal behavior on the part of pet owners leading to misconceptions about the behavior and inappropriate ways to resolve it.[86,170,193] A behavior problem is often a "terminal disease," so being able to help an owner can be important to saving the animal's life.[237] Prevention of a problem is usually easier than eliminating one, making the first kitten visits the most important. The entire veterinary staff should be educated about how to help new cat owners get started correctly. Handouts, books, and videotapes are good client education materials. Services that a clinic can make available to clients include preselection consultations, preventive behavior counseling by either the veterinarian or the veterinary technician, client education during "kitty kindergarten" classes, and preventive management products.[111]

Even with careful preventive measures, behavior problems can occur. One third of cats relinquished to animal shelters are there because of an unacceptable behavior.[193] The risk is greatest for cats younger than 6 months, those that were free to the owner, those that are a mixed breed, those that spent most of the day in a basement or garage, those that had behavior problems, and owners who had sought behavior advice but did not try it or found the advice not helpful or impractical.[170] Slightly more than half of pet owners have or would discuss a pet's problem with their veterinarian.[2,3,245] To help clients a veterinarian can first learn how to treat some of the most common behavior problems and gradually add others over time. Consulting with board-certified veterinary behaviorists or referring patients to them is an appropriate service for those more complicated cases. Housesoiling, damaging furniture, and aggression (particularly redirected or irritable aggression) are the most common problems.[2,103,244,245]

Behavior problems can be quite simple in their origins, such as pain-induced aggression when the cat's tail is pulled, or they can be very complex, as with aggression resulting from abnormal neurotransmitter function. On the surface both behaviors appear the same. Only when we can understand the causes at all levels will we really understand these problems (Figure 1-3), and that still remains a future goal. Appropriate workup of

Phenotype

    Neuroanatomy

        Neurophysiology/Neurochemistry

      Molecular

        Genotype

Figure 1-3 Levels of "causality." *(Modified from Overall KL:* Understanding repetitive, stereotypic behaviors: signs, history, diagnosis, and practical treatment. *Paper presented at American Veterinary Medical Association meeting, Pittsburgh, July 8, 1995.)*

a behavior case requires the establishment of a veterinarian-client-patient relationship to obtain all pertinent information. Although histories are important, information from appropriate physical examinations, including neurologic and orthopedic examinations, as well as interpretation of laboratory and special examination results, must be included in diagnostic considerations.

Several methods can be used to classify feline behaviors, with the simplest being to determine whether the behavior is normal or abnormal and acceptable or unacceptable.[15,17,106,239] Normal behaviors are those that are species specific. They may or may not be appreciated by the owner. Furniture scratching and urination (even outside the litter box) are examples of unacceptable normal behaviors. On the other hand, abnormal behaviors are those resulting from learning or from pathophysiologic processes. Psychogenic grooming and hypothyroid aggression would be included in this category. Not all individual cats will develop a behavior problem, much less the same problem behavior in the same environment. Environments are often blamed for stress or anxiety but serve to demonstrate that the threshold between normal and abnormal varies among individuals.[44]

Classification of behavior problems can also be done by the signs shown by the cat—descriptive classification. This scheme is currently the most often used because a problem generally falls into one of several categories. Examples include housesoiling-urination, excessive vocalization, and furniture scratching. Descriptive classification does not account for multiple causes of the same sign. As an example, "aggression" does not distinguish between fear-induced, intermale, and epileptic aggression.

Functional classifications are the most specific because they take environmental and physiologic factors into consideration. The list of specific problems becomes very long and difficult to keep in mind.[17] Functional diagnoses can relate to a stimulus-response relationship such as separation anxiety; disease, as in seizure-induced aggression; physiologic states such as fear-induced aggression; or other factors such as genetics or developmental conditions such as malnutrition. From a clinical approach it tends to be most useful to minimize the number of major categories by using signs and to put a functional diagnosis as a subcategory.

Four Major Functional Classifications of Behavior Problems

Feline behavior problems can be broadly classified by function into four categories.[14] Although these four categories could be applied to any animal, the frequency of each category varies among the species.

Stress-induced or frustration problems

The largest factor causing primary problems for the cat is stress or "frustration," which can be expressed in many forms for many reasons.[9,144] This is the largest category of behavior problems and one receiving a lot of attention recently because of drug therapy. Even with all the current attention on psychopharmacology, behavior modification or environmental change to manage the stress can still be successfully used with or without drugs. In fact, drug therapy alone is generally not sufficient or long-lasting without environmental change or behavior modification. All animals are creatures of habit, and unless a change is gradual, a break in routine can be very upsetting. The introduction of a new pet or family member, inconsistent punishment, a change in litter brands, or a lack of proper exercise will result in increasing tension. Reactions vary between individuals and within individuals at different times. Unfortunately for the cat, as for other animals, there is no normal innate pattern for the release of these stresses. Because frustration cannot be reasoned away by the animal, the resulting behavior is a normal pattern expressed in an inappropriate situation. Examples include urine marking, housesoiling, aggression, or a psychosomatic condition. The cat is still relatively independent of humans; however, as society asks that *F. catus* change, particularly relative to close social interactions with humans and other cats, the number of behavior problems will rise.

Problems resulting from improper socialization

Socialization is a process by which an animal learns to accept certain animal species, including its own, in close proximity, and it occurs most easily during a limited time span. Improper or inadequate socialization of a cat during its first few months of life can result in an individual that does not relate socially to other cats, the family dog, or people. The animal is handicapped in a social situation that is normal for most families and undergoes a great deal of stress if forced into such a situation.

Genetic-related problems

An animal's genetic makeup will affect behavioral inheritance. Fortunately, the cat's history has been good in one respect: Genetic behavioral problems are minimal. For this species, the minimal use of selective breeding has allowed it to maintain a diverse gene pool. Only 7% of cats are pedigreed as compared with 51% of dogs, indicating that human intervention is still minimal.[65,242] As cats undergo an increasing amount of selective breeding, the chances are good that the primary consideration will be for physical characteristics, not behavioral ones, as has occurred with dogs. This fails to produce cats that can better tolerate changes in society.

Behaviors resulting from medical conditions

Abnormal behavior in a domestic animal is usually a result of an organic state of neurologic or systemic origin. An owner takes the cat to a veterinarian because of an observed change in the animal's behavior, such as sneezing, lameness, or depression. The statement that "they just aren't acting right" shows the importance of behavior to an owner relative to the animal's overall health. Medical problems from leukemia to fever can present this way. Generally, a physical examination and some laboratory data are sufficient to provide a diagnosis. Just as frequent urination may indicate urinary calculi, interstitial cystitis, renal problems, or litterbox aversion, aggression may indicate thyroid dysfunction, local pain, generalized discomfort, or central nervous system abnormalities. In some cases it is easy to remember to connect a behavior and medical problem. Other times the medical relationship becomes a diagnostic challenge. Using the *degenerative, anomoly, metabolic, nutrition/neoplasia, infectious/inflammatory, trauma/toxin* (DAMN IT) scheme to consider differential diagnoses, every category has medically based conditions that must be included as causes of abnormal behavior.[112] Although not always the highest priority in a differential list, medical problems should always be considered. Much is still unknown about abnormal behaviors related to medical conditions, but there have been significant advances.

The Signalment

The signalment and name of the cat can provide useful hints about particular behavior problems. As an example, inappropriate urination in a young cat is more likely to be related to a box that is remotely located than it is to diabetes. Intact tomcats spray urine significantly more often than castrated males, and Persians have a higher incidence of litterbox problems than other breeds. The name is interesting too because derogatory ones can indicate a negative attitude toward the cat and a higher probability of treatment failure.

The Case History

For most behavior problems, the majority of information about the case will come from the history, so its importance cannot be overemphasized. The goal is to obtain an accurate description of all important aspects of the problems, including relevant information about the pet, the associated humans, and the environment.[97,235,237] It is also important to identify the immediate consequences, developmental factors, and other related problems that may be present.[238] The initial history-taking session, especially for chronic problems, will take more time than one for most medical problems, but it is crucial to the ultimate understanding of the behavioral complaint. Schedule an appropriate amount of time to devote to this owner and charge for your time.

One format used to take a behavioral history utilizes a list of specific questions, which can be useful to shorten the time of the initial assessment. A history form is one way to ensure that all pertinent data are obtained.[15,97,105,163] Some owners prefer an open format in which the owner discusses his or her perspective first, followed by additional questions to fill in missing information. This necessitates that the veterinarian organize the information somehow.[85] For the recently developed but less serious types of problems, the practitioner may be able to use a fairly structured questioning style. However, for the problem typically seen in a referral setting the owners want to describe the problem as they see it. Sessions should be structured enough so as to not miss important information, yet flexible enough to bring out the unexpected.[97]

The writing of the history for the patient's record can tax even the fastest note taker, but this technique gathers a lot of information that might otherwise be missed, ensures the owner of the veterinarian's interest in the pet, and helps the owner focus on specific events when more specific questioning follows. The history should include where the owners got the cat and if they know anything about its parents. Then fill in the details of its life history up to the present day. Some choose to ask about the latest episode first.[45,235] Others want the descriptions to occur in the order of occurrence. Questions during the owner's narrative can be asked but usually just for clarification of a point or two before the owner continues. After the owners have completed their segment, it is appropriate to ask for more details about specific episodes.[235] A rating scale can help quantify the seriousness of various episodes to the owner.[90] It should also be noted that different owners may have different perspectives about the problem or memories of the events. For this reason all the people involved should be present for this visit if possible.[45] Owners may also use incorrect terms for an event, such as *spraying* for *inappropriate urination,* so be sure they describe the specific behaviors and not just give the perception of what happened or why.[97]

Four general questions should be answered in any history-taking session—what, where, when, and when.[13,15] Based on the answers to these questions, many more specific questions help focus on the total scope of the problem.

What exactly happens?

This question should be first and may help determine whether the cat is clawing the furniture, spraying the house, or refusing to eat. Although the problem behavior is usually easy to define, "doing it all over the living room" will require multiple questions to actually define the "what." The history may also reveal other maladaptations of which the owner is unaware or to which he or she has already adjusted.

Where does the behavior occur?

For some behaviors, the *where* may be a simple answer such as on the Oriental rug in the dining room or on the owner's ankle. Many times, however, the answer is "all over the house." Careful questioning will often narrow down the location to one or two spots. To the owner the smell of urine or feces may be "all over" when the actual site of elimination is limited to one corner in the dining room.

The answer to *where* can also provide insight to causes. Events restricted to one area may indicate that a stressor is located nearby. The cat spraying near a window may be taunted by a neighbor cat that walks on the window ledge or that can be seen walking outside that window. Defecating next to the litter pan may indicate that a new type of litter is unacceptable to the cat.

When did the problem start?

This question is designed to determine how longstanding the problem is. For example, a 4-year-old cat that never used the litterbox will probably not start just because the owner is getting new carpeting. The "when did it start" questions might also help tie the start of a problem to another event occurring shortly before it. Acquisition of a new pet may initiate marking behavior by the resident cat, or aggression to the owners could begin after the birth of kittens. The length of time a problem has existed also helps from a prognostic standpoint of how long it will take to correct the behavior.

When does the behavior happen?

Many behavioral patterns have a precipitating event, such as aggression that occurs when the neighbor child pulls the cat's tail. In this case the problem is associated only with the child's presence. If an event occurs only while the owner is away, perhaps a friend or neighbor could be asked to see whether the event is occurring just after the owner leaves, throughout the owner's absence, or immediately before the owner's return. Some problems occur at certain times of the day. Others are related to either the presence or the absence of the owner. Additional information under this "when" heading will include frequency and duration of the average bout.[155] Knowing the schedule of the cat and the owner helps put this information into perspective, and may explain variations in the pattern of frequency and intensity.[155]

Another important part of the history is to determine what the pet's owners have already tried[45] and how they went about it. The knowledge that a specific therapy has already been appropriately tried means it need not be done again. In some types of problem cases, it can also help rule out certain things on a list of differential diagnoses. If a therapy has been tried but was not done for an appropriate length of time or compliance to the accepted protocol was poor, that therapy can be tried again with emphasis on the correct methods.

Physical Examination

After a complete history is obtained, the next step is a thorough physical examination. As is normally done, the animal is evaluated from body weight to temperature, respiration, and pulse. The abdomen is palpated and thorax ausculted. Particular emphasis may need to be placed on a neurologic evaluation, health of the eyes, musculoskeletal evaluation, skin lesions, and anal sacs. Physical problems should be noted and evaluated in the total context of the problem. Medical conditions can be common risk factors in cats presenting with behavior problems.[15,98,143,167] Medical conditions usually must be considered in the list of differential diagnoses for various problems, as is shown in later chapters. Common sense is also necessary during an examination. Every practice has its very aggressive cats that cannot be carefully examined and a behavior practice seems to collect more than its share. Because the highest priority must go to human safety, it may not be possible to do a detailed physical examination on every animal.

With a behavior case the physical examination becomes broader in scope. It includes how the cat interacts with other cats, new humans, and the hospital environment. Subtle cues like excessive alertness, crouched postures, aggression toward anything that moves, tail and ear postures, owner-cat interactions, abnormal gait, and reluctance to break eye contact provide a wealth of information that complement other physical findings. Allowing a nonaggressive patient to roam the examination room can provide insight about how the animal behaves and how the owners react.[45]

Differential Diagnoses

Information from the signalment, history, and physical examination allow the problem to be narrowed to a list of differential diagnoses. For behavior problems, the list of differential diagnoses often combines medical and behavioral problems. For example, a list of differentials for a cat urinating in the house could include feline lower urinary tract syndrome, urinary tract infection, kidney disease, diabetes mellitus, diabetes insipidus, hyperadrenocorticism, psychogenic polydipsia, unavailability of access to normal eliminative locations, marking behavior, and separation anxiety.

Special Tests

In performing the workup for a behavior problem, the veterinarian will use selected clinical tests based on the differential diagnoses chosen. Disease-related causes of behavior problems may require that additional information be obtained through special tests, or the tests may be needed to be sure a certain medication is appropriate. A complete blood count, biochemical profile, and urinalysis are the most commonly used of these tests. They are appropriate for the geriatric patient, particularly one presented for housesoiling,[98] or one to be placed on any of the human drugs currently used as extra-label treatments. Other tests for feline leukemia, feline immunodeficiency virus, or thyroid hormone levels might be appropriate. Radiographs with or without special contrast media, ultrasonography, electroencephalograms, electroretinograms, fundic examinations, cystograms, nuclear scans, computed tomography, and magnetic resonance imaging are needed in certain cases.

As with traditional medical problems, diagnoses can be ruled out based on the test results, with a resulting shift of the rank on the differential list. The veterinarian and client can work together to determine how far to look into a problem and in what order.

Diagnosis

As with any medical condition, a behavioral diagnosis is determined after considering all the information gathered. The most commonly used diagnostic approach is a mixture of classification schemes. For example, separation anxiety is functional, but the urination, defecation, and prolonged sucking are descriptive. An appropriate course of therapy can be prescribed only after a diagnosis is made.

Prognosis

Owners want to know the prognosis for the behavior problem and how long it will take to be "cured." Before a prognosis can be given or even a therapeutic plan devised, the veterinarian must determine the level of owner commitment.[97,113] For that it is helpful to ask each person what his or her feelings are about the cat[235] and what his or her goal is for the behavior program. If the therapeutic plan will involve a major commitment of time and effort, the owners need to know that up front rather than figure it out as they become discouraged. The more that is expected of the owner, the more difficult it will be and the more likely it is to fail.[154] They must be both willing and able to make the program work.[113] Several things have an impact on the prognosis of behavior therapy, including the etiology, duration, predictability, and type of problem; experience with the problem; danger; owner perception; owner compliance; ease of treatment; owner expectations; and response to therapy.[25,154] In assessing the cause, the veterinarian knows that the easiest to treat will be normal behaviors or simple learned ones shown by an individual. The toughest will be the abnormal, complex unlearned problem involving several animals.

Etiology is important. Untreatable medical causes of behavior changes, such as feline leukemia, have a poor prognosis. A simple change like cleaning a litterbox more often usually means a happy ending.

The duration of the problem is often related to how long it takes to treat the problem. This is especially true when learning is involved, because the animal will have to unlearn the unacceptable behavior and relearn the normal behavior.

Patterns of a problem can affect the outcome of a treatment program. If an occasional problem can be predicted because of a cofactor, removing the relationship or changing its context can be helpful. Feces that is only on the carpet Wednesday, Thursday, and Friday suggests the box is cleaned on Saturday. The cat is willing to tolerate a few days of buildup but after a few days the odor is no longer tolerated.

The type of problem dictates how treatable the condition is. Certainly past successes dealing with similar problems gives the veterinarian a better chance to be successful and a better prognostic perspective. Also, the more simple the solution, the greater is the likelihood of an acceptable outcome. When owners become fearful, as often happens with aggression, they may never trust the cat again even though the actual type of aggression would otherwise be treatable. Client and public safety is a factor that must be considered, and euthanasia may have to be the only "treatment" that is appropriate.

Assuming a correct diagnosis is made, individual variation can affect an outcome, as can owner compliance. When the therapy is a pill a day, compliance is reasonable. The more involved a behavior modification plan becomes, the lower the overall success rate will be. Owner expectations are also important. Some people are grateful for a small improvement, but others expect miracles overnight.

For behavior problems case follow-up is important. Recheck visits or phone calls help confirm that the therapeutic plan is progressing as expected. They reassure the owner that the veterinarian cares and provide an extra incentive to keep up the effort. Following up with the owner also provides an excellent learning experience about responses to various therapies to increase the level of expertise for the various types of problems.

INTRODUCTION TO TREATMENT OPTIONS

Once a diagnosis has been made for a behavior problem, an appropriate therapeutic regimen must be designed. Owners commonly want a magic pill or ultimate solution. Everyone wants a quick fix, but in the real world this seldom occurs. Primary influences on behavior include genetics, the environment, physiology, and experience.[237] As a result, behavior treatments can consist of drug therapy, behavior modification, client education, environmental manipulation, or some combination. Drug therapy alone is often unsatisfactory over the long term,[83] unless the main problem is primarily medical, such as hypothyroid aggression.

Client Education

Because one category of cat-owner interactions can be normal behavior that is unacceptable to the owner, the veterinarian is often required to educate the owner about what is normal for a cat. An animal cannot change a normal species-specific behavior, so the owners may have to change their expectations or find an alternative that allows both to have their way.[152] If a cat grooms itself at night, the owner may complain that the "slurping" noise is too loud. Because it would be difficult to get the cat to change its behavior, other alternatives may be acceptable. Some owners would learn to ignore the sound once they learned they could not make it stop. Others would not be willing to tolerate the noise and choose to keep the cat out of the bedroom. Teaching the client about what is normal for a cat provides a client service that can be particularly valuable as preventive and therapeutic.

Changing a behavior usually involves changing the environment too.[28] This requires client education about how to make the necessary changes. It could mean it will be necessary to remove a chair that is the frequent target of clawing or change a time schedule for interactions between owner and cat. In any case, owner compliance will be dependent on good client education.

Environmental Modification

For certain problems changing the environment may effect a behavior change. Because urine marking commonly happens where a cat sees other outdoor cats, the use of blinds, drapes, or shades may be helpful. Making one room a "cat room" and keeping the floor surface tiled may save the life of a cat that urinates on carpet. Changing the environment then can change some behaviors or the perception that a behavior is a problem. It is one more tool that can be used for feline behavior problems.

Behavior Modification

Behavior modification is the use of the principles of learning to cause a change in an individual. How an animal learns is discussed in greater detail in Chapter 2, but the various methods of behavior modification that can be used are discussed here. Because the results are usually not instantaneous, keeping the owner motivated can be challenging. Having weekly progress reports is one way; however, long-term treatments are often stopped when the problem has been minimized to a tolerable level.[132]

Behavior modification is an important part of many behavior problem therapies and must be applied appropriately to be effective. Punishment is a negative stimulus applied immediately after the start of a behavior, which decreases the likelihood that the behavior will reoccur. For cats punishment usually cannot come from the owner because the animal will wait until the owner leaves and then act. A plant sprayer, loud noise, or compressed air sprayer can be used for interactive punishment to get a longer range, particularly if the owner remains partially hidden or at least quiet.[18,78,80] Remote punishment that is activated by the cat itself or remotely by the owner is much more effective. A number of commercial products can be useful for remote punishment.[80,110] Remotely activated devices, sticky or noise gadgets, overturned mousetraps, and sensors that activate electric equipment would be included in such a list and are discussed further with specific problems. To be effective, punishers must be strong enough so habituation does not occur but not so strong as to create fear, appropriate in timing, and appropriate in type.[139]

Reinforcers increase the likelihood that a behavior will reoccur. Positive reinforcers, which we commonly call *rewards,* are positive things like food or petting that come to be associated with action. Negative reinforcers are negative stimuli that stop when a desired behavior occurs. These should not be confused with punishment because in this case the reward is the stopping of the reinforcers when a behavior is initiated. Both punishment and reinforcement must optimally occur within 30 seconds of the behavior.[216]

Conditioning

Classical conditioning is a process by which the cat learns to respond in a specific way when presented with a specific but unrelated stimulus. This type of learning begins when a specific stimulus results in a particular response (unconditioned stimulus [US], unconditioned response [UR]). At the same time the US is presented a totally neutral stimulus (NS) is also presented, and the UR occurs again. Eventually the NS alone will cause the response (now called a conditioned response).[216] The cat is conditioned to come running to the front door whenever it is opened if it was originally fed immediately after the owner came home. Negative lessons can also be learned. For example, a cat severely frightened by a loud noise or another cat might associate a person who also just happened to be present with that fearful event.[43] From then on the cat may be afraid of the individual. The general connection between the stimulus and the physical response is what is important.

A second type of conditioning, operant conditioning, involves the use of reinforcers to cause the behavior to be learned.[216] Several types of learning could be considered subtypes of operant conditioning. As an example, in trial and error learning a cat jumps on the counter and finds food; the result is a strong probability that the cat will repeat the behavior.

Counterconditioning

Counterconditioning is the use of learning to replace an unacceptable behavior with an acceptable one that is incompatible. Fear and eating are incompatible, so feeding treats as a fear-inducing stimulus comes gradually closer helps the cat dissociate the fear-stressor relation. A cat becomes afraid of a litterbox because the owner would catch it there to pill it. Giving the cat treats near the litterbox can teach that the area is safe again. Counterconditioning is often coupled with desensitization if the cat's behavior is associated with fear or excessive sensitivity.

Desensitization

When a cat shows an excessive amount of fear, sensitivity, or reactivity to a stimulus, it can be desensitized to that stimulus through learning.[43,238] This can be accomplished by either of two general concepts. One technique is through habituation, whereby the reaction-provoking stimulus is repeated until it no longer elicits a response. The second technique of desensitization introduces the stimulus but in such a small amount that no reaction occurs. Gradually the amount of stimulus is increased, but never so fast as to elicit a response. For example, consider the cat made afraid of the noise of a radio as the result of a particularly loud cymbal-crashing experience. The cat is exposed to very soft music at a level where there is no reaction. The volume is very gradually increased over many sessions until the fear is eliminated. This desensitization exposure to soft music can be paired with counterconditioning using food by playing the music at each meal. The combination can speed up the behavior-modification process if done properly.

Extinction

Another technique for behavior modification is extinction. Certain behaviors can be extinguished by removing all reinforcers. Cats quickly learn that they can get attention and food from an owner by waking that owner at 4:00 AM. The attention and food then reinforce that behavior. By stopping the attention the owner ensures that the behavior will gradually stop too, even though the cat may actually be more persistent or even aggressive at first. This is something owners should be warned about. Once the pet learns that the desired response is not going to happen, the behavior stops.

Flooding

Flooding is a learning technique that can make a problem significantly worse if not done properly. In this method the cat is exposed to the stimuli continuously until there is a major improvement in its reactions.[238] The key words here are *continuously* and *major*. If a cat is afraid of people, the owner could bring together several friends and have them sit in a circle with the cat physically restrained in the center. The people remain in that circle until the cat noticeably relaxes, however long that might be. Each successive trial becomes shorter in duration until the animal is no longer fearful of being in the company of people. If the sessions are stopped too soon, the fear is actually reinforced, and the problem is made worse instead of better.

Aversive conditioning

Aversive conditioning is the use of an obnoxious or negative experience that leads to the avoidance of a place, object, or behavior because of the association with the aversive experience. This could be due to a punishment that occurs immediately after the start of each behavior or due to negative reinforcement, which uses a negative stimulus to prevent the action in the first place. A cat that jumps onto a kitchen table is taught not to whenever it sees a sheet of paper extending over the side of the table. If two-sided sticky tape is placed on the table and part is allowed to hang over the edge, the cat will come to associate the piece it can see with the negative experience it has from jumping on the table.

Success in taste or smell aversion requires that the stimulus has been coupled with a previous bad experience. A foul-tasting product placed on an item that is targeted for chewing or licking is often ignored because its potency has been diluted. If the cat has had a significant oral dose previously, then the odor and mild taste bring back negative memories. For taste aversion, the cat is allowed to smell a foul-tasting substance such as a mixture of Tabasco and pepper sauce or a commercial product used to stop chewing. At the same time, a substantial dose is introduced into its mouth so the cat will associate the bad taste with a particular odor. From that point the smell of the substance, whether alone or mixed with household shortening for smearability, initiates an avoidance reaction. Thus the targeted object can be spread with hot sauce, and the oral habit can be broken. Another form of aversive conditioning smell aversion involves the use of a spray can. The owner shows the can to the cat, and while aiming the spray 90 degrees from the cat's face, the owner releases the spray while rapidly advancing the can toward the cat. The purpose is to scare the cat with the advancing, hissing spray can so that it associates the smell emitted with the threat. Then, with the cat absent, the owner sprays the targeted objects and allows the mist to settle before readmitting the cat to the room. These techniques vary in success because the amount of threat perceived by each cat and the offensiveness of the taste or odor chosen may differ widely.

Shaping

Shaping uses reinforcers for a natural behavior that somewhat resembles the behavior ultimately desired.[236] Gradually the criteria for the reward become stricter as the cat successfully masters the general behavior and works on the more specific aspects of the desired outcome.

Successive approximation

Successive approximation rewards graduated, successively closer approximations to the goal and is similar to shaping.[78] In this case the cat would be asked to be physically closer for each reward instead of behaviorally closer. For the animal hiding under the bed, small food treats would bring it closer to the edge of the bed each time and gradually out.

Drug Therapy

The use of drugs for behavior is nothing new, yet it remains a hot topic. Veterinarians and owners want to fix problems quickly and without a great deal of effort or time investment, so a pill would be nice. Veterinarians also are used to the medical treatment paradigm, so we are comfortable with prescriptions. In addition, many practitioners are not comfortable with behavior-modification techniques. Regardless of the cause of the interest in drug use for behavior problems, there remains a great deal to be learned.

As in all aspects of veterinary medicine, medication should be used only as an adjunct to treat the abnormal, not to suppress a normal behavior.[152] Drug use for behavior problems is still extra label, so owner consent is recommended. Clients must be available to monitor the drug effects initially,[162] so leaving that responsibility to someone else, such as might occur during a vacation, is not appropriate. This is to ensure it works appropriately and that no side effects develop. It should be remembered that a particular drug does not always work for a particular problem all of the time, and it does not work in all animals or at the same dose each time.[83]

Historically the first drug used to get rid of behavior problems probably was for euthanasia. Even today euthanasia solution remains the most used drug for behavior problems in cats surrendered to animal shelters. Fortunately a number of advances in neuropharmacology have taken place, and several more are currently being worked on. With the recent rush to try the tricyclic antidepressants (TCAs) and selective serotonin reuptake inhibitors (SSRIs), veterinarians are prescribing a number of drugs for many behavior problems. Unfortunately, in many cases a specific diagnosis was never determined. If the drug's use did result in improvement, it becomes impossible to know whether it was coincidental or to predict what situations are best suited for that drug. There has always been a tendency to try a new behavior drug on any or all types of problem behaviors. Usually, however, there was only a single drug at a time. Now a number of different drugs from various pharmacologic classifications are available. The most progress in understanding behavioral pharmacology comes from a scientific approach, either as an independent study or during drug trials, and these occur after a specific diagnosis is determined.

When a behavior problem is related to a specific medical entity, appropriate treatment may be obvious. Hypothyroid and hyperthyroid aggression and litterbox avoidance from pain of recently declawed feet are examples. Other drugs used in neuropharmacology should be looked at a little closer. The summary of drugs and doses used in cat problems, as currently cited in the literature, is found in Appendix E. This list will be ever changing as new knowledge is gained, and the reader is cautioned that it can be current only at one point in time.

An ideal drug would be effective at eliminating a problem, work on all patients, have no side effects, have a rapid onset of action, have a wide margin of safety, not impair normal motor or mental functions, have an intermediate half-life, and have a defined therapeutic blood level.[91,185] Unfortunately, the ideal drug does not exist, but the percentage of binding, active metabolites, half-life, and site of action for many drug groups are being identified and allow a better understanding of how therapeutic responses occur. Because cats are not small dogs, it is particularly important to understand a drug's metabolic pathway in each animal species.

All five major monoamine neurotransmitters (acetylcholine, dopamine, γ-aminobutyric acid [GABA], norepinephrine, and serotonin [5-HT]) are important in normal behavior. Abnormalities in their levels are thought to adversely affect these behaviors. In broad terms each neurotransmitter relates to specific behaviors. Dopamine is involved with psychomotor function in that its activation of D_1 receptors maintains movement, and activation of D_2 receptors initiates and allows repetition of movement, obviously being involved in the repetitive behaviors we call *stereotypies*.[101] Dopamine activation of the mesolimbic pathway receptors is said to mediate reward, incentive, motivation, learning, and response speed.[101] GABA is an inhibitory neurotransmitter that causes significant reduction in movement.[101] Norepinephrine is involved in mood regulation. Although normal levels mediate reward, arousal, and fear responses, excessive amounts result in mania.[101] Insufficient amounts are associated with depression.[101] Serotonin has a wide range of functions, which should be expected because there are so many receptor subtypes. For example, 5-HT_{1A} receptors mediate psychomotor responses; 5-HT_{2A} hallucinatory behavior; 5-HT_{2C} anxiety and appetite; and 5-HT_3 pain, anxiety, and sleep.[101] As these neurotransmitters work at the various synaptic transmission sites, they have several different modes of action using presynaptic or postsynaptic mechanisms. Presynaptic sites can be affected in seven ways (Figure 1-4).[149]

---

1. Availability of neurotransmitter precursors
     Direct administration of precursors
     Altered transport of precursors
     Altered delivery of precursors into the neuron
2. Neurotransmitter synthesis is affected by drugs or metabolites
3. Alteration of neurotransmitter storage vesicles
     Inhibited from forming
     Caused to release their content
4. Leakage of neurotransmitter reduces synthesis or release of additional amounts through feedback mechanisms
5. Blockage of the neurotransmitter's reuptake system
6. Inhibition of catabolic enzymes that normally metabolize neurotransmitters
7. Various combinations on neurotransmitter release from a neuron

---

Figure 1-4 Presynaptic alterations of neurotransmitter availability. *(Modified from Nutt JG, Irwin RP: Principles of neuropharmacology. II. Synaptic transmission. In Klawans HL, Goetz CG, Tanner CM, editors: Textbook of clinical neuropharmacology and therapeutics, ed 2, New York, 1992, Raven Press.)*

Postsynaptic events can also alter the reaction to neurotransmitters.[149] The first has to do with the receptors for each neurotransmitter. There are two families of receptors.[149] One family, like GABA$_A$ and nicotinic receptors, incorporates an ion channel into its structure, and the second uses guanine nucleotide–binding proteins (G proteins) to alter intracellular function. Within these two families there can be multiple receptor subtypes for each neurotransmitter. For example, more than 12 subtypes have been identified for serotonin.[36,39,70,134,209] In addition, a single neuron has receptors for several types of neurotransmitters and multiple subtypes for each. Another complication is that receptors can vary in sensitivity in different areas of the brain.[126]

A second type of postsynaptic alteration of neurotransmitters affects the various intraneuronal chemical components that are activated by neurotransmitters. Increasing or decreasing the sensitivity of postsynaptic responses is also possible.

With all the different locations at a synapse that react with the various neurotransmitters in so many ways, the multiple receptor subtypes, the interconnection of neural pathways, and the ability of external factors to alter neurochemicals, understanding normal brain function in any one species is extremely difficult.[134] The abnormal brain is even more difficult to understand. With the advent of psychopharmacology, drug actions on the central nervous system are becoming better understood. Drugs are also being designed to target specific neurotransmitters by actions at presynaptic and postsynaptic sites. Currently, a number of human drugs are being tried for behavior problems in animals, but there is a wide spectrum to be tried. An understanding of the broad categories and some representative drugs in each can result in a more rational selection. Serotonin, for example, is formed from tryptophan and degraded by monoamine oxidase (MAO). In addition to the brain, serotonin can be found in other cells of the body including the platelets and some cells of the intestinal wall.[209] After it is released into the interneuronal space, serotonin is picked up by the cell to be used again. TCAs inhibit this reuptake, resulting in a prolonged effect.[209] As would be expected, psychotropic drugs can have a number of side effects because of actions on other neurotransmitters or on neurotransmitters having other functions in the body. In general, they can potentiate cardiac arrhythmias, bring on seizures, affect thyroid hormones levels, and induce hepatic enzymes.[159] Weight gain is another effect that is associated with an increase in thirst and appetite.[159]

Antianxiety drugs

Anxiety is extremely difficult to quantify in animals, but as in humans, the threat that results in anxiety seems to come from within. In contrast, fear is related to a specific external event.[91] Panic attacks are described as acute anxiety of rapid onset, with a crescendo of symptoms of sympathetic overactivity.[208] They can last a few minutes to several hours.

Antianxiety drugs have been in use for many years. They can be grouped into two subgroups based on general actions.[91] The sedative hypnotics produce effects that start with sedation and progress toward sleep or hypnosis as the dose is increased. Other properties of these drugs include muscle relaxation, anticonvulsant properties, and development of tolerance and dependence.[91] Common examples used in veterinary medicine would include the barbiturates and benzodiazepines. The second subgroup, sedative autonomics, affect the peripheral autonomic nervous system, such as with anticholinergic blocking. The sedation produced is qualitatively different, at least in humans.[91] In addition, sedative autonomics tend to increase muscle tone, lower seizure thresholds, and minimize development of tolerance or dependence.[91] Habituation is a problem, partially because of the long half-lives and the active metabolites.[191] As is typical of many drugs with long half-lives, abrupt withdrawal should be avoided, even in animals.

The *benzodiazepines* have come to be the most popular of the antianxiety drugs in humans, probably because they have the most desirable attributes and fewest undesirable ones. The mechanism of action may account for this. Some postsynaptic benzodiazepine-specific receptors are functionally linked to $GABA_A$ receptors and to an associated chloride ion channel.[42,84,91,208,210] The benzodiazepines augment GABA as an inhibitory neurotransmitter to open the chloride ion channel, letting chloride into the neuron to cause hyperpolarization and decreased firing.[*] Low doses alleviate anxiety, agitation, and fear by actions on receptors in the limbic system, and high doses are associated with confusion via the hippocampus and cerebral cortex.[100,212] Affects also include being less reactive to the surroundings and stimuli, as well as mood elevation.[161] When given intravenously for 15 to 30 minutes, these drugs have associated amnestic effects,[161,194] and these may be associated with the poor ability to learn certain things while under the influence of these drugs.[153,164,166] Sedation, cortical depression, and muscle relaxation are side effects in humans who do not have a history of seizures.[212] In cats, side effects of diazepam include sedation, loss of inhibition for aggression, ataxia, increased appetite, weight gain, paradoxical excitation, and increased friendly behavior.[38,42,205] Diazepam has been associated with fatal idiopathic hepatic necrosis in both humans[221] and cats.[†] In cats, side effects are thought to be primarily associated with the active metabolite of diazepam, requiring hepatic oxidation, and one of the metabolites, N-desmethyldiazepam, is thought to be very lipophilic.[161,164] It is released over time, meaning it has a very long half-life.[95,164] Oxazepam, lorazepam, and temazepam have no intermediate metabolites and so may be somewhat safer in cats. They are used in humans with liver disease.[38] Long-term use of these drugs may induce physiologic and behavioral dependency, so acute withdrawal can result in increased tremors, twitches, anxiety, and activity levels.[37] They may also disinhibit normal agonistic responses, resulting in an increased likelihood of aggression, particularly in fearful situations.[212]

Buspirone, an *azapirone,* is considered to be about as effective in human generalized anxiety disorders as the benzodiazepines, although the onset of activity is at least 1 week.[38,39,212] Azapirones differ from the benzodiazepines by being less sedative, having minimal impairment on central sensory processing, not being effective against panic disorders, and not being useful for obsessive-compulsive problems.[19,39,100,208,212] Buspirone also differs from phenothiazines and TCAs.[166] Early studies indicate buspirone may be helpful in humans who have dementia with disruptive behaviors.[181] The mechanisms of action include being a serotonin type 1A partial agonist at the $5\text{-}HT_{1A}$ subtype postsynaptic receptor,[‡] which enhances serotonin transmission when serotonin levels are low.[47] In addition, buspirone acts as a full agonist at the

---

[*]References 37, 91, 100, 153, 161, 205, 212.
[†]References 95, 124, 161, 164, 166, 205, 212.
[‡]References 39, 84, 100, 166, 168, 212.

presynaptic autoreceptors,[208,210] resulting in symptomatic relief in certain anxiety states, having high resting serotonergic tone.[47] This can result in a cat that is more assertive.[153,165] Azapirones also interact with dopamine and noradrenergic neurotransmitter systems,[36,39,210] but most clinical effects are probably due to the serotonin activity.[36] Side effects in cats include increased aggression to other cats, mild sedation, increased affection to the owner, gastrointestinal symptoms, agitation after pilling, repeated vomiting, and tachycardia.[38,166]

Lithium is another human antidepressant drug that has been tried in problem animals.[183] It is thought to accelerate the presynaptic destruction of catecholamines, inhibit neurotransmitter release at the synapse, and reduce the sensitivity of the postsynaptic receptor.[91,100] Antimanic effects may be associated with lithium blocking the supersensitivity of dopamine neurons.[91] Its regulation of serotonin activity is complex, although well studied. Because it stabilizes serotonin levels, it may result in mood stabilization.[91] The chemical similarities with calcium and magnesium might increase membrane permeability and thus affect various enzyme systems.[91] As newer and safer drugs have become available, lithium has lost its popularity in human medicine. Its role in veterinary medicine is just beginning to be explored, primarily in dogs.

The most commonly used anxiolytic drugs in veterinary medicine today are phenobarbital, diazepam, and amitriptyline. Use of the first two is complicated somewhat because both drugs are narcotics and neither is a particularly good antianxiety agent in cats. Phenobarbital is useful as an antiseizure medication and therefore useful for behavioral manifestations of seizures. Diazepam works fairly well in cats, but liver problems have been associated with its use, so it has recently been losing favor. The third drug, amitriptyline, is a TCA and is discussed in the following section. Buspirone has been gaining popularity[84] but is not always the drug of choice if increased boldness is undesirable.

Antidepressant drugs

A number of drugs classified as antidepressant are currently receiving attention for behavior problems in animals, especially the tricyclics and SSRIs. Often, however, depression is not the specific problem being treated in veterinary medicine.

The *TCA* drugs are classified as mixed serotonin and norepinephrine reuptake inhibitors.[26,41] Drugs of this class probably work by attaching to and inhibiting the presynaptic serotonin transporter protein, thus inhibiting reuptake.[38,100,211] They block acetylcholine, dopamine, norepinephrine, and histamine receptors.[23,99,100] It is this last action that gives them antipruritic properties.[157,166] Amitriptyline has been tried the most in veterinary medicine, and clomipramine is approved for use in canine separation anxiety. In addition to TCA use as an antidepressant, physicians prescribe these drugs for anxiety, anxiety plus depression, panic disorders, and obsessive-compulsive disorders.[*] In cats, as in other animals, TCAs augment brain serotonin levels, which reduces the level of anxiety.[165] The effects of the tricyclics in treating obsessive-compulsive disorders may relate to cells in the dorsal horn of the spinal cord being modulated by the drug before stimulation, implicating an aberrant sensation.[157] Tricyclics differ among themselves most in the amount of sedation, with imipramine and clomipramine being

---

[*]References 57, 59, 157, 168, 208, 223.

quite low and amitriptyline among the highest.[91,158,180] This may be related to their antihistamine effects. Changing between them is of limited value, and failure to get a response to two tricyclics probably indicates the need to try a different class of drugs.[91] Clomipramine is the most serotonin selective of the TCAs, and its metabolite, desmethylclomipramine, inhibits norepinephrine reuptake.[41]

TCAs are metabolized by the liver by aromatic hydroxylation, demethylation, and glucuronide conjugation.[41,211] The metabolites are active too and are excreted through the bile and the kidneys.[41,115] Side effects are associated with anticholinergic properties, including mydriasis, hyperthermia, tachycardia, dry mouth, constipation, sedation, urinary retention, and arrhythmia.* The arrhythmias do not respond well to β-adrenergic receptor blocking drugs, so they are probably not directly attributable to enhanced norepinephrine effects.[182] Limited studies in cats and dogs have not demonstrated any change in electrocardiograms associated with either amitriptyline or clomipramine.[115,182] Nausea is common, and sexual dysfunction, seizures, and potentiation of concurrent thyroid conditions are also described.[41,57,99,157,164] The onset of action can be as long as 2 to 6 weeks.† An animal's owner may notice a change in the pet's behavior within a few days,[131] but this is most likely an antihistamine-induced response. The long duration of onset has to do with serotonin buildup at the neurotransmitter level, not with the drug's half-life. This means drug treatment should last at least 6 weeks before being considered a failure. Long-term use of the tricyclics apparently increases the sensitivity of postsynaptic serotonin receptors, partly because of the increased number of 5-HT$_{1A}$ binding sites.[126] The time it takes for this to occur is consistent with the delay in the onset of action relative to depression.[126]

Although classified as a TCA, carbamazepine is used primarily to treat psychomotor epilepsy and trigeminal neuralgia. In addition, it is often included in a broad category of mood stabilizers because it aids in the control of agitated and aggressive emotional states in humans.[199] Carbamazepine has been tried in fear-aggressive cats and may make them more docile and affectionate[199,212]; however, increased aggression toward other cats has been reported.[199] This drug also works presynaptically and postsynaptically on multiple neurotransmitter systems including serotonin, norepinephrine, glutamate, dopamine, GABA, and acetylcholine.[212] Side effects include transient dizziness, nausea, fatigue, blurred vision, dyspnea, ataxia, vomiting, defecation, dermatologic reactions, and, rarely, a blood dyscrasia.

MAO inhibitors (MAOIs) are also antidepressants but are not commonly used. Monoamine oxidase (MAO) is found in many body tissues, so most of the inhibitor drugs are nonspecific. In addition, several of these drugs inhibit MAO in a way that is not reversible, so they are potentially very toxic.[26,100] In presynaptic neurons, MAO is a mitochondrial enzyme involved in the deamination of catecholamines. This in turn reduces production of the neurotransmitter. Within the brain there are two naturally occurring types of MAOs: type A for norepinephrine and serotonin and type B for dopamine.[91,100,191] Although both types share dopamine and tyramine as substrates, MAO-A selectively either metabolizes or if in large amounts blocks serotonin and norepinephrine, and MAO-B selectively metabolizes benzylamine and/or β-phenylethylamine.[91,191,209] The newer MAOIs

---

*References 46, 99, 100, 131, 156, 158, 205, 208, 209, 211.
†References 38, 41, 115, 162, 205, 208.

have a higher affinity for either type A or type B. Most antidepressant effects are targeted for MAO-A.[209] Selegiline (L-deprenyl) is said to be more specific for MAO-B. This results in a decreased metabolism of dopamine, an increased synthesis and release of dopamine, and inhibition of dopamine reuptake.[41,60,92] Selegiline is also metabolized to amphetamine, which could account for some of its effects.[136,191] In humans, L-deprenyl is a parkinsonian drug; however, it is marketed as a treatment for canine hyperadrenocorticism and for cognitive disorders in geriatric dogs.[189,190] Some research has been done about its use in older cats.[114] Reported side effects include atropine-like responses, weight gain, hypotension, restlessness, vomiting, diarrhea, pruritus, diminished hearing, disorientation, and, rarely, liver damage.[60,209] This drug should not be used concurrently with TCAs or SSRIs, meperidine or other apodes, phenylpropanolamine, or other MOAIs. Selegiline should be stopped at least 2 weeks before starting a TCA or SSRI.[41,115]

SSRIs are drugs that work at presynaptic sites. This newer group of psychoactive drugs is often compared with the tricyclics, being approximately equal in antidepressant effects.[140,164,208,209] The SSRIs do have an advantage over TCAs in treating anxiety with depression.[140] The neurotransmitter serotonin is involved in depression and mood regulation,[140] so it is no surprise that the SSRIs have been reported to affect a number of behaviors and conditions, including obsessive-compulsive disorders.[89,214] In general, SSRIs work almost exclusively to enhance serotonin at the synaptic area, so there is no advantage to switching drugs within the group if one does not work. This enhancement lowers anxiety levels.[165] As with TCAs, it generally takes about 4 weeks to effect a change because serotonin builds up slowly.[41,164] Long-term use affects postsynaptic serotonin receptors by increasing postsynaptic adenosine monophosphate (AMP).[153] The drug clomipramine works as an SSRI,[115,159] but it is generally classified as a TCA because it is also a norepinephrine reuptake inhibitor.[140] Side effects of SSRIs in humans include nausea, muscle rigidity, anxiety, sexual dysfunction, insomnia, anorexia, diarrhea, nervousness, and headaches.[38,100,209,211,214] Aggression in previously nonaggressive dogs can occur,[41] so consideration of this possibility should be given to cats as well. Fluoxetine is the SSRI drug currently tried the most in cats. Concomitant use with a TCA or benzodiazepine may increase plasma levels of both and may prolong excretion.[164] They should not be used in conjunction with an MAOI and should be discontinued at least 5 weeks before beginning treatment with an MAOI.[41]

Sympathomimetic stimulants are classified as antidepressant drugs, although they are not considered particularly good ones. Children with attention deficit hyperactivity disorder are the human models, and the primary medications used are stimulants like amphetamine or methylphenidate. Secondary medications for those who do not tolerate the stimulants are usually TCAs.[228] Amphetamine works in part by being taken up into the vesicles of the nerve terminals, where it increases the release and blocks reuptake of biogenic amines, especially dopamine and norepinephrine.[73,191] The psychostimulant effects of this class of drugs are mediated at the dopamine synapse.[53,195] They receive minor use in veterinary behavior treatment of canine hyperkinesis.[15,16,24] Methylphenidate toxicosis has been reported in cats.[73] Other signs of peripheral sympathomimetic stimulation include hypertension and cardiac arrhythmias.[73]

Antipsychotic drugs

The phenothiazines, particularly acetylpromazine, promazine, and chlorpromazine, are the most commonly used antipsychotic and hypnotic drugs in veterinary medicine. In general, however, the group as a whole is not particularly effective in behavior therapy except as a hypnotic. The dose an animal receives is the primary determinant of how hypnotic the effect is. They are often prescribed to be given before long trips and to minimize destruction during thunderstorms or separation from the owner. Unfortunately, this is not their best use, because it is the sedation that is helpful rather than antianxiety action.[24,158] Side effects can be serious and must be considered before use is started. Differences in response to any of the antipsychotic drugs are largely due to route of administration and differences in individuals.[91] They are metabolized by the liver with metabolites excreted in the urine.[41] The side effects can include idiosyncratic reactions of excitement, altered hormonal balance, lowered seizure threshold, ataxia, depressed basal metabolic rate, reduced thermoregulation, and hypotension.[41,131] Anecdotally it is suggested that noise phobias may be exacerbated, as might be expected because startle reactions to noise are increased not reduced.[41] These drugs have also been reported to facilitate the onset of acute aggression.[41] At least some of these drugs are noncompetitive blockers that work at the nicotinic acetylcholine receptors[8] as dopamine agonists.[131,204] Others are dopamine receptor antagonists (haloperidol),[141] perhaps working directly or indirectly with serotonin.[188] The phenothiazines decrease the initiation of motor activity at the basal ganglia of the brain.[24]

β-Blocking drugs

The noradrenergic antagonists, which are β-adrenergic receptor blocking drugs, were first used as antipsychotic medications and from that were used to treat schizophrenia. These drugs may also serve as a membrane-stabilizing agent in higher doses.[91] β-Blocking drugs are metabolized by the liver and are highly lipid soluble.[42] Controlled studies indicate onset of action may be extremely prolonged.[29] In humans β-blockers, such as propranolol, have also been used to treat situational anxieties like stage fright because they tend to reduce the somatic manifestations like tremors and sweaty palms.[47,131] The effect happens at the adrenergic receptors on muscle spindles.[49] Side effects include bradycardia, depression, hypotension, and sleep disturbances.[42] Concurrent diseases such as cardiac abnormalities, diabetes, and hypothyroidism would usually make the use of β-blockers contraindicated.[42]

Hypnotic drugs

A number of different types of drugs are classified as hypnotic because of their properties of inducing or approaching the induction of sleep. Most groups of drugs under this heading that are significant for veterinary medicine are discussed elsewhere relative to their other uses in psychotherapy. The specific members in this list tend to be slightly more hypnotic than others in their group.

The *antihistamines* have received some interest in veterinary medicine, but controlled studies have not been performed to evaluate which if any behaviors are most positively affected by their use. The sedative effect on the central nervous system can be useful in situations that cause a mild apprehension, such as car trips. In humans histaminergic neurons are characterized by the presence of numerous markers for other neurotransmitter systems, making it difficult to study their specific functions. Researchers have identified three histamine receptor subtypes: H_1, H_2, and H_3, although most of the available antihistamines are H_1-receptor antagonists and affect the cortical activation and arousal mechanisms.[198] Several antidepressants and antipsychotic drugs also have a high affinity for H_1-receptors, probably accounting for their sedative properties.[198] Contraindications for use would be related to the anticholinergic or atropine-like effects, so caution is needed if certain problems exist like hyperthyroidism, urinary retention, or glaucoma.[158] New drugs in this group are being designed to minimize their H_1 affinity.

Opiate antagonists

Neurologically, three subtypes of opiate receptors have been identified: µ, δ, and κ.[21,164,191] Although distribution of the various receptors varies throughout the brain, most opiates work on multiple receptor subtypes. As with other psychotherapeutic drugs, opiate antagonists are used to block the receptors, although chronic use can result in an antagonist-induced receptor upregulation. Apparently over time there is an increase in the number of receptors, primarily µ, which is expressed behaviorally as a supersensitivity to the actions of opioids.[91] It has been well studied that opiates facilitate stimulation within the brain, perhaps by their actions on dopaminergic neurons.[230] Narcotic antagonists have been used in veterinary medicine to reverse the effects of narcotic drugs used as sedatives. More recently they have been used to try to control stereotypic behaviors such as self-mutilation under the theory that the action of the behavior is self-rewarding via the release of naturally occurring opioids (endorphins, enkephalins).[158,164] High doses of amphetamine-like drugs are associated with a stereotyped syndrome.[104] Most narcotic antagonists have short durations of action, so they are helpful as diagnostic aids rather than long-term therapies in animals. Pentazocine, a mixed narcotic agonist and antagonist, and naltrexone, a pure opioid antagonist, have been used for longer action.[158] In drug-naive cats naloxone will decrease food and water consumption and in high doses can cause vomiting, persistent vocalization, heavy salivation, mydriasis, and hissing.[61]

Progestins

Progestins were the primary drugs for treating behavior problems for several years. Their mode of action is due to their binding to cytosolic androgen receptors with direct inhibiting effects of the steroid 5α-reductase in neuroreceptors of the hypothalamus and limbic systems.[37,84,88] The steroid 5α-reductase is the same enzyme that converts testosterone to dihydrotestosterone by competitive inhibition, resulting in lower plasma testosterone levels.[88] They also have an antianxiety calming effect,[75] possibly by binding to specific hypothalamic nuclei that suppress the "pain and punishment" center.[88] For these reasons they have proven most useful for controlling undesirable male sexually dimorphic behaviors and problems where stress is a factor, with urine spraying fitting into both categories. A number of different side effects must be considered when making a decision to use either the injectable or oral progestins. An increase in appetite is a secondary effect seen in 25% of cats,* and it can sometimes be a desirable effect.

---

*References 79, 81, 85, 107, 131, 187.

Because food intake in cats can be significantly reduced with stress, progestins can be useful when the two problems coexist. More serious side effects include depression, lethargy, mammary nodules/hyperplasia/neoplasia, uterine hyperplasia/pyometra, depression of corticosteroid output, generalized epidermal atrophy, suppression of fibroblasts, immunosuppression of T-cell function, diabetes mellitus, feline acquired skin fragility, xanthomatosis, and acromegaly.[*] Because of the significance of these side effects and the availability of safer drugs, progestins are not commonly used any more.[166]

Other drugs

Cyproheptadine is an antihistaminic and antiserotonergic drug that also has anticholinergic and sedative effects.[201] Humans report sedation and a feeling of euphoria, which is perhaps the reason it has been successfully used for treating anorexia and urine spraying.[200,201]

Feline facial pheromone is a synthetic analog of the pheromone associated with the cheek area of cats. Because facial rubbing is a behavior expressed in apparently comfortable surroundings, the use of this pheromone can help reduce anxiety levels in cats associated with new environments, the introduction of strange or disliked cats, or other environmental stresses resulting in urine spraying.

Melatonin is being tried in animals with day-night reversals. In some cases it seems to be helpful, even in patients with cognitive dysfunction syndrome.[234] Melatonin is considered an inhibitor of hepatic cytochrome P-450 isoenzymes.[234] This could affect the concentration of other drugs that use the same pathway and would need to be considered in geriatric patients or patients with hepatic disease. There can be significant differences in response to various products, so a great deal of variation of results should be expected unless a specific product is used.[48,234]

REFERENCES

1. America is going to the cats, *DVM* 18:59, Aug 1987.
2. American Animal Hospital Association: AAHA pet owner survey results, *Trends Magazine* 9(2):32–33, 1993.
3. American Animal Hospital Association: Third annual pet owner survey fetches results, *Trends Magazine* 8(1):44–45, 1994.
4. American Animal Hospital Association: AAHA's fourth annual pet survey looks at human animal bond, *Trends Magazine* 11(2):30–31, 1995.
5. American Veterinary Medical Association Center for Information Management: *U.S. pet ownership & demographics sourcebook,* Schaumburg, Ill, 1993, American Veterinary Medical Association.
6. American Veterinary Medical Association Center for Information Management: *U.S. pet ownership & demographics sourcebook,* Schaumburg, Ill, 1997, American Veterinary Medical Association.
7. Anchel M: *Overpopulation of cats and dogs: causes, effects, and prevention,* New York, 1990, Fordham University Press.
8. Arneric SP, Sullivan JP, Williams M: Neuronal nicotinic acetylcholine receptors: novel targets for central nervous systems therapeutics. In Bloom FE, Kupfer DJ, editors: *Psychopharmacology: the fourth generation of progress,* New York, 1995, Raven Press.

[*]References 24, 30, 49, 52, 64, 79-82, 85, 88, 107, 131, 158, 164, 171, 172, 187, 202, 217.

9. Astrup C: Pavlovian concepts of abnormal behavior in man and animal. In Fox MW, editor: *Abnormal behavior in animals,* Philadelphia, 1968, WB Saunders.

10. Beadle M: *The cat: history, biology, and behavior,* New York, 1977, Simon & Schuster.

11. Beaver BG: The veterinarian's role in prescribing pets, *Vet Med Small Anim Clin* 69:1506, 1508, Dec 1974.

12. Beaver BV: *Animal behavior: pets and people, proceeding of the National Conference on Dog and Cat Control,* Denver, 1976, The American Humane Association.

13. Beaver BV: Behavioral histories, *Vet Med Small Anim Clin* 76(4):478, 480, 1981.

14. Beaver BV: Disorders of behavior. In Sherding RG, editor: *The cat: diseases and clinical management,* New York, 1989, Churchill Livingstone.

15. Beaver BV: *The veterinarian's encyclopedia of animal behavior,* Ames, 1994, Iowa State University Press.

16. Beaver BV: *Canine behavior: a guide for veterinarians,* Philadelphia, 1999, WB Saunders.

17. Borchelt PL, Voith VL: Classification of animal behavior problems, *Vet Clin North Am Small Anim Pract* 12:571–585, Nov 1982.

18. Borchelt PL, Voith V: Punishment, *Compend Contin Educ* 7:780–791, Sep 1985.

19. Boulenger JP, Squillance K, Simon P, et al: Buspirone and diazepam: comparison of subjective, psychomotor and biological effects, *Neuropsychobiology* 22:83–89, 1989.

20. Bradshaw JWS, Horsfield GF, Allen JA, et al: Feral cats: their role in the population dynamics of *Felis catus, Appl Anim Behav Sci* 65(3):273–283, 1999.

21. Brady LS: Opiate receptor regulation by opiate agonists and antagonists. In Hammer RP, editor: *The neurobiology of opiates,* Boca Raton, Fla, 1993, CRC Press.

22. Bronson RT: Age at death of necropsied intact and neutered cats, *Am J Vet Res* 42:1606–1608, Sep 1981.

23. Bruhwyler J, Chleide E, Rettori MC, et al: Amineptine improves the performance of dogs in a complex temporal regulation schedule, *Pharmacol Biochem Behav* 45(4):897–903, 1993.

24. Burghardt WF Jr: Behavioral medicine as a part of a comprehensive small animal medical program, *Vet Clin North Am Small Anim Pract* 21(2):343–352, 1991.

25. Burghardt WF Jr: Formulating a prognosis for behavioral therapy. Paper presented at American Veterinary Medical Association meeting, Minneapolis, July 18, 1993.

26. Burke MJ, Preskorn SH: Short-term treatment of mood disorders with standard antidepressants. In Bloom FE, Kupfer DJ, editors: *Psychopharmacology: the fourth generation of progress,* New York, 1995, Raven Press.

27. Cameron P, Pope C: Are pets harmful to the mental and physical health of our society? *Good Morning America Faceoff,* Dec 22, 1977.

28. Campbell WE: Environmental changes, *Mod Vet Pract* 58(3):275, 1977.

29. Casey DE: Tardive dyskinesia: pathophysiology. In Bloom FE, Kupfer DJ, editors: *Psychopharmacology: the fourth generation of progress,* New York, 1995, Raven Press.

30. Chastain CB, Graham CL, Nichols EE: Adrenocortical suppression in cats given megestrol acetate, *Am J Vet Res* 42(12):2029–2035, 1981.

31. Childs JE, Ross L: Urban cats: characteristics and estimation of mortality due to motor vehicles, *Am J Vet Res* 47:1643–1648, July 1986.

32. Clark JM: The effects of selection and human preference on coat colour gene frequencies in urban cats, *Heredity* 35:195–210, Oct 1975.

33. Clutton-Brock J: *Domesticated animals from early times,* Austin, 1981, University of Texas Press.

34. Collier GE, O'Brien SJ: A molecular phylogeny of the Felidae: immunological distances, *Evolution* 39(3):473–487, 1985.

35. Comfort A: Maximum ages reached by domestic cats, *J Mammal* 37:118–119, 1956.

36. Coop CF, McNaughton N: Buspirone affects hippocampal rhythmical slow activity through serotonin 1A rather than dopamine D_2 receptors, *Neuroscience* 40(1):169, 1991.

37. Cooper L, Hart BL: Comparison of diazepam with progestin for effectiveness in suppression of urine spraying behavior in cats, *J Am Vet Med Assoc* 200(6):797–801, 1992.

38. Cooper LL: Feline inappropriate elimination, *Vet Clin North Am Small Anim Pract* 27(3):569–600, 1997.

39. Coplan JD, Wolk SI, Klein DF: Anxiety and the serotonin 1A receptor. In Bloom FE, Kupfer DJ, editors: *Psychopharmacology: the fourth generation of progress,* New York, 1995, Raven Press.

40. Corson SA, Corson EO, Gwynne PH, Arnold LE: Pet-facilitated psychotherapy in a hospital setting. In Masserman JH, editor: *Current psychiatric therapies,* New York, 1975, Grune & Stratton.

41. Crowell-Davis SL: Psychopharmacology part I, *AAHA Scientific Proc* pp 12–15, March 10–14, 2001.

42. Crowell-Davis SL: Psychopharmacology part II, *AAHA Scientific Proc* pp 16–19, March 10–14, 2001.

43. Crowell-Davis SL, Barry K, Wolfe R: Social behavior and aggressive problems of cats, *Vet Clin North Am Small Anim Pract* 27(3):549–568, 1997.

44. Dallaire A: Stress and behavior in domestic animals: temperament as a predisposing factor to stereotypies, *Ann N Y Acad Sci* 697:269–274, Oct 29, 1993.

45. Danneman PJ, Chodrow RE: History-taking and interviewing techniques, *Vet Clin North Am Small Anim Pract* 12(4):587–592, 1982.

46. Dehasse J: Feline urine spraying, *Appl Anim Behav Sci* 52(3,4):365–371, 1997.

47. Dodman NH: Pharmacological treatment of behavioral problems in cats, *Vet Forum* pp 62–65, 71, April 1995.

48. Dodman NH: Personal communication, Feb 1, 2001.

49. Dodman NH, Shuster L: Pharmacologic approaches to managing behavior problems in small animals, *Vet Med* 89(10):960–969, 1994.

50. Dog and cat ownership, 1991–1998, *J Am Vet Med Assoc* 204(8):1166–1167, 1994.

51. Dorn C: Veterinary medical services: utilization by dog and cat owners, *J Am Vet Med Assoc* 156:321–327, Feb 1, 1970.

52. Eigenmann JE, Venker-van Haagen AJ: Progestogen-induced and spontaneous canine acromegaly due to reversible growth hormone overproduction: clinical picture and pathogenesis, *J Am Anim Hosp Assoc* 17(5):813–822, 1981.

53. Ernst M, Zametkin A: The interface of genetics, neuroimaging, and neurochemistry in attention-deficit hyperactivity disorder. In Bloom FE, Kupfer DJ, editors: *Psychopharmacology: the fourth generation of progress,* New York, 1995, Raven Press.

54. Excerpts from the Islamic teachings on animal welfare, *The Latham Letter* X:14, Summer 1989.

55. Faulkner LC: Pet population problem, *Calif Vet* 27(6):19, 38–39, 1973.

56. Feaver J, Mendl M, Bateson P: A method for rating the individual distinctiveness of domestic cats, *Anim Behav* 34:1016–1025, Aug 1986.

57. Feinberg M: Clomipramine for obsessive-compulsive disorder, *Am Fam Physician* 43(5):1735, 1991.

58. Feldmann BM: Why people own pets: pet owner psychology and the delinquent owner, *Gaines Dog Res Prog* 1:6, 8, Summer 1977.

59. Flament MF, Rapoport JL, Berg CJ, et al: Clomipramine treatment of childhood obsessive-compulsive disorder: a double-blind controlled study, *Arch Gen Psychiatry* 42:977–983, 1985.

60. Fortney WD: Behavioral problems in older dogs and cats, American Veterinary Medical Association Convention Notes. Available at www.avma.org/noah/members/convention/conv01/notes/04040603.asp.

61. Foster JA, Morrison M, Dean SJ, et al: Naloxone suppresses food/water consumption in the deprived cat, *Pharmacol Biochem Behav* 14(3):419–421, 1981.
62. Fox MW: *Understanding your cat,* New York, 1974, Coward, McCann, & Geoghegan.
63. Fox MW: The veterinarian: mercenary, Saint Francis—or humanist? *J Am Vet Med Assoc* 166:276–279, Feb 1, 1975.
64. Frank DW, Kirton KT, Murchison TE, et al: Mammary tumors and serum hormones in the bitch treated with medroxyprogesterone acetate or progesterone for four years, *Fertil Steril* 31(3):340–346, 1979.
65. Franti CE, Kraus JF: Aspects of pet ownership in Yolo County California, *J Am Vet Med Assoc* 164:166–171, Jan 15, 1974.
66. Fuller JL, Fox MW: The behavior of dogs. In Hafez ESE, editor: *The behavior of domestic animals,* ed 2, Baltimore, 1969, Williams & Wilkins.
67. Ganster D, Voith VL: Attitudes of cat owners toward their cats, *Feline Pract* 13:21–29, March/April 1983.
68. Gehrke BC: Results of the AVMA survey of US pet-owning households on companion animal ownership, *J Am Vet Med Assoc* 211(2):169–170, 1997.
69. Geisler J: New AAHA study: veterinary clients treat their pets more and more like people, *DVM Newsmagazine* 27(1):16S, 20S, 1996.
70. Glennon RA, Dukat M: Serotonin receptor subtypes. In Bloom FE, Kupfer DJ, editors: *Psychopharmacology: the fourth generation of progress,* New York, 1995, Raven Press.
71. Gorodetsky E: Epidemiology of dog and cat euthanasia across Canadian prairie provinces, *Can Vet J* 38(10):649–652, 1997.
72. Griffiths AO, Silberberg A: Stray animals: their impact on a community, *Mod Vet Pract* 56:255–256, April 1975.
73. Gustafson BW: Methylphenidate toxicosis in a cat, *J Am Vet Med Assoc* 208(7):1052–1053, 1996.
74. Hanson RL, Clark AP: Number of cat owners, *Feline Pract* 7:52, Sep 1977.
75. Hart BL: Behavioral effects of long-acting progestins, *Feline Pract* 4(4):8, 11, 1974.
76. Hart BL: Social interactions between cats and their owners, *Feline Pract* 6(1):6, 8, 1976.
77. Hart BL: Children and pets: an interview with a child psychiatrist, *Feline Pract* 8(1):8, 10, 12, 1978.
78. Hart BL: Problem solving, *Feline Pract* 9(1):8, 10, 1979.
79. Hart BL: Evaluation of progestin therapy for behavioral problems, *Feline Pract* 9(3):11–14, 1979.
80. Hart BL: Behavioral therapy with mousetraps, *Feline Pract* 9(4):10, 12, 14, 1979.
81. Hart BL: Problems with objectionable sociosexual behavior of dogs and cats: therapeutic use of castration and progestins, *Compend Contin Educ Small Anim* 1:461–465, 1979.
82. Hart BL: Progestin therapy for aggressive behavior in male dogs, *J Am Vet Med Assoc* 178(10):1070, 1981.
83. Hart BL, Cooper LL: Integrating use of psychotropic drugs with environmental management and behavioral modification for treatment of problem behavior in animals, *J Am Vet Med Assoc* 209(9):1549–1551, 1996.
84. Hart BL, Eckstein RA, Powell KL, Dodman NH: Effectiveness of buspirone on urine spraying and inappropriate urination in cats, *J Am Vet Med Assoc* 203(2):254–258, 1993.
85. Hart BL, Hart LA: *Canine and feline behavioral therapy,* Philadelphia, 1985, Lea & Febiger.
86. Heidenberger E: Housing conditions and behavioral problems of indoor cats as assessed by their owners, *Appl Anim Behav Sci* 52(3,4):345–364, 1997.
87. Heiman M: Man and his pet. In Slovenko R, Knight JA, editors: *Motivations in play, games and sports,* Springfield, Ill, 1967, Charles C Thomas Publisher.
88. Henik RA, Olson PN, Rosychuk RA: Progestogen therapy in cats, *Compend Contin Educ Pract Vet* 7(2):132–136, 140–141, 1985.

89. Heninger GR: Indoleamines: the role of serotonin in clinical disorders. In Bloom FE, Kupfer DJ, editors: *Psychopharmacology: the fourth generation of progress,* New York, 1995, Raven Press.

90. Hewson CJ, Luescher UA, Ball RD: Measuring change in the behavioral severity of canine compulsive disorder: the construct validity of categories of change derived from two ratings scales, *Appl Anim Behav Sci* 60(1):55–68, 1998.

91. Hollister LE: *Clinical pharmacology of psychotherapeutic drugs,* ed 2, New York, 1983, Churchill Livingstone.

92. Houpt KA: Cognitive dysfunction in geriatric cats. In August JR, editor: *Consultations in feline internal medicine,* vol 4, Philadelphia, 2001, WB Saunders.

93. Houpt KA: Behavioral genetics of cats and dogs, American Veterinary Medical Association Convention Notes. Available at www.avma.org/noah/members/convention/conv01/notes/04010101.asp.

94. HSUS: Pet overpopulation, *Can Pract* 19(2):21, 1994.

95. Hughes D, Moreau RE, Overall KL, VanWinkle TJ: Acute hepatic necrosis and liver failure associated with benzodiazepine therapy in six cats, 1986–1995, *J Vet Emerg Crit Care* 6(1):13–20, 1996.

96. Huidekopper RS: *The cat,* New York, 1895, D. Appleton & Company.

97. Hunthausen W: Collecting the history of a pet with a behavior problem, *Vet Med* 89(10):954–959, 1994.

98. Hunthausen WL: Rule out medical etiologies first in geriatric behavior problems, *DVM* 22(7):24, 1991.

99. Johnson LR: Tricyclic antidepressant toxicosis, *Vet Clin North Am Small Anim Pract* 20(2):393–403, 1990.

100. Julien RM: *A primer of drug action: a concise nontechnical guide to the actions, uses, and side effects of psychoactive drugs,* ed 7, New York, 1995, WH Freeman and Company.

101. Kamerling SG: Drugs and animal behavior, American Veterinary Medical Association Convention Notes. Available at www.avma.org/noah/members/convention/conv01/notes/04050101.asp.

102. Karsh EB, Turner DC: The human-cat relationship. In Turner DC, Bateson P, editors: *The domestic cat: the biology of its behavior,* New York, 1988, Cambridge University Press.

103. Keeping the pets in line, *Vet Forum* pp 60–66, Sep 1997.

104. Kelly PH: Drug-induced motor behavior. In Iversen LL, Iversen SD, Snyder SH, editors: *Handbook of psychopharmacology,* vol 8, *Drugs, neurotransmitters, and behavior,* New York, 1977, Plenum Publishing.

105. Knol BW: Behavioural problems in dogs. Problems, diagnoses, therapeutic measures and results in 133 patients, *Vet Q* 9(3):226, 1987.

106. Knol BW: Social problem behavior in dogs: etiology and pathogenesis, *Vet Q* 16(51):505, 1994.

107. Knol BW, Egberink-Alink ST: Treatment of problem behavior in dogs and cats by castration and progestogen administration: a review, *Vet Q* 11(2):102, 1989.

108. Kolata RJ, Kraut NH, Johnston DE: Patterns of trauma in urban dogs and cats; a study of 1,000 cases, *J Am Vet Med Assoc* 164:499–502, March 1, 1974.

109. Kretchmer KR, Fox MW: Effects of domestication on animal behaviour, *Vet Rec* 96:102–108, Feb 1, 1975.

110. Landsberg G: Products for preventing or controlling undesirable behavior, *Vet Med* 89(10):970–977, 980–983, 1994.

111. Landsberg G: Providing behavior services to clients, Friskies PetCare Symposium, *Small Anim Behav Proc* pp 32–36, Oct 4, 1998.

112. Landsberg GM: Veterinarians as behavior consultants, *Can Vet J* 31(3):225, 1990.

113. Landsberg GM: Techniques for solving behavior problems. Paper presented at American Veterinary Medical Association meeting, Minneapolis, July 17, 1993.

114. Landsberg GM: Behavior problems of older cats, *Proc Am Vet Med Assoc* pp 317–320, 1998.

115. Landsberg GM: Clomipramine—beyond separation anxiety, *J Am Anim Hosp Assoc* 37(4):313–318, 2001.

116. Lehman HC: The child's attitude toward the dog versus the cat, *J Genet Psychol* 35:62–72, 1928.

117. Levine BN: Practice today: small animal pet population trends and demands for veterinary service, *AAHA Trends* 1(3):24–31, 1985.

118. Levinson BM: Pets: a special technique in child psychotherapy, *Ment Hyg* 48:243–248, 1964.

119. Levinson BM: Household pets in residential schools: their therapeutic potential, *Ment Hyg* 52:411–414, July 1968.

120. Levinson BM: Interpersonal relationships between pet and human being. In Fox MW, editor: *Abnormal behavior in animals,* Philadelphia, 1968, WB Saunders.

121. Levinson BM: *Pet-oriented child psychotherapy,* Springfield, Ill, 1969, Charles C Thomas Publisher.

122. Levinson BM: Pets and old age, *Ment Hyg* 53:364–368, July 1969.

123. Levinson BM: Pets and environment. In Anderson RS, editor: *Pet animals and society,* London, 1974, Baillière Tindall.

124. Levy JK, Cullen JM, Bunch SE, et al: Adverse reaction to diazepam in cats, *J Am Vet Med Assoc* 205(2):156–157, 1994.

125. Luke C: Animal shelter issues, *J Am Vet Med Assoc* 208(4):524–527, 1996.

126. Maes M, Meltzer HY: The serotonin hypothesis of major depression. In Bloom FE, Kupfer DJ, editors: *Psychopharmacology: the fourth generation of progress,* New York 1995, Raven Press.

127. Mahlow JC, Slater MR: Current issues in the control of stray and feral cats, *J Am Vet Med Assoc* 209(12):2016–2020, 1996.

128. Major research set on man-animal role, *DVM* 9:1, 5, Feb 1978.

129. Manning AM, Rowan AN: Companion animal demographics and sterilization status: results from a survey in four Massachusetts towns, *Anthrozoös* V (3):192–201, 1992.

130. Marchand C, Moore A: Pet populations and ownership around the world, *Waltham International Focus* 1:14–15, 1991.

131. Marder AR: Psychotropic drugs and behavioral therapy, *Vet Clin North Am Small Anim Pract* 21(2):329–342, 1991.

132. Marshall MA, Hart BL: Behavior modification technique, *Can Pract* 6(4):8, 10, 1979.

133. Matheson C: The domestic cat as a factor in urban ecology, *J Anim Ecol* 13:130–133, Nov 1944.

134. Mench JA, Shea-Moore MM: Moods, minds and molecules: the neurochemistry of social behavior, *Appl Anim Behav Sci* 44(2–4):99–118, 1995.

135. Mestel R: Ascent of the dog, *Discover* p 90, Oct 1994.

136. Milgram NW, Ivy GO, Head E, et al: The effect of L-deprenyl on behavior, cognitive function, and biogenic amines in the dog, *Neurochem Res* 18(12):1211–1219, 1993.

137. Miller DD, Staats SR, Partlo C, Rada K: Factors associated with the decision to surrender a pet to an animal shelter, *J Am Vet Med Assoc* 209(4):738–742, 1996.

138. Miller J: The domestic cat: perspective on the nature and diversity of cats, *J Am Vet Med Assoc* 208(4):498–502, 1996.

139. Mills DS: Using learning theory in animal behavior therapy practice, *Vet Clin North Am Small Anim Pract* 27(3):617–635, 1997.

140. Montgomery SA: Selective serotonin reuptake inhibitors in the acute treatment of depression. In Bloom FE, Kupfer DJ, editors: *Psychopharmacology: the fourth generation of progress*, New York, 1995, Raven Press.

141. Moon BH, Feigenbaum JJ, Corson PE, Klawans HL: The role of dopaminergic mechanisms in naloxone-induced inhibition of apomorphine-induced stereotyped behavior, *Eur J Pharmacol* 61:71–78, 1980.

142. Morey DF: The early evolution of the domestic dog, *Am Scientist* 82(4):336, 1994.

143. Morgan RV, editor: *Handbook of small animal practice*, New York, 1988, Churchill Livingstone.

144. Mosier JE: Personal communication, 1970.

145. MVP Staff Report: outlook for the 70's, *Mod Vet Pract* 51:39–47, Oct 1970.

146. Nassar R, Mosier JE: Feline population dynamics: a study of the Manhattan, Kansas feline population, *Am J Vet Res* 43:167–170, Jan 1982.

147. Nassar R, Mosier JE, Williams LW: Study of the feline and canine populations in the greater Las Vegas area, *Am J Vet Res* 45:282–287, 1984.

148. New JC Jr, Salman MD, King M, et al: Characteristics of shelter-relinquished animals and their owners compared with animals and their owners in U.S. pet-owning households, *J Appl Anim Welfare Sci* 3(3):179–201, 2001.

149. Nutt JG, Irwin RP: Principles of neuropharmacology. II. Synaptic transmission. In Klawans HL, Goetz CG, Tanner CM, editors: *Textbook of clinical neuropharmacology and therapeutics*, ed 2, New York, 1992, Raven Press.

150. O'Brien SJ: The family line, *National Geographic* 191(6):77–85, 1997.

151. Olson PN, Johnston SD: New developments in small animal population control, *J Am Vet Med Assoc* 202(6):904–909, 1993.

152. Overall K: Choose medication last when trying to treat feline behavioral disorders, *DVM* 26(3):24S, 26S, 27S, 1995.

153. Overall K: *Neurochemistry of anxiety and aggression.* Paper presented at Western Veterinary Conference, Las Vegas, February 21, 2000.

154. Overall K: The success of treatment outcomes, *APDT Newsletter* pp 11–12, Jan/Feb 2001.

155. Overall KL: Part 1: A rational approach: recognition, diagnosis, and management of obsessive-compulsive disorders, *Canine Pract* 17(2):40–44, 1992.

156. Overall KL: Part 2: A rational approach: recognition, diagnosis, and management of obsessive-compulsive disorders, *Canine Pract* 17(3):25, 1992.

157. Overall KL: Part 3: A rational approach: recognition, diagnosis, and management of obsessive-compulsive disorders, *Canine Pract* 17(4):39, 1992.

158. Overall KL: Practical pharmacological approaches to behavior problems. *Purina Specialty Review: Behavioral Problems in Small Animals* p 36, 1992.

159. Overall KL: Use of clomipramine to treat ritualistic stereotypic motor behavior in three dogs, *J Am Vet Med Assoc* 205(12):1733, 1994.

160. Overall KL: Understanding repetitive, stereotypic behaviors: signs, history, diagnosis, and practical treatment. Paper presented at American Veterinary Medical Association meeting, Pittsburgh, July 8, 1995.

161. Overall KL: Drug therapy for spraying cats, *Feline Pract* 24(6):40–42, Nov/Dec 1996.

162. Overall KL: Prescribing Prozac means taking thorough medical, behavioral history, *DVM* 27(11):2S, 24S, 1996.

163. Overall KL: *Clinical behavioral medicine for small animals*, St Louis, 1997, Mosby–Year Book.

164. Overall KL: Pharmacologic treatments for behavior problems, *Vet Clin North Am Small Anim Pract* 27(3):637–665, 1997.

165. Overall KL: Managing an aggressive cat, *Vet Med* 93(12):1051–1052, Dec 1998.

166. Overall KL: Behavioral pharmacology, *Proc Am Anim Hosp Assoc*, pp 65–75, 2000.

167. Owren T, Matre PJ: Somatic problems as a risk factor for behavior problems in dogs, *Vet Q* 16(51):505, 1994.

168. Pato MT, Piggott TA, Hill JL, et al: Controlled comparison of buspirone and clomipramine in obsessive-compulsive disorder, *Am J Psychiatry* 148:127–129, 1991.

169. Patronek GJ, Beck AM, Glickman LT: Dynamics of dog and cat populations in a community, *J Am Vet Med Assoc* 210(5):637–642, 1997.

170. Patronek GJ, Glickman LT, Beck AM, et al: Risk factors for relinquishment of cats to an animal shelter, *J Am Vet Med Assoc* 209(3):582–588, 1996.

171. Pemberton PL: Feline and canine behavior control: progestin therapy. In Kirk RW, editor: *Current veterinary therapy,* vol VII, *Small animal practice,* Philadelphia, 1980, WB Saunders.

172. Pemberton PL: Feline and canine behavior control: progestin therapy. In Kirk RW, editor: *Current veterinary therapy,* vol VIII, *Small animal practice,* Philadelphia, 1983, WB Saunders.

173. Pet estimates vary, *The NACA News* 6:1, June/July 1984.

174. Pet owners blissfully ignorant, survey says, *Vet Pract News* 12(11):8, 2000.

175. Pet pause, *Advantage* 1(1):2, 1991.

176. Podberscek AL, Blackshaw JK: Reasons for liking and choosing a cat as a pet, *Aust Vet J* 65:332–333, 1988.

177. Podberscek AL, Blackshaw JK, Bodero DAV: An evaluation of human-cat associations, *Aust Vet Pract* 18(1):16–20, 1988.

178. Pond G: *The complete cat encyclopedia,* New York, 1972, Crown Publishers.

179. Price EO: Behavioral aspects of animal domestication, *Q Rev Biol* 59(1):1–32, 1984.

180. Rann R: Target animal safety in dogs and cats with clomipramine, *AVSAB Newsletter* 19(2):3, 1997.

181. Raskind MA: Alzheimer's disease: treatment of noncognitive behavioral abnormalities. In Bloom FE, Kupfer DJ, editors: *Psychopharmacology: the fourth generation of progress,* New York, 1995, Raven Press.

182. Reich M, Overall KL: Assessment of anti-anxiety medication on canine and feline patients: potential for cardiac side effects and correlation with intermediate metabolite levels. Paper presented at American Veterinary Society Animal Behavior meeting, Baltimore, July 27, 1998.

183. Reisner I: Use of lithium for treatment of canine dominance-related aggression: a case study, *Appl Anim Behav Sci* 39:190, 1994.

184. Remfry J: Feral cats in the United Kingdom, *J Am Vet Med Assoc* 209(4):520–523, 1996.

185. Richelson E: Pharmacology of antidepressants—characteristics of the ideal drug, *Mayo Clin Proc* 69:1069, 1994.

186. Robinson R: Cat. In Mason IL, editor: *Evolution of domesticated animals,* New York, 1984, Longman.

187. Romatowski J: Use of megestrol acetate in cats, *J Am Vet Med Assoc* 194(5):700–702, 1989.

188. Roth BL, Meltzer HY: The role of serotonin in schizophrenia. In Bloom FE, Kupfer DJ, editors: *Psychopharmacology: the fourth generation of progress,* New York, 1995, Raven Press.

189. Ruehl WW: Rationale to develop the investigational drug L-deprenyl for use in pet dogs, *Am Vet Soc Anim Behav Newsletter* 15(1):4, 1993.

190. Ruehl WW, DePaoli AC, Bruyette DS: L-Deprenyl for treatment of behavioral and cognitive problems in dogs: preliminary report of an open label trial, *Appl Anim Behav Sci* 39:191, 1994.

191. Ryall RW: *Mechanisms of drug action on the nervous system,* ed 2, New York, 1989, Cambridge University Press.

192. Salman MD, Hutchison J, Buch-Gallie R, et al: Behavioral reasons for relinquishment of dogs and cats to 12 shelters, *J Appl Anim Welfare Sci* 3(2):93–106, 2000.

193. Salman MD, New JG Jr, Scarlett JM, et al: Human and animal factors related to the relinquishment of dogs and cats in 12 selected animal shelters in the United States, *J Appl Anim Welfare Sci* 1(3):207–226, 1998.

194. Scharf MB, Sachais BA: The pharmacology of disordered sleep. In Klawans HL, Goetz CG, Tanner CM, editors: *Textbook of clinical neuropharmacology and therapeutics*, ed 2, New York, 1992, Raven Press.

195. Schatzberg AF, Schildkraut JJ: Recent studies on norepinephrine systems in mood disorders. In Bloom FE, Kupfer DJ, editors: *Psychopharmacology: the fourth generation of progress*, New York, 1995, Raven Press.

196. Schneider R: Observations on overpopulation of dogs and cats, *J Am Vet Med Assoc* 167(4):281–284, 1975.

197. Schneider R, Vaida ML: Survey of canine and feline populations: Alameda and Contra Costa counties, California, 1970, *J Am Vet Med Assoc* 166(5):481–486, 1975.

198. Schwartz JC, Arrang JM, Garbarg M, Traiffort E: Histamine. In Bloom FE, Kupfer DJ, editors: *Psychopharmacology: the fourth generation of progress*, New York, 1995, Raven Press.

199. Schwartz S: Carbamazepine in the control of aggressive behavior in cats, *J Am Anim Hosp Assoc* 30(5):515–519, 1994.

200. Schwartz S: Use of cyproheptadine to control urine spraying and masturbation in a cat, *J Am Vet Med Assoc* 214(3):369–371, 1999.

201. Schwartz S: Use of cyproheptadine to control urine spraying in a castrated male domestic cat, *J Am Vet Med Assoc* 215(4):501–502, 1999.

202. Scott DW, Miller WH Jr, Griffin CE: *Muller & Kirk's small animal dermatology*, ed 5, Philadelphia, 1995, WB Saunders.

203. Searle AG: Gene frequencies in London's cats, *J Genet* 49:214–220, Dec 1949.

204. Seeman P: Dopamine receptors. In Bloom FE, Kupfer DJ, editors: *Psychopharmacology: the fourth generation of progress*, New York, 1995, Raven Press.

205. Seksel K: Feline urine spraying. In Houpt KA, editor: Recent advances in companion animal behavior problems, International Veterinary Information Service, Oct 11, 2000. Available at www.ivis.org.

206. Selby LA: Family life cycle as related to cat, dog ownership, *DVM* 9:20–22, Feb 1978.

207. Serpell JA: The domestication and history of the cat. In Turner DC, Bateson P, editor: *The domestic cat: the biology of its behaviour*, New York, 1988, Cambridge University Press.

208. Shader RI, Greenblatt DJ: The pharmacotherapy of acute anxiety: a mini-update. In Bloom FE, Kupfer DJ, editors: *Psychopharmacology: the fourth generation of progress*, New York, 1995, Raven Press.

209. Shanley K, Overall K: Rational selection of antidepressants for behavioral conditions, *Vet Forum* p 30, Nov 1995.

210. Shull-Selcer EA, Stagg W: Advances in the understanding and treatment of noise phobias, *Vet Clin North Am Small Anim Pract* 21(2):353–367, 1991.

211. Simpson BS, Simpson DM: Behavioral pharmacotherapy. I. Antipsychotics and antidepressants, *Compend Contin Educ Pract Vet* 18(10):1067–1081, 1996.

212. Simpson BS, Simpson DM: Behavioral pharmacotherapy. II. Anxiolytics and mood stabilizers, *Compend Contin Educ Pract Vet* 18(11):1203–1213, 1996.

213. Smith RC: *The complete cat book*, New York, 1963, Walker & Company.

214. Sommi RW, Crismon ML, Bowden CL: Fluoxetine: a serotonin-specific, second-generation antidepressant, *Pharmacotherapy* 7(1):1, 1987.

215. Speck RV: Mental health problems involving the family, the pet, and the veterinarian, *J Am Vet Med Assoc* 145:150–154, July 15, 1964.

216. Spreat S, Spreat SR: Learning principles, *Vet Clin North Am Small Anim Pract* 12(4):593–606, 1982.

217. Stabenfeldt GH: Physiologic, pathologic and therapeutic roles of progestins in domestic animals, *J Am Vet Med Assoc* 164(3):311–317, 1974.

218. Suehsdorf A: The cats in our lives, *National Geographic* 125:508–541, April 1964.

219. Swingler RC: Educational value of classroom pets, *Educ Dig* 31:50–52, Feb 1966.

220. Teclaw R, Mendlein J, Garbe P, Mariolis P: Characteristics of pet populations and households in the Purdue Comparative Oncology Program catchment area, 1988, *J Am Vet Med Assoc* 201(11):1725–1729, 1992.

221. Tedesco FJ, Mills LR: Diazepam (Valium) hepatitis, *Dig Dis Sci* 27(5):470–472, 1982.

222. The state of the American pet. Ralston Purina Web site. Available at www.purina.com/institute/survey.asp.

223. Thorén P, Åsberg M, Cronholm B, et al: Clomipramine treatment of obsessive-compulsive disorder. I. A controlled clinical trial, *Arch Gen Psychiatry* 37:1281–1285, 1980.

224. Thornton GW: The welfare of excess animals: status and needs, *J Am Vet Med Assoc* 200(5):660–662, 1992.

225. Todd NB: Cats and commerce, *Sci Am* 237:100–107, Nov 1977.

226. Todd NB: An ecological, behavioral genetic model for the domestication of the cat, *Carnivore* 1:52–60, 1978.

227. Top 10 reasons for relinquishment identified, *J Am Vet Med Assoc* 210(9):1256, 1997.

228. Towbin KE, Leckman JF: Attention deficit hyperactivity disorder in childhood and adolescence. In Klawans HL, Goetz CG, Tanner CM, editors: *Textbook of clinical neuropharmacology and therapeutics,* ed 2, New York, 1992, Raven Press.

229. Turner DC, Rieger G: The influence of house cats on human moods in comparison with the influence of human partners, Abstract book from *9th International Conference on Human-Animal Interactions,* p 89, 2001.

230. Unterwald EM, Kornetsky C: Reinforcing effects of opiates—modulation by dopamine. In Hammer RP, editor: *The neurobiology of opiates,* Boca Raton, Fla, 1993, CRC Press.

231. vanAarde RJ, Blumenberg B: Genotypic correlates of body and adrenal weight in a population of feral cats *Felis catus, Carnivore* 2(2,3):37–45, 1979.

232. Veterinary health care market for cats, *J Am Vet Med Assoc* 184:481–482, Feb 15, 1984.

233. Veterinary service market for companion animals, 1992. I. Companion animal ownership and demographics, *J Am Vet Med Assoc* 201(7):990–992, 1992.

234. Virga V: Personal communication, Feb 2, 2001.

235. Voith VL: Anamnesis, *Mod Vet Pract* 61(5):460, 1980.

236. Voith VL: You, too, can teach a cat tricks (examples of shaping, second-order reinforcement, and constraints on learning), *Mod Vet Pract* 62:639–642, Aug 1981.

237. Voith VL, Borchelt PL: Introduction to animal behavior therapy, *Vet Clin North Am Small Anim Pract* 2(4):565–570, 1982.

238. Voith V, Borchelt P: Fears and phobias in companion animals, *Compend Contin Educ* 7:209–219, March 1985.

239. Voith VL, Marder AR: Introduction to behavior disorders. In Morgan RV, editor: *Handbook of small animal practice,* New York, 1988, Churchill Livingstone.

240. Wayne RK, Benveniste RE, Janczewski DN, O'Brien SJ: Molecular and biochemical evolution of the carnivora. In Gittleman JL, editor: *Carnivore behavior, ecology, and evolution,* Ithaca, NY, 1989, Cornell University Press.

241. Weigel I: Small cats and clouded leopards. In Grzimek HCB, editor: *Grzimek's animal life encyclopedia,* vol 12, New York, 1975, Van Nostrand Reinhold.

242. Wilbur RH: *Pets, pet ownership and animal control: social and psychological attitudes, 1975: proceedings of the National Conference on Dog and Cat Control,* Denver, 1976, The American Humane Association.

243. Wood GL: *Animal facts and feats,* Garden City, NY, 1972, Doubleday & Company.

244. Woodbury D: Fido's no longer in the doghouse, *Trends Magazine* XIV(2):42–43, 1998.
245. Woodbury D: Risking life or limb for Fido, *Trends Magazine* XV(2):30–31, 1999.
246. Zasloff RL: Cats and their people: a (nearly) perfect relationship, *J Am Vet Med Assoc* 208(4):512–516, 1996.
247. Zaunbrecher KI, Smith RE: Neutering of feral cats as an alternative to eradication programs, *J Am Vet Med Assoc* 203(3):449–452, 1993.
248. Zeuner FE: *A history of domesticated animals,* New York, 1963, Harper & Row.

ADDITIONAL READINGS

Anderson RK, Fenderson DA, Schuman LM, et al: *A description of the responsibilities of veterinarians as they relate directly to human health, report for Bureau of Health Manpower,* Washington, DC, 1976, US Department of Health, Education, and Welfare.

Antelyes J: Pets and mental health—but whose? *Mod Vet Pract* 54:69, 72, 73, Aug 1973.

Arendt J, Minors DS, Waterhouse JM: *Biological rhythms in clinical practice,* Boston, 1989, Wright.

Arkow P: New statistics challenge previously held beliefs about euthanasia: a new look at pet overpopulation, *The Latham Letter* XIV(2):1, 10–11, 1993.

Beaver BVG: Feline behavioral problems, *Vet Clin North Am* 6:333–340, Aug 1976.

Bierma NH: Prescription pet, *Cats* 34:10–11, March 1977.

Biologist sees link of pets with health, *DVM* 10:30, Jan 1979.

Borchelt PL, Tortora DF: Animal behavior therapy: the diagnosis and treatment of pet behavior problems, *Proceedings of the American Animal Hospital Association,* 1979.

Boudreau JC, Tsuchitani C: The cat *Felis catus.* In Boudreau JC, Tsuchitani C, editors: *Sensory neurophysiology,* New York, 1973, Van Nostrand Reinhold.

Brunner F: The application of behavior studies in small animal practice. In Fox MW, editor: *Abnormal behavior in animals,* Philadelphia, 1968, WB Saunders.

Bryant D: *The care and handling of cats,* New York, 1944, Ives Washburn.

Budge RC, Spicer J, St. George R, Jones BR: Compatibility stereotypes of people and pets: a photograph matching study, *Anthrozoös* 10(1):37–46, 1997.

Buffington CAT: External and internal influences on disease risk in cats, *J Am Vet Med Assoc* 220(7):994–1002, 2002.

Bustad LK, Gorham JR, Hegreberg GA, Padgett GA: Comparative medicine: progress and prospects, *J Am Vet Med Assoc* 169:90–105, July 1976.

Catanzaro TE: Behavior management as an income center, *Vet Forum* pp 50, 52, May 1994.

Colbert EH: *Evolution of the vertebrates,* ed 2, New York, 1969, John Wiley and Sons.

Corson SA, Corson EO, Gwynne PH: Pet facilitated psychotherapy. In Anderson RS, editor: *Pet animals and society,* Baltimore, 1975, Williams & Wilkins.

Council for Science and Society: *Companion animals in society,* New York, 1988, Oxford University Press.

Drewitt MStGN: Cats at war: a letter to the editor, *Vet Rec* 93:351, 1973.

Eleftheriou BE, Scott JP: *The physiology of aggression and defeat,* New York, 1971, Plenum Publishing.

Ewer RF: *The carnivores,* Ithaca, NY, 1973, Cornell University Press.

Fox MW: Influence of domestication upon behavior of animals, *Vet Rec* 80:696–702, 1967.

Fox MW: The place and future of animal behavior studies in veterinary medicine, *J Am Vet Med Assoc* 151:609–615, Sep 1967.

Fox MW: Ethology: an overview. In Fox MW, editor: *Abnormal behavior in animals,* Philadelphia, 1968, WB Saunders.

Fox MW: The influence of domestication upon behavior of animals. In Fox MW, editor: *Abnormal behavior in animals,* Philadelphia, 1968, WB Saunders.

Fox MW: Psychomotor disturbances. In Fox MW, editor: *Abnormal behavior in animals,* Philadelphia, 1968, WB Saunders.

Fox MW: The behavior of cats. In Hafez ESE, editor: *The behavior of domestic animals,* ed 3, Baltimore, 1975, Williams & Wilkins.

Fraser AF: Behavior disorders in domestic animals. In Fox MW, editor: *Abnormal behavior in animals,* Philadelphia, 1968, WB Saunders.

French ED, Vasquez SA, George R: Behavioral changes produced in the cat by acute and chronic morphine injection and naloxone precipitated withdrawal, *Eur J Pharmacol* 57(4):387–397, 1979.

Hart BL: Genetics and behavior, *Feline Pract* 3:5, 8, Feb 1973.

Hart BL: The medical interview and clinical evaluation of behavioral problems, *Feline Pract* 5(6):6, 8, 1975.

Hart BL: Behavioral aspects of selecting a new cat, *Feline Pract* 6(5):8, 10, 14, 1976.

Hart BL: Water sprayer therapy, *Feline Pract* 8(6):13–16, 1978.

Hart BL: Prescribing cats, *Feline Pract* 10(1):8, 10, 12, 1980.

Hart BL, Cliff KD: Interpreting published results of extra-label drug use with special reference to reports of drugs used to correct behavior in animals, *J Am Vet Med Assoc* 209(8):1382–1385, 1996.

Hatcher MG: In defense of the cat, *J Am Vet Med Assoc* 160:802, 805, March 1972.

Hemmer H: *Domestication: the decline of environmental appreciation,* New York, 1990, Cambridge University Press.

Jacobs DL: Behavior modification technique, *Feline Pract* 8(2):6, 1978.

Kleiman DG, Eisenberg JF: Comparisons of canid and felid social systems from an evolutionary perspective, *Anim Behav* 21:637–659, Nov 1973.

Kling A, Kovach JK, Tucker TJ: The behavior of cats. In Hafez ESE, editor: *The behavior of domestic animals,* ed 2, Baltimore, 1969, Williams & Wilkins.

König J: Surplus dogs and cats in Europe. In Allen RD, Westbrook WH, editors: *The handbook of animal welfare,* New York, 1979, Garland STPM Press.

Levinson BM: Influence of pets on families, *J Am Vet Med Assoc* 156:639, March 1970.

Levinson BM: Pets, child development, and mental illness, *J Am Vet Med Assoc* 157:1759–1766, Dec. 1, 1970.

Levinson BM: Man and his feline pet, *Mod Vet Pract* 53:35–39, Nov 1972.

Levinson BM: *Pets and human development,* Springfield, Ill, 1972, Charles C Thomas Publisher.

Levinson BM: Forecast for the year 2000. In Anderson RS, editor: *Pet animals and society,* London, 1974, Baillière Tindall.

Levoy RP: Important things to learn about new clients, *Vet Med Small Anim Clin* 73:224–226, Feb 1978.

Liberg O: Spacing patterns in a population of rural free roaming domestic cats, *Oikos* 35(3):336–349, 1980.

Littlejohn A: An approach to clinical veterinary ethology, *Br Vet J* 125:46–48, Jan 1969.

McMillan FD: Development of a mental wellness program for animals, *J Am Vet Med Assoc* 220(7):965–972, 2002.

Moss LC: Psychoneurosis—a veterinary problem, *J Am Vet Med Assoc* 114:1–2, Jan 1949.

MVP Staff Report: Euthanasia: an act of compassion or one of expediency? *Mod Vet Pract* 56:395–400, June 1975.

National shelter census results revealed, *J Am Vet Med Assoc* 210(2):160–161, Jan 1997.

Norton S, deBeer EJ: Effects of drugs on the behavioral patterns of cats, *Ann N Y Acad Sci* 65:249–257, 1956.

O'Brien SJ, Nash WG: Genetic mapping in mammals: chromosome map of domestic cat, *Science* 216:257–265, April 1982.

Oppriecht L: AAHA's public relations program, *Trends Magazine* 1(3):9–10, 1985.

Patronek GJ, Rowan AN: Determining dog and cat numbers and population dynamics, *Anthrozoös* 8(4):199–205, 1995.

Pet day at the Falls nursing home, *Shoptalk* 24:4–5, May 1976.

Placidi GF, Tognoni G, Pacifici GM, et al: Regional distribution of diazepam and its metabolites in the brain of the cat after chronic treatment, *Psychopharmacology* 48:133–137, 1976.

Pond G, Calder M: *The longhaired cat,* New York, 1974, Arco Publishing.

Rudorfer MV: Challenges in medication clinical trials, *Psychopharmacol Bull* 29(1):35–44, 1993.

Sambraus HH: Applied ethology—its task and limits in veterinary practice, *Appl Anim Behav Sci* 59(1–3):39–48, 1998.

Schmidt JP: Psychosomatics in veterinary medicine. In Fox MW, editor: *Abnormal behavior in animals,* Philadelphia, 1968, WB Saunders.

Seal US: Carnivora systematics: a study of hemoglobins, *Comp Biochem Physiol* 31:799–811, Dec 1969.

Seksel K, Lindeman MJ: Use of clomipramine in the treatment of anxiety-related and obsessive-compulsive disorders in cats, *Aust Vet J* 76(5):317–321, 1998.

Selby LA, Rhoades JD, Irvin JA, et al: Values and limitations of pet ownership, *J Am Vet Med Assoc* 176(11):1274–1276, 1980.

Shebar S, Schoder J: The pet burial business, *Dog Fancy* 7:22–25, April 1977.

Shull EA: Psychopharmacology in veterinary behavioral medicine, *Friskies PetCare Small Anim Behav* p 1–14, 1997.

Survey reveals bond between owners and pets, *J Am Vet Med Assoc* 209(12):1985, 1996.

Szasz K: *Petishism: pets and their people in the western world,* New York, 1969, Holt, Rinehart & Winston.

Tallan HH, Moore S, Stein WH: Studies on the free amino acids and related compounds in the tissues of the cat, *J Biol Chem* 211:927–939, 1954.

Thrusfield MV: Demographic characteristics of the canine and feline population of the UK in 1986, *J Small Anim Pract* 30(2):76–80, 1989.

Top cats: good medicine for emotionally handicapped, *Vet Econ* 15:14, Aug 1974.

Turner DC: Treating canine and feline behaviour problems and advising clients, *Appl Anim Behav Sci* 52(3,4):199–204, 1997.

Voith V, Borchelt P: History taking and interviewing, *Compend Contin Educ* 7:432–435, May 1985.

Wolpe J: Parallels between animal and human neuroses, *Proc Annu Am Psychopathol Assoc* 55:305–313, 1967.

Worden AN: Abnormal behavior in the dog and cat, *Vet Rec* 71:966–978, Dec 26, 1959.

2

Feline Behavior of Sensory and Neural Origin

Studying the senses of an animal is extremely difficult because we as humans are limited by our own sensory capacities. It is difficult to understand that which cannot be experienced. Mammalian senses differ greatly, developing primarily to meet biologic needs. Thus the importance of each will vary among the species. The cat has served as a scientific model for neuroanatomic studies, so we are fortunate to know more about its senses and neurologic connections than those of most other animals.

THE SENSES

Comparative development of the senses is shown in Appendix B.

Sense of Vision

External visual system development

Like the young of several other species, the newborn kitten is care dependent at birth and for several weeks thereafter. This immature state is reflected in the visual system, which needs postnatal time for development. At birth the kitten's ocular development is approximately equivalent to that of a 5-month-old human fetus. Continued development happens even though the eyes are sealed until 5 to 14 days after birth (mean 8 days).[92,172,212] At first the eye opens only slightly, but by 17 days (mean 9 days) both eyes are completely open (Figure 2-1). Several factors can influence when the opening begins. Early handling can accelerate this process by approximately 24 hours.[81,112] Other factors include genetic influences from the sire, exposure to light (dark reared open earlier), sex of the kitten (females open earlier than males), and age of the mother (young mothers result in earlier opening).[172] Anatomic changes in vascularization occur in about 3 weeks and result in a sudden improvement in the kitten's visual optics.[251] Although visual electrical potentials can be recorded from the cortex of the brain as early as 4 days of age and the first electroretinogram can be recorded at day 6, neither becomes adultlike until week 9 or 10.[76]

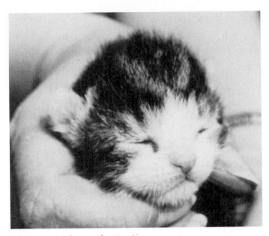

Figure 2-1 A 7-day-old kitten with eyes beginning to open.

A few reflexes associated with vision appear before the opening of the eyes. The palpebral reflex starts as a slow blink response during the first 3 days of life, becoming adultlike by the ninth day. The light blink reflex develops as early as day 50 of gestation or as late as day 13 of postnatal life (mean 6 days postnatal life). Although the palpebral reflex continues, the light blink reflex disappears around 21 days, probably because of the development of acute pupil control. Pupillary response generally appears within 24 hours after the eyes open, taking 2 or 3 days to develop normal speed. Until this time the kitten usually tries to turn its head away from the light source.

Visual acuity develops independently of the opening of the eyes.[268] Visual pursuit first occurs as an eye-turning and head-turning action at about 11 days, when kittens first visually follow people and moving objects. Visual acuity, measured in terms of visual angles, gradually improves from a 180-minute arc around 16 days to a 43-minute arc about 21 days, and then to an 11-minute arc around 25 days.[268] Between 22 and 28 days (mean 25 days) visual placing reactions of the forelimbs first occur and are significantly related to good visual acuity.[53,268] There is a sixteenfold overall increase of visual acuity between 2 and 10 weeks of age.[235]

Depth perception initially appears a few days after the eyes open (mean 13 days) and is well developed by 4 weeks of age. With continued maturation of the visual system, the kitten gradually increases the use of its eyes for behaviors such as avoiding objects and finding food, with good binocular vision by 47 days.[261] There is an accompanying sudden onset of light-seeking behavior at 2 months of age.[61] By this time the kitten has adult sight capacities, even though the visual system continues its development for another 2 months.[92,160]

Eye color starts changing around 23 days of age, but early handling can speed this up slightly.[112]

External visual system characteristics

Physical features of the typical eye are species specific. In the cat the dimensions of the globe are 20 to 22 mm in the anteroposterior direction, 19 to 20.7 mm on the vertical axis, and 18 to 21 mm transversely. This makes the adult cat slightly myopic (+4.73S).[76,208] Because of eye shape and pupil extremes, both the lens and the cornea of cats are larger and more highly curved than their counterparts in the human.[32,71] The cornea composes up to 30% of the outer layer of the eye.[208] The tapetum lucidum is relatively thick at 2 μm, with an average of 12 to 15 layers.[47,208,266] The more superficial layers of the tapetum tend to reflect shorter wavelengths; deeper layers reflect longer wavelengths.[47] The retinal fovea (macula, area centralis), the area of most acute vision, cannot be identified before 5 weeks of age.[76] In the adult, it is located a mean distance of 3.42 mm dorsolateral from the center of the optic disc.[26,56] Although cones are most concentrated here, this area in the cat is relatively large and indefinite because both cones and rods are present.[19,52,138,141,280] In the human, there are only cones in the area of the fovea. Each feline eye has a blind spot on the dorsolateral retina at 13 degrees lateral.[26,260]

Because the feline adult visual and behavioral characteristics are closely related, it is important to note the anatomic adaptations that make night hunting possible. As a result of the large lens and cornea, the eye can collect more light, there is a larger visual field, and a relatively large portion of the retina is activated.[208] The tapetum lucidum reflects light within the eye for maximal stimulation of the rods in the retina. In addition to the many low-threshold rods (rod/cone ratio is 25:1 as compared with 20:1 in humans), the cat eye also has more layers of sensitive cells in the retina.[72,114] These retinal differences allow cats to use up to 50% more of the available light than humans and have vision in one sixth the illumination needed by humans. The cat has an absolute brightness threshold of 1.32×10^{-7} millilamberts.[175]

Other changes occur to protect the eye from being overstimulated by sunlight. The ability of the pupil to become a very narrow slit rapidly is typically found in nocturnal animals that also bask in the sun.[266] While the tapetum reflects light, the remainder of the fundus is heavily pigmented, particularly in the lower half. This protects the sensitive retina from overhead glare.[207] In addition, the rods have the ability to adapt so that they do not saturate with light before the cones take over vision in higher light intensities.[249]

Visual acuity is most accurate at 75 cm but is compromised for night-hunting abilities.[138,238] The visual acuity of the cat matures from slightly more than one cycle per degree at 35 days of age to five to six cycles per degree at 4 months, to eight to nine cycles per degree as an adult.[72,142,180,274] These figures are 10% those of humans.[29,72] The low level of visual acuity is due to three internal factors: Reflection by the tapetum lucidum blurs the image; the increased number of rods decreases the resolution of the image by lowering the visual stimulus threshold; and the lens loses one half to one third of its capacity for accommodation.[266] Accommodation does, however, relate to the significance of the viewed subject.[69] Although some retinal ganglion cells are comparable to those in humans, the brain is apparently unable to use incoming information to the same degree.[226] In spite of its slight myopia the cat shows a marked ability to notice movement, a necessity in hunting behaviors.[19,69] Thresholds to recognize real movement are as little as a 0.4-cm/sec movement.[153]

The iris has a prominent bulging shape and can change colors during sympathetic stimulation.[139,240]

The cat is generally considered color blind. There are cones present in the retina and there are a few spectral opponent ganglia.[257] Considering the anatomy as a whole, however, cat eyes are not specialized for color vision. Experimental evidence shows that cats can perceive only limited color. The photopic wavelength sensitivity is dichromat, meaning the cat is most sensitive around two wavelengths. At long wavelengths, they are most responsive at 554 nm, a greenish yellow, which is maximally sensitive to the cat's most common cones.[167] At the shorter wavelength, cats respond around 447 nm, in the blue area.[167] It also seems necessary that background illumination be greater than 3.0 cd/m^2 so as not to be a factor in getting appropriate test results.[167] It is generally agreed that color vision, although possible, is of little natural importance to the cat. Further evidence of this is suggested by the relatively low number of cones compared with rods in the retina as a whole.[280] Brightness is of much greater significance than color in visual discrimination, allowing the cat to detect luminance differences of only 10% to 12%.[274] They can perceive illumination at one fifth the threshold of humans.[132]

Binocular vision is important for hunting success of this predator because its prey tend to be small and quick. Because of eye position and head shape, each eye has a visual field between 155 and 208.5 degrees, of which 90 to 130 degrees overlap the visual field of the opposite eye to produce binocular vision (Figure 2-2).[19,52,72,229,232] The remaining 73- to 173-degree field behind the head is a blind area. To provide this much binocular vision, the median plane of the eye is at an angle of only 4 to 9 degrees from that of the body.[52,72] In kittens this alignment of the optic axes is quite divergent, but it becomes almost parallel within a few months.[228,264] About 40% of the cats studied show no convergence of both eyes while examining close objects, although with certain lifestyles such as hunting insects, this percentage may decrease (Figure 2-3).[138]

Internal visual system characteristics

The optic nerve of the cat has between 112,000 and 147,000 myelinated axons, a number that is approximately equal to the number of ganglion cells in the retina.[245,246] Of these, 60% to 65% decussate at the optic chiasm.[19,51,56,208,266] Those fibers from areas medial to the retinal fovea cross to the opposite cerebral hemisphere, whereas those lateral to it do not decussate.[56] Once they reach the brain, the impulses are generally received by ordered sections of the visual cortex (Figure 2-4).[239] The cortex area is apparently important in integration of bilateral stimuli. Depth discrimination of prey is governed by this integration, the corpus callosum, and by the possibility that different cortical units are optically excited by objects on different sides and at different distances.[12,67,73]

Form discrimination by cats is based primarily on size differences, orientation of shapes, and general form. These general forms are basically open or closed, such as an O shape as opposed to a V shape, or a slot in contrast to a post. Neurons in the visual cortex appear selectively sensitive to orientation, length, width, and movement, and their reaction to these stimuli is based on early visual orientation.[87,185,217] Four fifths of these cells are influenced independently by both eyes, although not necessarily in equal amounts.[135] There is evidence that the central nervous system has physiologic mechanisms to differentiate newness of a stimulus, which is an extremely valuable feature for a predator.[248]

Visual acuity develops gradually as the nervous system of the neonate matures, and its development requires light stimulation during the first 3 months, peaking between 28 and 35 days.[61,136,184,281] Form and light exposure during this critical period are necessary for normal cell development and vision as an adult.[136,256] Deprivation of these

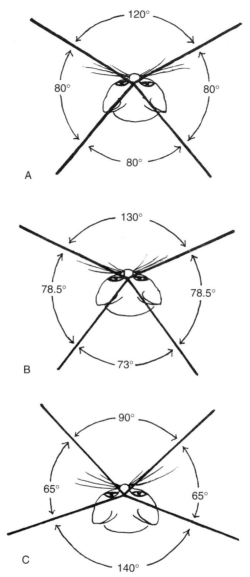

Figure 2-2 Visual fields of binocular, uniocular, and blind vision. (**A** data from Beadle M: *The cat: history, biology, and behavior,* New York, 1977, Simon & Schuster; **B** data from Ewer RF: *The carnivores,* Ithaca, NY, 1973, Cornell University Press; **C** data from Sherman SM: *Brain Res* 49:25–45, Jan 15, 1973.)

stimuli, achieved experimentally by suturing the eyelids closed or by dark rearing, results in a loss of visual acuity, even to the point of behavioral blindness. Divergent strabismus also develops.[228] When one eye is deprived of early vision, the associated visual field is abnormal. It responds only to objects in the monocular field, oblivious to those that it should share as binocular vision with the normal eye.[230,231] Concurrently, varying

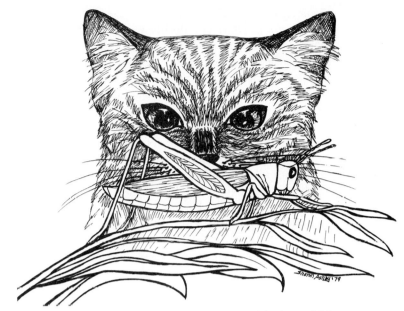

Figure 2-3 Small-prey hunting may require convergence of the lines of sight.

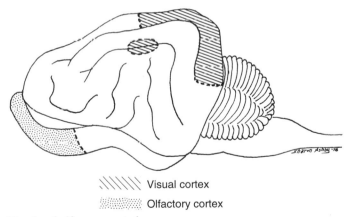

////// Visual cortex

:::::: Olfactory cortex

Figure 2-4 Visual and olfactory cortical areas.

histologic changes occur in the cells of the visual cortex. Thus monocular deprivation is not compensated for by the nonsutured eye either behaviorally, physiologically, or histologically.* Enucleation results in an extensive reorganization within the cortical area so that the remaining eye is innervating the entire visual cortical and subcortical regions.[27] Eye movements, body movement, and a view of the forelimbs are also believed to be important for development of visual motor skills.[125,126]

*References 88, 94, 96, 120, 209, 229, 241, 242, 253, 255.

As a model for neurologic investigations, the brain of the cat has been extensively studied. The dorsal lateral geniculate nucleus is the first stop for visual information. The top layer (A) receives input from the contralateral eye. The next layer (A1) receives its information from the ipsilateral eye and is shorter in length.[242] The medial part of layer A overlies all of layer A1, and the combined segment is associated with binocular vision. The lateral portion of layer A represents the monocular portion of the contralateral eye.[96,242] Lesions of the marginal and posterolateral gyri result in deficits in the discrimination of form and in the ability to learn mazes.[48] The visual cortex receives input from the lateral geniculate relative to patterns and appears to be the first step in perceptual generalization.[133] Each of the six laminae of the visual cortex's area 17 (striate cortex) is laid out in a specific order,[200] and these are bilaterally symmetric.[134] This area is thought to be involved in binocular vision.[24] Retinal lesions result in a change in both primary and secondary visual cortex.[149] The visual cortex has been experimentally removed and the animal evaluated with regard to visual deficits. Despite major ablations of the cortex, long-term impairment of visual performance is minimal. Bilateral removal of the occipital lobes does result in apparent blindness, although the cat does retain discrimination of light intensity.[207] Visual learning is also associated with the superior colliculus and pretectal areas of the brain.[206] Maturation begins here about day 15 and continues until at least day 25.[195]

Although color vision is not well developed, certain parts of the brain have been identified as being related to this function. The ventral lateral geniculate nucleus has areas within it that respond differently to colors, particularly blue.[140]

The Siamese visual system

External appearances are not the only variations from normal that accompany Siamese eyes. The characteristic crossing of the eyes does not appear until 6 to 8 weeks of age and is not present in all Siamese cats. Abnormal retinocerebral connections are typical of all albino animals, whether cross-eyed or not, and are associated with albino, Himalayan (Siamese), and occasionally chinchilla (Burmese) feline color genes.[19,95] The visual field is normal, but the cats react to visual stimuli as if each eye does not see past the median plane (Figure 2-5).[95,173,234] As a result, these cats have difficulty locating objects in space. In the normal animal, visual input from the left eye goes to the top layer A of the left lateral geniculate nucleus and to the second layer A1 of the right lateral geniculate nucleus, whereas right eye input goes to the top A layer of the right lateral geniculate nucleus and to the second A1 layer of the left lateral geniculate nucleus. In the Siamese cat, hemispheric vision is such that fewer fibers decussate at the optic chiasm,[51] and the fibers are misdirected. Each eye has fibers going to the appropriate position on the top A layer but of the contralateral side. In addition, each eye lacks some fibers going to the top layer of the ipsilateral lateral geniculate nucleus.[19,95,137,225,234] Non–cross-eyed Siamese and heterozygous albino cats show abnormal optic fiber decussation to a lesser degree.[95,165] In the esotropic (cross-eyed) Siamese cats, essentially no cells exhibit binocular interaction. The orthophoric (non–cross-eyed) Siamese cats have 40% of the cells exhibiting binocular interaction, compared with 80% in normal cats.[45] The receptive field size for Siamese cats is also one third larger, and direction selectivity of the striate cortex neurons is significantly less.[45] The Siamese cat has a narrower contrast sensitivity compared with other cats.[28,225] In addition, they have less than half the number of Y cells in the retinal ganglion.[28,225]

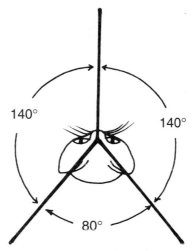

Figure 2-5 The visual field of Siamese cats lacks a binocular area.

Sense of Audition

Auditory development

Development of hearing in the kitten is not complete at birth, which is evidenced by the fact that the external auditory canal begins to open only between 6 and 14 days of age (mean 9 days), being completed by day 17 (Figure 2-6). This is followed by a deepening and increasing concavity of the pinna until day 31.[196] Electronically the earliest evoked potential of the auditory system can be recorded at 2 to 3 days of age, and kittens initially hear sound of 100 dB SPL in the range of 500 to 2000 cycles per second (cps).[201] By day 6, the range has expanded to cover 200 to 6000 cps.[201] The development of the auditory startle response to sharp noise is generally present by day 7 but can be variable.[196] Kittens begin orienting toward a sound as early as the seventh day and use this orientation for investigation by 13 to 16 days.[196,261] Sound recognition of littermates or people follows during the third or fourth week and is coordinated with the appearance of the conditioned defense response: an arched-back, hissing response, which will stabilize during the fifth week.[81,261,263]

Auditory characteristics

The auditory capabilities of the cat are not completely known. It has been suggested that this sense is more important to the cat than vision,[123,143] as might be reasonable for a night hunter. The lower audible frequencies are probably between 20 and 55 cps, and from those frequencies up to 4000 cps, the cat's hearing ability is approximately the same as the human's. Maximal sensitivity is between 250 and 35,000 cps, at 20 dB or fewer.[202] Although the upper limit of audition is said to be approximately 78,000 cps at 60 dB SPL, the actual limit may be closer to 100,000 cps.* The use of different instrumentation has shown that cochlear activity is present at these high frequencies, but

---

*References 72, 124, 201, 202, 276, 278.

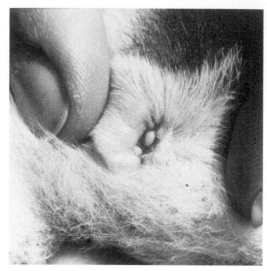

Figure 2-6 A 6-day-old kitten with the external auditory canals beginning to open.

whether the cat can actually hear these sounds is still unknown.[278] This acute perception may be significant because social interactions between a rodent female and her young use frequencies of 17,000 to 148,000 cps, typically 80,000 cps or lower.[122,201,218] Inexperienced kittens will attack baby mice if stimulated by the squeak of the female mouse, indicating they can hear the sound and will instinctively react.[85,114] The range of hearing in humans is approximately 20 to 19,000 cps.[122,276]

The cat can accurately hear one tenth to one fifth of a tone difference at higher pitches but only about half of a tone change at lower frequencies.[19,72,240] Cats are also capable of distinguishing the difference of click rates of four per second versus six per second.[50] With age some peripheral auditory capability is lost, especially in higher ranges.[19,72,102]

Sound reception and interpretation

As a nocturnal hunter the cat must rely on the sense of hearing to locate prey. Sound localization and maximal reception are primarily functions of the cup-shaped pinna, particularly at high frequencies.[77] Ear position does alter sound perception. Maximal interaural intensity differences are produced by sounds of at least 20,000 cps, located 20 to 40 degrees from the frontal midline.[178] This also happens for lower sounds from the periphery. Because the pinna can rotate approximately 180 degrees and acts as a funnel, it may introduce or at least amplify complex variations in sound quality with relation to the source, an important factor in localization.[32,72] Unless coming from directly ahead or behind, the sound arrives at slightly different times at each ear. This varies from 25 to more than 80 μsec and helps with sound localization.[93]

Within the ear the tympanic bulla is large, thus increasing acoustic resonance.

The feline cochlea differs from that of the human in length, density of cells, and absolute thresholds. The length is approximately two thirds that of a human cochlea, even though there is a much greater range of sounds to which to respond.[68,276]

Although there are only 12,300 hair cells in the cat's cochlea, compared with 23,500 in the human, they connect to more ganglion cells.[68]

From the ganglion cells, approximately 40,000 cochlear nerve fibers carry impulses to the brain, and this is 10,000 more than are seen in humans.[19,58,68,72,132] Each nerve fiber has a "best" frequency that sets it off at the lowest threshold.[205] For a tone, 68% of the units are either excited or inhibited. The rest respond only with an onset spike.[5] These sound impulses travel a well-defined neural pathway to the auditory cortex, being analyzed there and along the way.[243,248] The superior colliculus is involved in sound location.[11,178] This makes it responsible for coordinating eyes, ears, and head direction via responses to visual, auditory, and somatosensory stimulation.[178] The organization of incoming frequencies to the auditory cortex is not tonographic.[70] Although the auditory fibers are the only sensory fibers completely myelinized at birth, the auditory system continues to undergo maturation, as evidenced by decreasing peak latencies of cortical evoked potentials, until the minimal adult refractory interval of approximately 1 ms between discharges is reached.[58,146,189,254] This rate of central nervous development is faster than that of the visual system.[92] Studies in conscious cats indicate that other areas of the brain may also be involved with electrical potentials from sound, particularly in areas immediately surrounding the auditory cortex.[91,145,205]

In addition to the movable pinna, auditory neurons play a significant role in sound localization, which is 75% accurate to an angle of approximately 5 degrees, only 2 degrees less accurate than for the human.[19,72,122,190] However, in cats this ability does decrease at the lower and higher frequencies.[93] Certain neurons respond to contralateral stimuli but are inhibited by stimuli of the same frequency presented biaurally.[31,36,213] This occurs in a direct projection from the cochlear nucleus to the contralateral trapezoid nucleus, and then to the lateral superior olive area.[90] Other neurons respond to different latencies of the stimuli between the ears. Still others may be affected by differences in stimulus intensity between the two sides.[36,174,191,213] All seem to respond easier to change in a sound from high to low frequency than in the other direction.[176] This is consistent with the natural tendency in vocalization.

As with the visual system, the effects of ablation of the cortical portions of the auditory system have been studied (Figure 2-7). Although amplitude and frequency discrimination in the adult can generally be affected to varying degrees, localization of sound is most severely impaired by this procedure.

Hearing loss in cats has also been attributed to certain drugs, particularly the aminoglycosides. Kanamycin affects hair cells at the basal end of the cochlea and results in loss of high-frequency perception, and neomycin can cause damage to the auditory function of the eighth cranial nerve.[22,32] Deafness can also result from prolonged administration of streptomycin.[22]

Sense of Gustation

The sense of taste has been studied less than the other senses, perhaps because it has proven more difficult to evaluate. Taste buds are found on the vallate, fungiform, and occasionally foliate papillae of the tongue, as well as on the epiglottis, soft palate, lips, buccal walls, and pharynx.[32,37] By stimulating these taste buds with chemicals known to produce certain tastes in humans and recording from afferent nerves or the presylvian

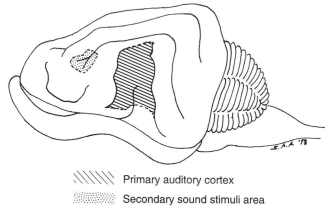

\\\\\\\   Primary auditory cortex

░░░░░░   Secondary sound stimuli area

Figure 2-7 Auditory cortical areas.

gyrus, the primary center for taste reception, researchers have arrived at a few probabilities concerning the sense of taste in the cat.[56,162] The apex and anterolateral margins of the tongue show the most sensitivity to salt.[204] The base and posterolateral portions are the most sensitive to bitter, and all regions except the middorsum are sensitive to acid.[204]

Within the first day of life, the kitten can distinguish sodium chloride in milk and by the tenth day shows definite responses to salt and bitter, with possible responses to sweet and sour.[53,203] The adult cat responds to chemicals associated with salt, sour, and bitter, with maximal sensitivity to the three taste stimuli occurring at 30° C, the normal temperature of the tongue.[187] Response to sweet is minimal at best. Considering foods eaten naturally by cats, one is not surprised that sweetness is not a major part of the cat's taste spectrum, although some individual cats may develop a strong liking for foods with high sugar content.

Three types of taste fibers have been identified in the efferent nerves. One responds to acid, a second to acid and salt, and a third to acid and bitter.[204] Threshold concentrations vary for different fibers of any one type, and the discharge is of the slowly adapting type.[204] Water fibers, maximally receptive to water, have been described in the chorda tympani. They are proposed to extend taste sensitivity to salt solutions.[46]

Neurologic studies indicate that the limbus of the brain is concerned with the memory of past gustatory experiences.[56]

Sense of Olfaction

Olfactory development

The sense of smell is highly developed at birth, and within the first 2 days, kittens show a strong avoidance reaction to offensive odors.[20,53,160] Olfaction is well developed at this early age because of its importance in guiding the young animal to the mammary gland for nursing. By 3 days of age, each kitten establishes a preferred nipple position and primarily uses odor to identify and follow previous paths to the specific nipple.[214,215] Distress caused by removing the young kitten from its home area, which contains the concentrated odors of the queen and the kittens, can be quieted by providing the smell of the area, even without physical contact. If placed near the home area, a kitten will crawl to it, guided by smell, and then fall asleep.[83,84,100,215] The gradual building of olfactory cues from the home area provides odor orientation when the kitten begins to explore outside areas.[216] As vision develops, especially after 3 weeks of age, olfactory cues become less important but may have already influenced later stimulus preferences.[80]

Olfactory characteristics

In the adult, scent is used for identification during the typical behavioral approach of familiar cats—first face to face then face to anus. Epithelia of the anal sacs in felids contain sebaceous tissue that can give off oils unique to that of other carnivores, which have only apocrine glands.[6] Scents are also used to explore and habituate to new environments.[1] Certain odors cause an immediate response and are called *releasers*. Moth balls, for example, cause avoidance. Companies have tried to use releasers such as methyl nonyl ketone and cinnamic aldehyde repellents for garbage bags with only limited success.[221,285] Primers, such as the cat's own urine, are odors having a delayed effect or those that are not behaviorally obvious.[66] Olfactory cues appear to be used to acquire information about the environment, for intercat communication, and perhaps in predetection.[199] The pheromone associated with scent glands along the cheeks have been synthesized artificially, and the associated odor has a calming effect on most cats. This actually verifies the importance of odors in a cat's world, because humans cannot detect the specific pheromone smell. Home areas and familiar smells are also reassuring to cats, so leaving a cat in the bottom of the carrier after the top has been removed can facilitate handling.

In regard to size, the nasal olfactory area of the cat is larger than its corresponding area in the human.[19] In addition, the olfactory bulb is relatively larger and contains approximately 67 million cells, about 15 million more cells than are found in the human but far fewer than are present in the dog (see Figure 2-4).[19,113] Because cats use smell behaviorally but not for tracking prey, these findings are not surprising.

Vomeronasal olfactory system

Central olfactory pathways eventually connect to the amygdala area of the brain, a factor of significance when considering the second olfactory system of the cat.[7,62] Immediately caudal to the incisor teeth is a papilla onto which open two nasopalatine canals. These canals allow the slow passage of odors from the mouth to the vomeronasal organ, a chemoreceptive structure located within the cartilage of the nasal septum. The nature of the stimulus access suggests that this system responds to nonvolitive cues, including pheromones.[30,128,158] There may also be selective responses, such as almost exclusive response to male or female urine.[128] The vomeronasal organ (organ of Jacobson) is lined with two types of receptors that differ from receptors in other olfactory cells. The vomeronasal organ has seven transmembrane receptors coupled to guanosine triphosphate–binding protein that appear to activate inositol 1,4,5-trisphosphate signaling, as opposed to cyclic adenosine monophosphate.[158] Unlike other sensory neurons, ones associated with the vomeronasal organ do not adapt under prolonged stimulus exposure.[128] The vomeronasal olfactory system also has central pathways different from those of olfactory epithelium. Impulses first travel to the glomerular layer of the accessory olfactory bulb.[99] Eventually they go to the amygdala and stria terminalis,[99] interacting with areas of the hypothalamus associated with sexual, feeding, maternal defensive, and social behaviors, as well as neuroendocrine secretions.

Flehmen is the behavior associated with the inhalation of odors into the nasopalatine canals. Beginning as early as 6 weeks, a cat will sniff a particular odor source, such as urine, often touching it with its nose and perhaps its tongue.[160] The head is then raised with the lips drawn back, nose wrinkled, and mouth partially open for inhalation (Figure 2-8). Flehmen behavior enlarges the openings of the nasopalatine ducts, also activating a pumping/suction mechanism to deliver odors to the vomeronasal organ.[99] This behavior is similar to that seen in ruminants and horses; however, the philtrum of the feline upper lip prevents its complete elevation. Flehmen, also called *lip curl* or *gape,* is most commonly displayed by tomcats.

Plant-induced olfactory behavior

Fourteen chemicals of diverse biologic origin, including certain plants, are known to affect the behavior of the cat when their fragrances are inhaled. The three chemical groups from these compounds include the 7-methylcyclopentapyranones, 7-methyl-2-pyridines, and 4-methylbenzofuranones.[258] A few of the more common plants include matatabi (*Actinidia polygama,* oriental vine, silvervine), valerian *(Valeriana officinalis),* cat thyme *(Teucrium manum),* bush honeysuckles *(Loniero tortorico capri foliaceae),* buckbean (*Menyanthes triboliata,* bog myrtle), and the most famous, catnip (*Nepeta cataria,* catmint). Reactions to catnip are often speculated to be hallucinogenic because humans who have smoked it report effects similar to those produced by marijuana. The active ingredient, *cis-trans*-nepetalactone, is a monoterpene that can be detected at levels as low as one part in 10^9 to 10^{11}.[6] After approaching the catnip plant, the cat will smell it and may lick, chew, or eat it. After head shaking, gazing, and salivating, the cat may rub its head on the catnip, usually while holding it in the forepaws. The skin over its back frequently twitches. As the intensity of the response increases the cat will roll on its side holding the catnip in its paws. There may also be animated leaping. The response generally lasts 5 to 15 minutes, with the most intense response lasting a mean

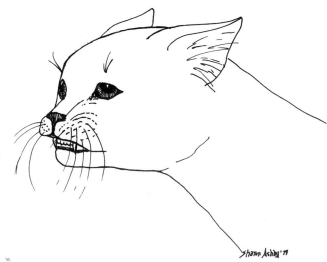

Figure 2-8 Flehmen by a cat.

of 2.7 minutes.[21,107,121] Satiation lasts at least one hour. It has also been speculated but is not widely accepted that catnip's odor activates central areas associated with estrous behavior because the behavioral response of the cat is similar to that during certain phases of female estrus.[107]

There is a great deal of individual variation in reactions to catnip, and 30% to 50% of the cats studied do not respond at all.[32,111,113] Although the response is inherited by means of an autosomal dominant gene, it is also modified by age and experience.[19,30,32,107,121] Those cats showing a decreased reaction to catnip include kittens younger than 2 months, fearful animals, and those under stress. Estrus can extend the response, and prolonged (regular, long-term) use of the drug has led to a chronic state of partial unawareness of surroundings.[21,147]

Sense of Touch

External tactile development

Like olfaction the sense of touch is fairly well developed at birth, probably because it too plays a role in orientation of the neonate. Developing fetuses are responsive to tactile sensations by 24 days of gestation and exhibit flexor withdrawal to the toe pinch by 37 days.[92,284] Therefore it is not surprising that tactile response is present at birth, and cutaneous pain reaction appears within the first 4 days after birth.[20,53] Homeostatic mechanisms do not function well at birth; therefore, kittens are responsive to temperature influences, and huddling is necessary for survival. For this reason, rooting behavior, the pushing of the head into warm objects, is present up to 16 days of age (mean day of ending is 8 days) (Figure 2-9). The auriculonasocephalic reflex, a turning of the head when the side of the face is touched (Figure 2-10), and Galant's reflex, a turning of the head and trunk when the flank region is touched (Figure 2-11), occur in kittens but not consistently between individuals. During the first week both thermal and olfactory cues help kittens find home base equally well.[83] There is then a shift of increasing importance toward olfaction. Physical contact with the dam has a calming effect on young kittens. When kittens are reunited with the queen after a separation,

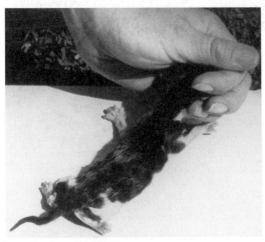

Figure 2-9 The rooting reflex in a day-old kitten.

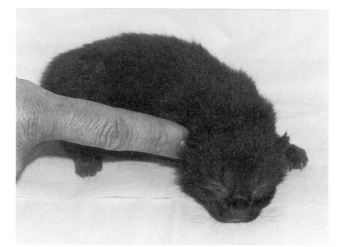

Figure 2-10 The auriculonasocephalic reflex is directed toward the cervical touch stimulus by a day-old kitten.

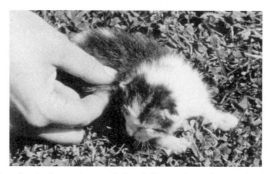

Figure 2-11 Galant's reflex is directed toward the abdominal touch stimulus by a 7-day-old kitten.

they bury their heads in her fur. This behavior may be carried over to the adult cat that can be calmed by having its face covered with a pair of hands.[14] Odor may be slightly more important at this older age because the technique generally works better if the cat's owner covers its face.

Tactile placing of the forelimb appears during the first 5 days, almost 3 weeks before visual placing occurs (Figure 2-12). Then, as late as 6 weeks, kittens still show a preference for tactile determination of depth, using vision only secondarily.[220] The difference between dependence on the two senses represents the difference in time required for the completion of connections with the motor cortex.[268]

External tactile characteristics

In adults, areas of tactile dermatomes have been well mapped, but skin sensitivity varies. Pinkus' plates, specialized tactile pads or touch areas, have been found covering the skin at a rate of 7/cm to 25/cm by the seventh week of age.[19,37,151] The cat's face

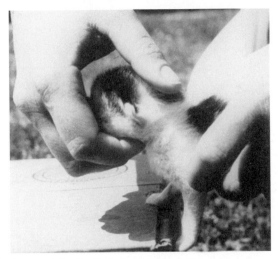

Figure 2-12 Tactile placing of the forelimbs in a 7-day-old kitten.

is approximately one third as sensitive to radiant heat as a human face, although the nasal area can respond to minute changes, as little as a 0.2° C rise or 0.5° C decrease.[19,155,156,157] Response in the remainder of the body requires a level of heat change that would be painful to humans, from 6° to 9° C.[34,154,156,157] Humans report pain at 44° C, whereas cats react between 51° and 54° C.[155] This lack of sensitivity on the trunk accounts for the cat's ability to sit on a stove or radiator, apparently comfortable, even though its hair may singe. Prolonged exposure to high environmental temperatures (25° to 30° C) results in hypoexcitability, and at temperatures more than 30° C the cat exhibits panting, hyperexcitability, and circling. Cold exposure increases somatic rage (bared teeth) and circling.[89] Sensitivity can also vary by age and by the type of nerve ending activated. On the footpads 40% of the fibers are slow to adapt in both adults and kittens. They take a deflection of approximately 0.5 mm to plateau.[74] The remaining 60% are fast-adapting fibers, which in adults are more sensitive and responsive than in kittens.[74]

Response to touch varies among breeds and individuals. In general, however, cats prefer to be held firmly but not tightly to be sure of their support; they usually prefer gentle stroking to patting. Occasionally a cat will resent being handled near the base of the tail and will turn to confront the source of stimulation or will twitch the tail and skin of the lumbar region. Also, cats generally do better with minimal restraint, so giving an intramuscular injection is often possible while holding only the cat's pelvic limb.

Tactile vibrissae

As a nocturnal hunter the cat may use touch for stalking or for measuring location. In this regard the special vibrissae transmit sensory information only.[192] Each vibrissa is contained in a follicle approximately five times larger than that associated with regular hairs.[4] Each has at least one associated sebaceous gland and is attached to striated muscle for voluntary control.[4] The follicles have blood-filled sinuses and various types

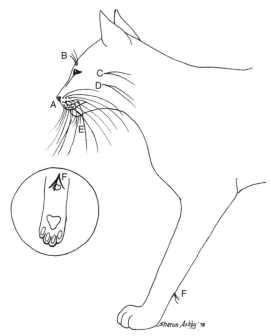

Figure 2-13 Location of facial and carpal vibrissae. **A,** Mystacial tufts; **B,** superciliary tuft; **C,** genal tuft one; **D,** genal tuft two; **E,** mandibular tuft; **F,** carpal vibrissae.

of nerve receptors.[4] Impulses have been demonstrated with as little as a 2-mg weight or 5-Å directional movement when the direction of movement of these sinus hairs is opposite the natural slant.[49,75] In this way an animal can detect wind and air currents reflected from nearby objects. The loss of these hairs makes the cat more dependent on vision. Facial vibrissae, or whiskers, are located in specific areas (Figure 2-13). Large areas of mystacial vibrissae are present in rows on each upper lip. The dorsal two rows of mystacial vibrissae move independently of the ventral two rows, and their positions vary with movement and behavior.[19] A large superciliary tuft is located above each eye. Genal tuft one is ventral to the base of each ear, and a genal tuft two is ventral to each genal tuft one near the angle of the mandible. There is a poorly developed mandibular (submental) tuft on the chin.[4,19,72] While the cat is walking, the whiskers project craniolaterally to scan a wide angle. When at rest the cat moves them caudolaterally for a much narrower area. During a greeting, defense, or sniff, these tactile hairs are folded back along the side of the head.[37,275]

Carpal (ulnar carpal) vibrissae are structurally identical to cranial vibrissae and are found on the caudal surface of the forearm immediately proximocaudal to the carpus. Because the associated nerves are sensitive to a proximal displacement of the tactile hair, it has been speculated that their presence is related to the use of the forelimbs for functions other than ambulation, such as capturing prey.[23,192,193]

Pain is another tactile-associated response. The pain threshold is the point at which the perception of tissue damage or insult occurs.[233] The level of tolerance to painful stimuli varies with individuals.

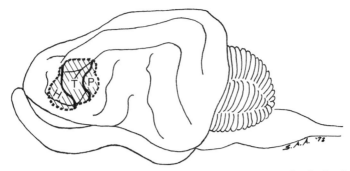

Figure 2-14 Somatic sensory cortical areas. *H*, Somatic sensory cortex for the head; *T*, somatic sensory cortex for the thoracic limb; *P*, somatic sensory cortex for the pelvic limb.

Internal tactile characteristics

Cerebral studies have mapped cortical locations of touch-sensitive areas, with few differences found between the young and the adult cat (Figure 2-14).

Unexplained Senses

Certain behaviors are probably related to neurologic capabilities, although the exact relationship has not been defined.

Earthquake prediction

Before some earthquakes, cats have been reported to undergo behavioral changes. Behavior typical of extreme fear or excitement, including restlessness and piloerection, may be seen in cats even though electric instruments do not perceive environmental changes.[9,114] Exactly what the cat detects is unknown, but speculations include variations in electromagnetic fields, atmospheric electrostatic charges, air pressure, ultrasonic or subsonic emissions, the earth's level, water levels, and gaseous emissions.[114] In a comparison of reactions in two similar quakes, the vast majority of animal reactions occurred for the one with a relatively shallow hypocenter, occurring on a strike-slip fault.[168]

Homing behavior

Cats often go back to a previous home after a move, especially if the old location is nearby. This behavior demonstrates the importance of a territory to a cat. Individuals are said to "run away" during this search, especially if they become lost. Some cats reportedly can travel great distances returning to an old home, and many such trips have been documented. The homing ability is apparently independent of memory, because cats often take a direct route instead of retracing a path. In addition, this directional orientation is not blocked by anesthesia.[273] Careful investigations have documented extended trips by cats to meet owners at new locations as far as 1500 miles from the original home.[210] Care must be exercised in studying such travels to be sure that the same cat arrives as the one who left. Great similarities in behaviors and physical characteristics can be misleading and are not positive proof of identification. Microchips, tattoos, or rabies tags are necessary for positive identification.

FELINE PLAY BEHAVIOR

Of all developmental behaviors associated with kittens, play is probably the most familiar. Play assumes a wide variety of patterns and functions. A broad definition of *play* is as follows: behaviors of specific patterns performed in disconnected and varying groupings, during which each action develops its own spontaneous, exuberant, action-specific energy, and is not directly useful.

Play Behavior Development

At about 2 weeks self-play begins with attempts to bat moving objects. This play progresses with a kitten's muscle coordination, so at about 3 weeks of age, social play appears as oriented pawing and occasional biting. Within another few weeks interactions with littermates and specific patterns appear. Certain sequences are more common at specific ages.[13] By day 35 stalking, chasing, and arching of the back are seen; wrestling appears at day 43.[81,261] Climbing and balancing on ledges starts around day 48.[170] Leaping is more variable in time of development, ranging from day 17 to 43.[81]

Play serves many purposes. Each of the numerous types of play can produce several results. Physical fitness is the most obvious benefit derived. Furthermore, when the kitten becomes independent, certain species-specific behaviors, such as hunting, must be mature enough to allow its survival. Play permits the acquisition of endogenous pattern coordination, timing, physical coordination, and central nervous system maturation. In addition, play behaviors provide a method for kittens to explore their environment and make social contacts, which decrease the probability of serious fighting later.

Social Play

Social play involves two or more cats, and it has eight associated categories of behavior. These behaviors are most prevalent during weeks 4 through 16, and the decline of social play is related to the decreased preference for social contact and the need for dispersal.[42,130,265,277] Until week 12, there are no gender differences in the play of kittens, but during the next 4 weeks, differences are seen based on the kitten's play partner. Female kittens that play with male kittens become more malelike in their play.[55] Early weaning and all-male groups have been associated with a higher frequency of social play by kittens.[42,171] Initially the various social play postures are highly correlated with each other, but this interrelation is largely lost by 12 weeks.[41]

"Belly-up" describes a posture of dorsal recumbency with the thoracic limbs making a pawing motion while the pelvic limbs tread (Figure 2-15). The mouth is often open, exposing the teeth. Belly-up, first seen between days 21 and 23, is specific to social play but may occasionally be seen during mating.[81] At 6 weeks of age, this behavior occurs during 13% of the social play and at 12 weeks occupies 16% of social play.[277]

"Stand-up" involves one kitten standing over a second kitten that is in a belly-up posture (Figure 2-16). These two social play patterns appear together 67% of the time. With heads oriented in the same direction, the kittens may paw and bite each other.

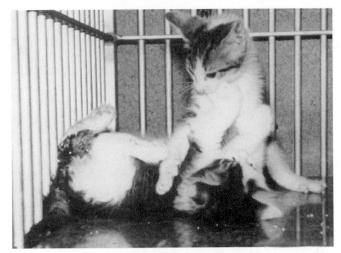

Figure 2-15 "Belly-up" play posture shown by the kitten in dorsal recumbency.

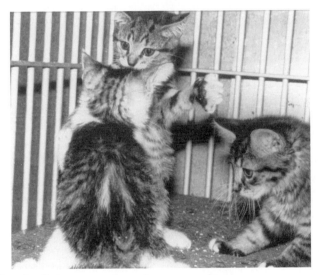

Figure 2-16 "Stand-up" play posture shown between two kittens.

Stand-up play first appears at about 23 days of age. After this point, up to 15% of social play is devoted to stand-up play.[277]

A third type of social play, "side-step," develops at about 32 days of age and occupies 20% of playtime by 6 weeks of age. It involves one kitten showing a lateral body position, including a slight body arch and an upward curve in the tail, to a second kitten (Figure 2-17). Arching peaks at about 6 weeks.[41] The posturing kitten then walks laterally toward the second kitten or circles around it.[277] This lateral posturing contains many of the same positions later used in distance-increasing silent communication.

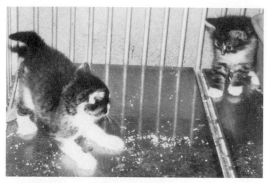

Figure 2-17 The lateral body position of "side-step."

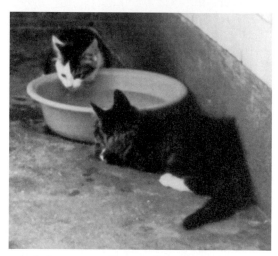

Figure 2-18 The crouched play posture of "pounce."

In the "pounce" the kitten crouches low with the pelvic limbs underneath its body and its tail straight back (Figure 2-18). Initially the weight is shifted forward and back by the pelvic limbs, which then provide a sudden forward thrust toward the other kitten. This particular social play begins between days 33 and 35 and occupies 42% of a 6-week-old kitten's play behavior. By 12 weeks, 5% less time is devoted to it.[277]

From a sitting position, the kitten shifts its weight to its hindquarters, thereby raising its forelimbs perpendicular to the body. By extending the pelvic limb joints into a stationary bipedal position, the kitten assumes the "vertical stance" or "rearing" posture (Figure 2-19). Appearing at about 35 days of age, this posture does not occupy a large portion of play until about 12 weeks of age, when it occurs during approximately 25% of the playtime.[277]

"Chase" is the social play of pursuit and flight, which develops between 38 and 41 days of age (Figure 2-20).[277] This type of activity continues to steadily increase over the next 7 weeks.[41] Kittens eventually spend a considerable amount of the play period in pursuit of one another, although at times one kitten runs, and the second fails to follow.

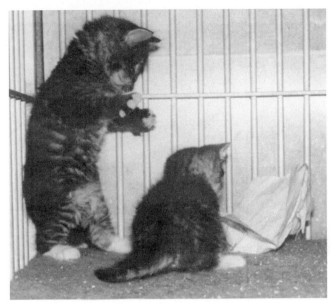

Figure 2-19 The "vertical stance" play posture directed toward another kitten and a paper.

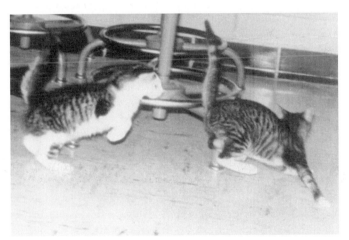

Figure 2-20 "Chase."

About 5 days after the appearance of chase the "horizontal leap" develops. With body postures like those associated with side-step play, the kitten suddenly leaps off the ground.[277]

The last of the eight social play categories to develop is "face-off." By 48 days two kittens sit looking at each other, intensely leaning forward. Simultaneously they direct paw movements at each other's face. Frequently, however, only one of the kittens participates in a solitary version of the game (Figure 2-21).[277]

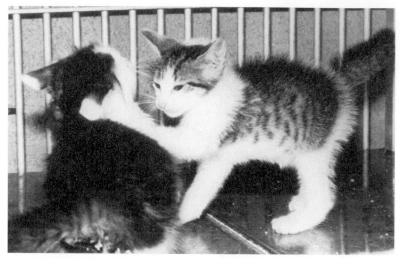

Figure 2-21 Unilateral "face-off" from a standing position.

Individual Play

Play behaviors associated with predatory behavior take different forms and may be self-rewarding because kittens will perform them for long periods, even to the point of exhaustion. Isolated kittens play more individually and play with their mothers more than those raised with littermates; object play occurs more often in kittens if the mother was on a rationed diet.[16,18,97,177] Object play increases dramatically around 50 days of age in both male and female kittens without littermates or in female kittens with male littermates.[15,17] In adult cats, there also seems to be an increased likelihood of play with small objects, especially if the cat has not eaten for several hours.[98] Object play may be important as training for solitary hunting, perhaps less so for developing motor skills as for learning important aspects of the situations that accompany the hunt.[64]

Games of prey perfect some hunting skills and provide exercise. The game "mouse" involves leaping on a small movable object, such as a ball, and securing it with the forepaws while doing body acrobatics (Figure 2-22). In other versions, the paw is used to bat the object. Occasionally two kittens join in this game; one holds the "mouse" as the other bats at it, alternating paws. "Bird" involves intercepting flying objects and bringing them into the mouth (Figure 2-23). Intense interest is directed toward the interception of objects that take off from the ground or that fly from one point to another. Kittens that chase the beam of a flashlight or a laser pointer are good examples of how intense a game of "bird" can become. As skills progress, kittens undertake the game of "rabbit," in which they ambush large moving objects, such as another cat (Figure 2-24). To succeed is to bring the object to the ground and use the neck bite. Two cats will often alternate between stalking and being chased, but with age the game can become very rough, so the cat prefers a younger or less-animated playmate.[32,81]

In addition to living and inanimate things, play behavior can be directed toward imaginary objects. During "hallucinatory" play, the kitten leaps at a wall to catch an imaginary object or bats and chases imaginary objects along the ground (Figure 2-25).[81] A kitten may

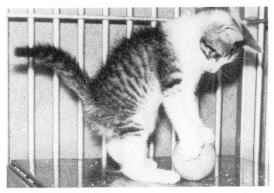

Figure 2-22 "Mouse" played with a ball.

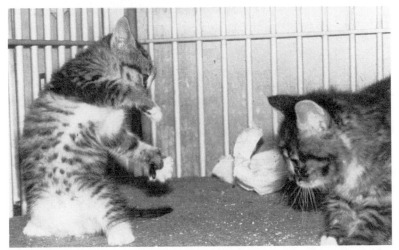

Figure 2-23 An unsuccessful attempt to catch a piece of paper in the game of "bird."

express another form of this behavior usually in the early evening by suddenly jumping up with dilated pupils and running wildly around the house as if chasing an invisible kitten.

By 6 months novel objects will attract playful interaction, and the cat exhibits a corresponding reduction in self-play and inactivity.[57] The type of toy has a profound effect on whether the activity will continue. Balls are the most desirable play objects.[57] Object play may actually be highly linked to predatory behavior, because the more similarities between the object and natural prey, the more predatory-like the play.[64] Stress and increasing age suppress play behavior, and adult cats show almost none.

FELINE LEARNING

Development of Learning

Learning is a change in behavior as the result of an individual's experience.[252] It contrasts with instinctive behavior, which involves inherited, species-specific patterns. Although learning behavior in cats, as in other animals, does involve certain genetically determined characteristics of the nervous and musculoskeletal systems, it remains an individual process. Kittens can learn immediately after birth, usually via sensory input. By at least 10 days of age kittens learn to locate a preferred teat for nursing, primarily through trial and error with the sense of smell. It has been experimentally shown that at this age they are also capable of learning to avoid or escape offensive situations (active avoidance).[10,71] Passive avoidance occurs when the kitten can identify environmental cues associated with a noxious stimulus and completely avoid the situation. This type of learning occurs sometime between 25 and 50 days.[54]

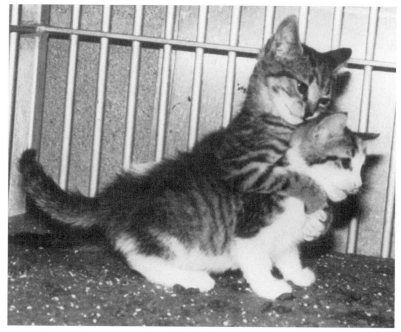

Figure 2-24 The top kitten is using the lower one as the target in a game of "rabbit."

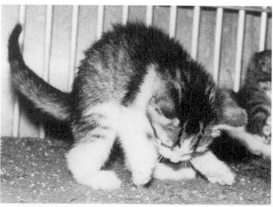

Figure 2-25 "Hallucinatory" play.

In certain situations the cat demonstrates a behavior somewhat unique to the species—observational learning. The queen is responsible for much of this stimulus-controlled response by her kittens. Kittens often do not exhibit an observed behavior immediately after observing the queen perform it, but by 9 or 10 weeks of age, they will suddenly perform the act with the same directness as an individual that has performed it many times.[44,211] The importance of imitation is probably variable, depending on the particular action involved.[3,25,127] Instinctive imitation, such as the learning of hunting behaviors, is important to mental development and self-preservation. In contrast, the imitation of many voluntary acts requires several observations to learn and a reward to perform. To retain the connection between a previous learning experience and its external stimuli, a cat may imitate the act even though the stimulus is no longer present.[25] For example, a cat trained to pull a string for a food reward will continue pulling at a nonexistent string. It is more significant to the cat to watch another cat acquire a response than it is to watch one perform a skill that has already been learned.[172] Kittens can use observational learning to push a lever for food but never develop the same skill through trial and error.[172] One extreme example of observational learning is an orphaned kitten that was raised with dogs and learned to lift its leg to a tree by observing its male dog companion doing so (Figure 2-26).

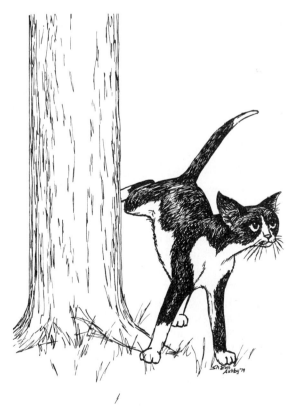

Figure 2-26 Observational learning by an orphaned kitten that learned from a male dog companion.

At 8 weeks of age the kitten still lacks a stable attention span, so learning is difficult to evaluate. However, kittens have been shown to be capable of solving specific types of problems.[33,270] Individuals of this age can solve oddity sets by choosing the different shape from a group with several similar figures. Probability problems have also been solved. (For example, if a cat is to choose a dark-colored dish for a food reward most of the time, but once in a while the food is in the light-colored dish, the kitten will go to the dark-colored dish first based on probability.) The kitten can also learn to select choices that had previously been incorrect and leave previously correct responses alone (such as learning to choose a triangle shape for a reward when the reward was previously received for choosing a circle shape). Motivation at this age is probably a limiting factor in experimental studies. Food and play behaviors are effective incentives for early learning. For example, the kitten must learn which species are prey.[40] Pain has also been an effective motivator, but success is dependent on the difficulty of the problem's discrimination (e.g., choosing between a dark color and a light color versus choosing between yellow and yellow-green).[60,179]

Certain types of early experiences allow for latent learning—that is, learning that is not immediately obvious. Between 5 and $6\frac{1}{2}$ weeks of age, human handling is effective in developing an individual that shows much less fear of strangers in later life, and early activity-encouraging environments tend to produce less active kittens that are mainly affected by novel stimuli.[81,97,161,172,282] Discipline begun before 6 weeks results in a generalized learned response that lasts into adulthood, and that which is started later is effective on the cat only in the specific incident.[81]

Characteristics of Learning

Adult cats have been used as experimental models of learning, with vision being the primary modality studied. Discrimination between patterns of different shapes can be learned whether or not the shape differences are paired with other cues such as brightness.[237,271] Even for the adult cat the learning of oddity sets is possible although difficult.[109,269] Teaching cats to stay out or off of certain places is exceedingly difficult unless people are present to serve as a negative cue. Search techniques in strange areas tend to be random, although each area is searched only once.[101] This indicates a high degree of trial-and-error learning. Transfer learning also occurs in cats[272]: The animal uses information from one problem to solve a second problem. For example, a circular form selected from square figures in one oddity set will be generalized to a dull object placed among illuminated objects in a second problem.

Motivational factors are an important part of adult learning and behavioral choice.[223] Avoidance learning is widely used with adults and kittens. The cat can be taught by the owner yelling and throwing things at it or picking the cat up on the dorsum of its neck or by its chest and gently shaking it. Picking the cat up and shaking it has the advantage of discomfort without pain. Affection and attention or lack thereof, food, and stimulus strength have been successful motivational factors. With proper motivation and a great deal of patience, a cat can be taught several tricks, such as sitting up, rolling over, or giving "high fives" (Figure 2-27). Training sessions must be of short duration, generally not more than 5 minutes per session, for two or three sessions per day.

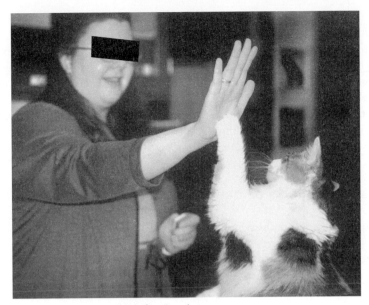

Figure 2-27 A cat trained to do "high fives" with its paw.

It is easiest to start with a task that uses a natural behavior, such as jumping on something or getting an object from under a cover; however, shaping, which is placing the cat in the desired position, can also be successful. Through successive approximation from an initial behavior that is gradually increased for the reward, a cat can be taught such behaviors as using a cat door and a toilet. Once the given task has been performed correctly, it should be repeated for reinforcement. The latency period between performance and reward can also affect the learning. Reinforcement is optimally given within a half second of initiation; however, with a 30-second delay cats are still 68% correct.[262,273] Discipline too must be applied immediately, at an appropriate strength, and in a form understood by the cat. Intrinsic motivational factors certainly exist, such as itch reduction from scratching, but they are extremely difficult to evaluate.[217]

Intelligence

The intelligence of *Felis catus* is often discussed and compared with that of other animals,[267] with these comparisons usually based on certain learned behaviors, such as how quickly each species can paw at a lever in response to a stimulus. Lever pushing using a foot is inherently easy for horses, dogs, and cats; however, the nose-pushing dolphin, chicken, and elephant would do less well. For perspective, one should also note that there is much controversy regarding the definition of intelligence and how to measure it, even in humans. Not until this controversy is settled can intelligence in animals be measured. Considering the motivational differences between individuals and species, the inherent differences in natural behavioral patterns, and the various physical limitations of individuals and species makes the task particularly difficult.

The Brain and Learning

Studies of the central nervous system's involvement in learning have been quite variable. The hippocampus is probably the most important part of the brain for learning because of its control over attention spans and its relationship to learning habits requiring discrimination.[2,8] It has been theorized that the maturation of this brain area transforms an exuberant juvenile into a placid adult.[8] The caudate nuclei play a role in adapting to changes in learned patterns.[166] Other brain areas have also been studied for learning, with experimental results often related to the sensory areas' studies.

NEUROLOGIC ORIGINS OF BEHAVIOR

Development of the central nervous system during the first several weeks of life is considerable (Figure 2-28), but even kittens of the same age and litter can have significant differences structurally and functionally.[219] Electroencephalograms do not become adultlike until the end of the first month.[219] In the first 3 weeks of life the spinal gray matter undergoes a marked proliferation of a fine fiber meshwork, pericellular plexus, and end bulbs.[283] This parallels the appearance of motor control in the limbs. The incompletely developed neonatal brain is extremely resistant to hypoxia. Because their brain cells use anaerobic glycolysis when deprived of oxygen, individuals tested have survived for more than 20 minutes with no ill effects. This is probably why young kittens are said to be so difficult to drown.[19,279]

Although the brain has been extensively studied with respect to the specific senses, numerous studies have also been conducted to show the interrelationships between

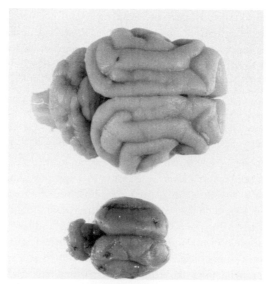

Figure 2-28 The brain of a newborn kitten is physically and functionally less developed than that of an adult.

the neural areas and the behavioral functions of each. Stimulation of one sense can stimulate cortical neurons associated with other senses. Peripheral stimuli have been hypothesized to activate a common central association system, which projects equally to all sensory cortical fields.[250] That would explain why a sharp noise or a sudden pain can also be perceived as a flash of light.

In considering the role of the brain in behavior, one invariably discusses the limbic system. Although some authors are more inclusive, most agree that the limbic system is composed of the limbic lobe and associated subcortical nuclei. The limbic lobe comprises the following: parahippocampal gyri, cingulate gyri, subcallosal gyri, hippocampus, and dentate gyri. The associated subcortical nuclei include the amygdaloid complex, hypothalamus, epithalamus, septal nuclei, and rostral thalamic nuclear areas. Several complicated tracts with specific behavioral functions have been defined within the limbic system. An example of such a tract is the Papez circuit (hippocampus to fornix, to mammillary body, to rostral thalamic nucleus, to cingulate gyrus, to cerebral cortex), which deals with emotion.[144]

The limbic system integrates information from internal and external sources and influences the *internal* (physiologic) and *external* (behavioral) responses.[182] Within the limbic system specific areas also have particular functions. The cingulate gyri are thought to be involved in the functional organization of associated behaviors because they have been shown to maintain a lack of aggression and to have a role in psychomotor seizures.[56,169,182] More thoroughly studied and complex, the hippocampus functions in very broad behavioral contexts, including emotion, attention mechanisms, personality, recent memories, internal physiologic changes, submissive behavior patterns without response to social threat, and psychomotor seizures.[56,144,152,194] The amygdaloid complex mainly modulates the activity of the hypothalamus and is particularly involved with the regulation of agonistic behavior. Agonistic behavior is generally divided into four aggression components: flight, defense, predatory attack, and offensive attack, which includes a ragelike response. In addition, the amygdaloid complex regulates hypothalamic output with respect to activity patterns, water consumption, and food intake.

As the most studied portion of the limbic system, the hypothalamus has diversified functions. The various parts control water balance, appetite, predatory attacks, sexual behavior, and the sleep-wake cycle. Some emotions are also associated with this area, including fear, anger, aggression, and rage, with its defensive threat postures. The septal nuclei of the limbic system regulate sensory stimuli to prevent hyperreactivity, moderate water consumption, and control emotional responses. In the latter situation, the septal nuclei suppress aggressive behaviors of either amygdaloid or hypothalamic origin. Sensory input into the thalamus is directed to specific cortical areas, making this area the chief sensory integrating mechanism.[144] The thalamus also regulates states of consciousness and the hypothalamus.[144,181]

The brain directly affects the response behaviors of injury or illness. Behavioral responses to pain can include changes in temperament (e.g., flight, aggressiveness, excitability), lack of movement, unusual responses to the owner, self-mutilation, vocalization, and hiding.[233] Responses associated with fever are also neurologic in origin.[116,117,118] Depression is one method used to conserve energy that would otherwise be lost by movement. Anorexia also reduces the amount of movement for energy and body heat conservation and has the added benefit of reducing the intake of iron, depriving iron-using bacteria of their nutrition.

Numerous other neural-behavioral interrelationships have been investigated with less-specific conclusions drawn. Information about specific neurotransmitters is discussed relative to drug therapy because that is where most psychopharmacologics work. Other neural-behavior connections will be dealt with in the chapters that follow.

SENSORY AND NEURAL BEHAVIOR PROBLEMS

Behavior Problems and the Senses

Problem behaviors involving the cat's senses occur in a few types of circumstances. Cats that are stroked a great deal have shown persistent mobilization of the third eyelid, indicative of vagal nerve overstimulation.[43,222] Recovery requires a separation of owner and cat for a prolonged period.

Fearful behaviors associated with auditory or visual stimuli account for approximately 5% of cat cases that are referred to a specialist.[259] Sharp, particularly loud, noises can startle a cat. So too can the sudden appearance of objects. It would be interesting to compare the frequency of such problems with the inherent personality of affected cats.

White, blue-eyed cats, except those with Burmese or Siamese dilutions, are usually deaf. In affected individuals, degeneration of the organ of Corti starts at about 5 days of age, so the kitten never hears. An occasional colored spot on a basically white cat can result in one ear with normal hearing. As with most deaf cats, bilaterally affected individuals exhibit characteristic hyperalertness. Several months after affected cats received intracochlear implants, cortical activity was established that resembled the activity present in a hearing cat.[159] The gene producing this blue-eyed, deaf cat is also responsible for the absence of the reflective tapetal area of the eye, so nocturnal vision is also reduced.

Behavior Problems and Development

Malnutrition can have a particularly strong influence on neonatal learning abilities. Kittens born to severely undernourished queens have poor brain development and their physical maturation is also delayed. They are more reactive to external stimuli and less responsive to other cats. Males play more aggressively, and females show more climbing behavior.[197] The increased emotionality results in increased vocalization and poor bonding with the queen.[86] Deprivation may result in changes in food-related emotional behaviors.[106] The mildly deprived male kitten's brain undergoes compensatory growth if he is returned to an adequate plane of nutrition.[236] With more severe deprivation during the early postnatal period, such as occurs at a 20% nutritional plane for the nursing mother, neuron development and learning ability are permanently affected.[106] Runts in a normal litter may suffer neurologically because of nutritional problems, in addition to being susceptible to possible psychologic difficulties induced by intimidation from littermates.[106]

Early separation from the mother, at 2 weeks of age, for example, can affect a kitten. Commonly the amount of random, non–goal-oriented activity increases.[224] These kittens are more emotional in various situations and are slower to calm down later.[224] Hand-reared and orphaned kittens do not learn appropriate play behavior, especially relative to roughness and bite inhibition. Therefore their aggressive play must be corrected early.

Stress-Related Behavior Problems

Generalized stress

Stress is probably the most common cause of behavior changes in cats. Hospitalization or other variations in environment, forced confinement, physical trauma, crowding, changes in routine, changes in schedule, unpredictable handling, continued exposure to high-frequency sounds (like those from some television remote controls), prolonged anticipatory waiting, mourning, and restraint are but a few causes of stress. Signs of abnormalities caused by these stresses vary even more than the causes because they affect a number of body systems. Included in this gamut of signs are convulsions, hysteroepilepsy, sudden depigmentation, fear, restlessness, excitability, depression, changes in taste preferences, anorexia, aversion to locations, catatonia, eliminations, fever, vomiting, diarrhea, shyness, colic, hair loss, bronchospasm, ulcers, paroxysmal hypotonia, aggression, psychologic neutering, excessive grooming, and nongrooming. The cat spends more time awake and alert, yet active exploratory and play behaviors are suppressed. It attempts to hide.[39] In general these signs can be classified as inhibitory or excitatory.[79] The signs in the cat, however, are generally of a narrower spectrum than are those seen in the dog or human. Stress can produce intense sympathetic stimulation, which in turn can extend to the neurosecretory hypothalamus and the hormone system, particularly the adrenal glands. Thus, under prolonged stressful conditions the cat's resistance to disease usually decreases.[115] Sympathetic system changes may be particularly severe in older cats, and the failure of the cat to adapt can result in a very rapid psychologic and physiologic decline.[79,183] Anxiety disorders in cats are similar to some in humans,[198] making interesting parallels in diagnosing and treating them.

Several methods for controlling stress-related problems are available. If the cat's environment cannot be changed, a small dark enclosure such as a paper box or sack can provide security. Even giving the cat its own room will provide a small territory where life can be quiet and routine. Drug therapy is widely used and is most effective when it is important to alleviate mental anxiety. At the same time, it is critical to also modify the environment to eliminate the source of the stress or to desensitize the cat using behavioral modification. After several weeks, the drug dosage may be gradually reduced until it is no longer needed. The phenothiazine derivatives and haloperidol of the butyrophenone derivatives are neuroleptics and can reverse impaired thought processes in psychotic humans.[104,150] The benzodiazepine family, including oxazepam and diazepam, are effective in cases of human anxiety and nervousness where psychosis is not a major problem.[104,150] They also dissociate the stressor from the environment. Tricyclic antidepressants, selected serotonin reuptake inhibitors, and azaperone have been useful in the long-term management of stress-related problems.[104] In any case in which drugs are used, it is important to remember that any drug can produce pronounced individual reactions, particularly when long-term drug therapy is indicated. For short-term treatment of anxiety, particularly if anorexia is part of the problem, progestins can be used.[103]

Cats that show extreme displeasure with veterinarians during an office call may have learned to associate the sight of a syringe or a white coat with pain. The remedy may simply be to hide the syringe while approaching the cat, distracting it with a food treat,[108] working with the cat surrounded by the familiar scents of the bottom half of its carrier (Figure 2-29), or using the synthetic facial pheromone on a towel or clinician's hands.

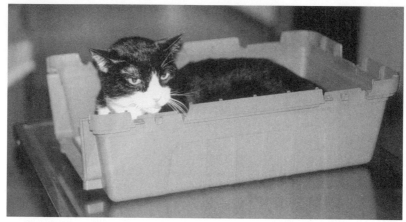

Figure 2-29 A cat can often be examined more easily if it remains in the bottom of its carrier, surrounded by familiar smells.

The same principles of eliminating the stimulus cue that causes stress and distraction can work successfully for a wide range of situations.

Psychogenic shock

Cats, particularly nervous individuals, are particularly vulnerable to psychogenic shock. This condition can be initiated by preparation for surgery; war conditions; or severe fights with other cats, dogs, or humans.[21,43,148] Affected cats tend to hide in dark corners, showing depression, salivation, anorexia, pupil dilation, and hyperesthesia.[21,148,286] Hallucinatory behavior such as jumping into the air to catch imaginary objects has also been reported in affected adults.[148,286] The shock syndrome may have developed as a method for survival, because the lack of motion inhibits an attack by a predator.[21] Treatment is the same as that for any shock condition.

Inappropriate Behaviors

Certain natural behaviors of the adult cat appear at inappropriate times, and artificial environments are causing the incidence of this abnormality to increase. Each normal behavior pattern is allotted a given amount of natural energy.[252] If one of these normal behavior patterns is not expressed over a period because an appropriate stimulus is lacking, the energy produced for it builds up within the individual. Cats kept in tidy homes often do not have the opportunity to stalk and kill prey. As these energies build up, the threshold stimulus to initiate the behavioral expression decreases to the point that very minor stimuli can result in the behavior in situations that seem inappropriate. The motion of human feet can initiate a prey-killing attack directed at the ankles. When hearing the mail carrier, a cat may wait under the indoor mail slot to attack the incoming mail. Even after being hit on the head by a large magazine or catalog the cat may continue the inappropriate prey-killing attack. For other cats, the barren environment could result in masturbation, excessive digging motions around the outside of the food bowl or litter box, and aggressive extremes in play behavior because of the lack of sexual, normal digging, and play activities, respectively. Kittens raised with minimal social play will bite more often and harder than those that were allowed to interact with littermates.[97] Although they can play well by themselves, their social skills are rudimentary. Rhythmic pacing, head swinging, and prolonged sniffing of the air in one location can also be seen when the cat's normal energies are not released.[82,265] These behaviors are displacement activities and are managed most easily by encouraging activity, generally play, with another cat or a toy. Owners need to divert these behaviors early so that they do not become the repetitive behaviors called *stereotypies*.

Behavior Problems and the Brain

Abnormalities in the central nervous system are not completely understood, but certain generalizations can be made. Irritative lesions such as encephalitis and atrophying scar tissue are commonly unilateral.[59,105,110] Suppressive changes of parts of the central nervous system are generally bilateral and thus often involve a midline lesion.[105,110] Included in the latter category are septal or ventral hypothalamic lesions, which precipitate aggression, hyperreactivity, and increased or decreased ingestive behavior; amygdala lesions, which prevent male copulatory behavior; and hippocampal abnormalities, which cause staring, excessive grooming, excessive vocalization, and seizures.[38,59,65,105] Localized twitching of the skin, along with tail lashing, urination, and vocalization, may be focal motor seizures, manifestations of one of the other cat diseases, toxins, or feline hyperesthesia syndrome.[119] The latter is discussed in Chapter 10.

Several feline diseases or medical conditions are also associated with behavior changes. Although some are obvious, as with polydipsia/polyuria in diabetes mellitus, others are not. Feline leukemia virus (FeLV) is often associated with tumor formation, typically lymphosarcoma. When the brain is affected, behavior changes can occur and may proceed to more classic neurologic signs. Even without tumors, abnormal behaviors in FeLV-positive cats may not be responsive to treatment. The feline immunodeficiency virus (FIV) can also cause behavior abnormalities. Most commonly these include depression or higher activity levels, social withdrawal, housesoiling, decreasing ability to walk on narrow ledges, and unusual aggression.[63,244] It is important to check the FeLV and FIV status of cats with behavior problems. The noneffusive form of feline infectious peritonitis (FIP) often affects the nervous system. Unfortunately for the cat, FIP is rapidly progressive, so other organ systems are also quickly affected. Feline ischemic encephalopathy is a poorly understood condition in which a portion of one cerebral hemisphere is ischemic.[227] Behavior changes and aggression are common presenting signs and may be residual concerns even if the cat survives. Motor deficits, seizures, visual deficits, and circling can also occur. Supportive care, corticosteroids for edema, and anticonvulsants for seizures are the reported treatments.[227] Simple partial seizures are partial seizures with a normal state of consciousness.[188] When these are characterized by intermittent, repetitive abnormal behavior, they are referred to as *behavioral, temporal lobe, limbic lobe*, or *psychomotor seizures*.[188] Experimental simulation of these in different areas of the brain results in a variety of behavior changes including quick glancing; searching movements; reduced responses to external stimuli; staring; fear or defensive reactions with piloerection; salivation; pupillary dilation, growling, and hissing; uncharacteristic tameness; rhythmic chewing, licking, and swallowing; and nonresponsive running (i.e., continued running without heed to owner calling, loud noise, etc.).[188]

Geriatric humans, dogs, cats, and rodents develop diffuse β-amyloid plaques within their brain. Aging also reduces serotonin levels and cholinergic activity. There is an increase in monoamine oxidase B (MAO-B), which leads to reduced dopamine and adrenergic levels, which lead to lowered cerebral perfusion and the production of free radicals.[78,163] Cognitive dysfunction associated with those changes is different in cats from that in dogs. Increased vocalization is the most common complaint. Other signs include housesoiling; sleep-cycle disturbances; decreased appetite and affection; and increased irritability, aggression, disorientation, wandering, and overgrooming.[78,131,163,164] Selegiline is a veterinary label drug for canine cognitive dysfunction that has also shown promising results in geriatric cats.[164] By irreversibly inhibiting the activity of MAO-B, selegiline protects the metabolism of dopamine, hydrogen peroxide, and maybe other cytotoxic free radicals.[78,131] Propentofylline, a xanthine derivative, and nicergoline increase cerebral blood flow and have been used to treat canine cognitive dysfunction.[131] Recently certain types of pet foods have been enriched with antioxidants to significantly reverse many of the clinical signs of cognitive dysfunction.

It is no surprise that drugs can alter the mental state of the cat. The one most commonly noted in this regard is ketamine hydrochloride. When used in combination with xylazine, it has been reported to cause hallucinations during recovery.[186] Ketamine hydrochloride is also known to produce hallucinations, irritability, and mental confusion in humans and may cause similar reactions in cats, particularly if the anesthetic recovery period includes many external stimuli. That could account for individual cats becoming extremely withdrawn for varying periods after anesthetization.

Behavior Problems and Genetic Variations

Temperament has been genetically linked to the sire in cats.[197] In addition, kittens from excitable/reactive litters are less likely to have their behavior modified by early handling.[197] Breed variations in behavior and reactions to situations are not well known. In general, cat lines that have undergone a great deal of concentrated inbreeding or line breeding may experience more behavior problems: Abyssinian, Russian blue, and Siamese cats often exhibit excessive restlessness, nervousness, and an unreliable disposition.[35,247] Persians are twice as likely to be presented for housesoiling, but are only half as likely to have a problem with aggression.[129] White spotting on cats is associated with a higher incidence of behavior problems when compared with non–white-spotted cats presented to the same hospital.[129] At Texas A&M, the white-spot pattern was associated with cats that tended toward extremes of tolerance for handling rather than having a typical graduated scale of tolerance.

REFERENCES

1. Adamec RE, Stark-Adamec C, Livingston KE: The expression of an early developmentally emergent defensive bias in the adult domestic cat *(Felis catus)* in non-predatory situations, *Appl Anim Ethol* 10:89–108, March 1983.
2. Adey WR: Hippocampal states and functional relations with corticosubcortical systems in attention and learning, *Prog Brain Res* 27:228–245, 1967.
3. Adler HE: Some factors of observational learning in cats, *J Genet Psychol* 86:159–177, 1955.

4. Ahl AS: The role of vibrissae in behavior: a status review, *Vet Res Commun* 10(4):245–268, 1986.

5. Aitkin LM, Prain SM: Medial geniculate body: unit responses in the awake cat, *J Neurophysiol* 37:512–521, 1974.

6. Albone ES, Shirley SG: *Mammalian semiochemistry: the investigation of chemical signals between mammals,* Somerset, NJ, 1984, John Wiley & Sons.

7. Allison AC: The morphology of the olfactory system in vertebrates, *Biol Rev* 28:195–244, May 1953.

8. Altman J, Brunner RL, Bayer SA: The hippocampus and behavioral maturation, *Behav Biol* 8:557–596, May 1973.

9. Animal behavior may predict earthquakes, *Vet Med Small Anim Clin* 73:834–836, June 1978.

10. Bacon WD: Aversive conditioning in neonatal kittens, *J Comp Physiol Psychol* 83:306–313, May 1973.

11. Barinaga M: Neurons tap out a code that may help locate sounds, *Science* 264(5160):775, 1994.

12. Barlow HB, Blakemore C; Pettigrew JD: The neural mechanism of binocular depth discrimination, *J Physiol* 193:327–342, Nov 1967.

13. Barrett P, Bateson P: The development of play in cats, *Behavior* LXVI(1–2):106–120, 1978.

14. Barrett RP: The "calming response," *Feline Pract* 7:46, Jan 1977.

15. Bateson P: Discontinuities in development and changes in the organization of play in cats. In Immelmann K, Barlow GW, Petrinovich L, Main M, editors: *Behavioral development,* Cambridge, 1981, Cambridge University Press.

16. Bateson P, Mendl M, Feaver J: Play in the domestic cat is enhanced by rationing of the mother during lactation, *Anim Behav* 40:514–424, Sep 1990.

17. Bateson P, Young M: The influence of male kittens on the object play of their female siblings, *Behav Neural Biol* 27:374–378, 1979.

18. Bateson P, Young M: Separation from the mother and the development of play in cats, *Anim Behav* 29:173–180, Feb 1981.

19. Beadle M: *The cat: history, biology, and behavior,* New York, 1977, Simon & Schuster.

20. Beaver BV: Reflex development in the kitten, *Appl Anim Ethol* 4:93, March 1978.

21. Beaver BVG: Feline behavioral problems, *Vet Clin North Am* 6:333–340, Aug 1976.

22. Beaver BVG, Knauer KW: The ear. In Catcott EJ, editor: *Feline medicine and surgery,* ed 2, Santa Barbara, 1975, American Veterinary Publications.

23. Beddard FE: Observations upon the carpal vibrissae in mammals, *Proc Zool Soc* 1:127–136, 1902.

24. Berkley MA, Sprague JM: Behavioral analysis of the role of geniculocortical system in form vision. In Cool SJ, Smith EL, editors: *Frontiers in visual science,* New York, 1977, Springer-Verlag.

25. Berry CS: An experimental study of imitation in cats, *J Comp Neurol Psychol* 18:1–26, Jan 1908.

26. Bishop PO, Kozak W, Vakkur GJ: Some quantitative aspects of the cat's eye: axis and plane of reference, visual field co-ordinates, and optics, *J Physiol* 163:466–502, Oct 1962.

27. Bisti S, Trimarchi C: Visual performance in behaving cats after prenatal unilateral enucleation, *Proc Natl Acad Sci U S A* 90(23):11142–11146, 1993.

28. Blake R: Spatial vision in the cat. In Cool SJ, Smith EL, editors: *Frontiers in visual science,* New York, 1977, Springer-Verlag .

29. Blake R, Cool SJ, Crawford MLJ: Visual resolution in the cat, *Vision Res* 14:1211–1217, Nov 1974.

30. Bland KP: Tom-cat odor and other pheromones in feline reproduction, *Vet Sci Commun* 3:125–136, 1979.

31. Boudreau JC, Tsuchitani C: Binaural interaction in the cat superior olive S segment, *J Neurophysiol* 31:442–454, May 1968.

32. Boudreau JC, Tsuchitani C: *Sensory neurophysiology,* New York, 1973, Van Nostrand Reinhold.

33. Boyd BO, Warren JM: Solution of oddity problems by cats, *J Comp Physiol Psychol* 50:258–260, June 1957.

34. Brearley EA, Kenshalo DR: Behavioral measurements of the sensitivity of cat's upper lip to warm and cool stimuli, *J Comp Physiol Psychol* 70:1–4, Jan 1970.

35. Bryant D: *The care and handling of cats,* New York, 1944, Ives Washburn, Inc.

36. Burkhardt D, Schleidt W, Altner H: *Signals in the animal world,* New York, 1967, McGraw-Hill.

37. Burton M: *The sixth sense of animals,* New York, 1973, Taplinger Publishing.

38. Caplan M: An analysis of the efforts of septal lesions on negatively reinforced behavior, *Behav Biol* 9:129–167, Aug 1973.

39. Carlstead K, Brown JL, Strawn W: Behavioral and physiological correlates of stress in laboratory cats, *Appl Anim Behav Sci* 38(2):143–158, 1993.

40. Caro TM: The effects of experience on the predatory patterns of cats, *Behav Neural Biol* 29:1–28, 1980.

41. Caro TM: Predatory behaviour and social play in kittens, *Behaviour* 76:1–24, 1981.

42. Caro TM: Sex differences in the termination of social play in cats, *Anim Behav* 29:271–279, 1981.

43. Chertok L, Fontaine M: Psychosomatics in veterinary medicine, *J Psychosom Res* 7:229–235, 1963.

44. Chesler P: Maternal influence in learning by observation in kittens, *Science* 166:901–902, 1969.

45. Chino YM, Shansky MS, Jankowski WL: Response properties of striate neurons in area 17 of Siamese cats. In Cool SJ, Smith EL, editors: *Frontiers in visual science,* New York, 1977, Springer-Verlag.

46. Cohen MJ, Hagiwara S, Zotterman Y: The response spectrum of taste fibers in the cat: a single fiber analysis, *Acta Physiol Scand* 33:316–332, 1955.

47. Coles JA: Some reflective properties of the tapetum lucidum of the cat's eye, *J Physiol* 212:393–409, 1971.

48. Cornwell P, Overman W: Behavioral effects of early rearing conditions and neonatal lesions of the visual cortex in kittens, *J Comp Physiol Psychol* 95(6):848–862, 1981.

49. Craig D: Personal communication, 1977.

50. Cranford JL, Igarashi M, Stramler JH: Effect of auditory neocortex ablation on identification of click rates in cats, *Brain Res* 116:69–81, 1976.

51. Creel DJ: Visual system anomaly associated with albinism in the cat, *Nature (Lond)* 231:465–466, June 18, 1971.

52. Crescitelli F: *The visual system in vertebrates,* New York, 1977, Springer-Verlag.

53. Cruickshank RM: Animal infancy. In Carmichael L, editor: *Manual of child psychology,* New York, 1946, John Wiley and Sons.

54. Davis JL, Jensen RA: The development of passive and active avoidance learning in the cat, *Dev Psychobiol* 9(2):175–179, 1976.

55. Deag JM, Manning A, Lawrence CE: Factors influencing the mother-kitten relationship. In Turner DC, Bateson PPG, editors: *The domestic cat: the biology of its behaviour,* Cambridge, 1988, Cambridge University Press.

56. DeLahunta A: *Veterinary neuroanatomy and clinical neurology,* Philadelphia, 1977, WB Saunders.

57. deMonte M, LePape G: Behavioural effects of cage enrichment in single-caged adult cats, *Anim Welfare* 6(1):53–66, 1997.

58. De Reuck AVS, Knight J: *Hearing mechanisms in vertebrates,* Boston, 1968, Little, Brown and Company.

59. Dhume RA, Gogate MG, deMascarenhas JF, Sharma KN: Functional dissociation within hippocampus: correlates of visceral and behavioral patterns induced on stimulation of ventral hippocampus in cats, *Indian J Med Res* 64:33–40, Jan 1976.

60. Dodson JD: The relation of strength of stimulus to rapidity of habit-formation in the kitten, *J Anim Behav* 5:330–336, July/Aug 1915.

61. Dodwell PC, Timney BN, Emerson VF: Development of visual stimulus-seeking in dark-reared kittens, *Nature* 260:777–778, April 29, 1976.

62. Doty RL: *Mammalian olfaction reproductive processes and behavior,* New York, 1976, Academic Press.

63. Dow SW, Dreitz MJ, Hoover EA: Exploring the link between feline immunodeficiency virus infection and neurologic disease in cats, *Vet Med* 87(12):1181–1184, 1992.

64. Egan J: Object-play in cats. In Bruner JS, Jolly A, Sylva K, editors: *Play: its role in development and evolution,* Charmondsworth, Middlesex, 1976, Penguin Books.

65. Egger MD, Flynn JP: Effects of electrical stimulation of the amygdala on hypothalamically elicited attack behavior in cats, *J Neurophysiol* 26:705–720, Sep 1963.

66. Eisenberg JF, Kleiman DG: Olfactory communication in mammals, *Annu Rev Ecol Syst* 3:1–32, 1972.

67. Elberger AJ: The effect of neonatal section of the corpus callosum on the development of depth perception in young cats, *Vision Res* 20:177–187, 1980.

68. Elliott DN, Stein L, Harrison MJ: Discrimination of absolute-intensity thresholds and frequency-difference thresholds in cats, *J Acoust Soc Am* 32(3):380–384, 1960.

69. Elul R, Marchiafava PL: Accommodation of the eye as related to behaviour in the cat, *Arch Ital Biol* 102:616–644, 1964.

70. Evans EF, Ross HF, Whitfield IC: The spatial distribution of unit characteristic frequency in the primary auditory cortex of the cat, *J Physiol* 179:238–247, 1965.

71. Ewer RF: Further observations on suckling behaviour in kittens, together with some general considerations of interrelations of innate and acquired responses, *Behaviour* 17:247–260, 1961.

72. Ewer RF: *The carnivores,* Ithaca, NY, 1973, Cornell University Press.

73. Ewert JP: *Neuroethology,* New York, 1980, Springer-Verlag.

74. Ferrinston DG, Rowe MJ: Functional capacities of tactile afferent fibres in neonatal kittens, *J Physiol* 307:335–353, Oct 1980.

75. Fitzgerald O: Discharges from the sensory organs of the cat's vibrissae and the modification of their activity by ions, *J Physiol* 98:163–178, May 14, 1940.

76. Flynn JT, Flynn TE, Hamasaki DI, et al: Development of the eye and retina of kittens. In Cool SJ, Smith EL, editors: *Frontiers in visual science,* New York, 1977, Springer-Verlag.

77. Flynn WE, Elliott DN: Role of the pinna in hearing, *J Acoust Soc Am* 38:104–105, 1965.

78. Fortney WD: Behavioral problems in older dogs and cats, American Veterinary Medical Association Convention Notes. Available at www.avma.org/noah/members/convention/conv01/notes/04040603.asp.

79. Fox MW: New information on feline behavior, *Mod Vet Pract* 56:50–52, April 1965.

80. Fox MW: Neurobehavioral development and the genotype-environment interaction, *Q Rev Biol* 45:131–147, June 1970.

81. Fox MW: The behaviour of cats. In Hafez ESE, editor: *The behaviour of domestic animals,* ed 3, Baltimore, 1975, Williams & Wilkins.

82. Fox MW: Personal communication, 1977.

83. Freeman NCG, Rosenblatt JS: The interrelationship between thermal and olfactory stimulation in the development of home orientation in newborn kittens, *Dev Psychobiol* 11(5):437–457, 1978.

84. Freeman NCG, Rosenblatt JS: Specificity of litter odors in the control of home orientation among kittens, *Dev Psychobiol* 11(5):459–468, 1978.

85. Galambos R: Processing of auditory information. In Brazier MAB, editor: *Brain and behavior,* vol 1, Washington, DC, 1961, American Institute of Biological Sciences.

86. Gallo PV, Werboff J, Knox K: Protein restriction during gestation and lactation: development of attachment behavior in cats, *Behav Neural Biol* 29:216–223, 1980.

87. Ganz L, Fitch M: The effects of visual deprivation on perceptual behavior, *Exp Neurol* 22:638–660, Dec 1968.

88. Ganz L, Haffner ME: Permanent perceptual and neurophysiological effects of visual deprivation in the cat, *Exp Brain Res* 20:67–87, 1974.

89. Giammanco S, Paderni MA, Carollo A: The effect of thermic stress on the somatic reaction of rage and on rapid circling turns in the cat, *Arch Int Physiol Biochem* 84:787–799, Oct 1976.

90. Glendenning KK, Hutson KA, Nudo RJ, Masterton RB: Acoustic chiasm. II. Anatomical basis of binaurality in lateral superior olive of cat, *J Comp Neurol* 232:261–285, 1985.

91. Goldstein MH Jr, Knight PL: Comparative organization of mammalian auditory cortex. In Popper AN, Fay RR, editors: *Comparative studies of hearing in vertebrates,* New York, 1980, Springer-Verlag.

92. Gottlieb G: Ontogenesis of sensory function in birds and mammals. In Tobach E, Aronson LR, Shaw E, editors: *The biopsychology of development,* New York, 1971, Academic Press.

93. Gourevitch G: Directional hearing in terrestrial mammals. In Popper AN, Fay RR, editors: *Comparative studies of hearing in vertebrates,* New York, 1980, Springer-Verlag.

94. Guillery RW: The effect of lid suture upon the growth of cells in the dorsal lateral geniculate nucleus of kittens, *J Comp Neurol* 148:417–422, 1973.

95. Guillery RW: Visual pathways in albinos, *Sci Am* 230:44–54, May 1974.

96. Guillery RW, Stelzner DJ: The differential effects of unilateral lid closure upon the monocular and binocular segments of the dorsal lateral geniculate nucleus in the cat, *J Comp Neurol* 139:413–422, 1970.

97. Guyot GW, Cross HA, Bennett TL: The domestic cat. In Ro MA, editor: *Species identity and attachment: a phylogenetic evaluation,* New York, 1980, Garland STPM Press.

98. Hall SL, Bradshaw JWS: The influence of hunger on object play by adult domestic cats, *Appl Anim Behav Sci* 58(1,2):143–150, 1998.

99. Halpern M: The organization and function of the vomeronasal system, *Annu Rev Neurosci* 10:325–362, 1987.

100. Halpin ZT: Individual odors among mammals: origins and functions, *Adv Study Behav* 16:39–70, 1986.

101. Hamilton GV: A study of trial and error reactions in mammals, *J Anim Behav* 1:33–66, Jan/Feb 1911.

102. Harrison J, Buchwald J: Auditory brainstem responses in the aged cat, *Neurobiol Ageing* 3(3):163–171, 1982.

103. Hart BL: Psychopharmacology in feline practice, *Feline Pract* 3(3):6, 8, 1973.

104. Hart BL: Drug choice in feline psychopharmacology, *Feline Pract* 3(4):8, 10, 1973.

105. Hart BL: The brain and behavior, *Feline Pract* 3(5):4, 6, 1973.

106. Hart BL: Behavior of the litter runt, *Feline Pract* 4(5):14–15, 1974.

107. Hart BL: The catnip response, *Feline Pract* 4(6):8, 12, 1974.

108. Hart BL: Handling and restraint of the cat, *Feline Pract* 5(2):10–11, 1975.

109. Hart BL: Learning ability in cats, *Feline Pract* 5(5):10, 12, 1975.

110. Hart BL: The medical interview and clinical evaluation of behavioral problems, *Feline Pract* 5(6):6, 8, 1975.

111. Hart BL: Quiz on feline behavior, *Feline Pract* 6(3):10, 13, 1976.

112. Hart BL: Behavioral aspects of selecting a new cat, *Feline Pract* 6(5):8, 10, 14, 1976.

113. Hart BL: Olfaction and feline behavior, *Feline Pract* 7(5):8–10, 1977.

114. Hart BL: Sensory capacities and behavioral feats, *Feline Pract* 7(6):8, 10, 12, 1977.

115. Hart BL: Psychosomatic aspects of feline medicine, *Feline Pract* 8(4):8, 10, 12, 1978.

116. Hart BL: Animal behavior and the fever response: theoretical considerations, *J Am Vet Med Assoc* 187(10):998–1001, 1985.

117. Hart BL: Behavior of sick animals, *Vet Clin North Am Small Anim Pract* 3(2):383–391, 1987.

118. Hart BL: Biological basis of the behavior of sick animals, *Neurosco Biobehav Rev* 12(2):123–127, 1988.

119. Hart BL, Beaver B, Wastlhuber J, Parker AJ: Seizure activity, *Feline Pract* 15(4):35–36, 1985.

120. Hata Y, Stryker MP: Control of thalamocortical afferent rearrangement by postsynaptic activity in developing visual cortex, *Science* 265:1732–1735, Sep 16, 1994.

121. Hatch RC: Effect of drugs on catnip *(Nepeta cataria)*-induced pleasure behavior in cats *Am J Vet Res* 33:143–155, Jan 1972.

122. Heffner HE: Auditory awareness, *Appl Anim Behav Sci* 57(3–4):259–268, 1998.

123. Heffner HE, Heffner RS: Auditory perception. In Phillips C, Piggins DEL, editors: *Farm animals and the environment,* New York, 1992, CAB International.

124. Heffner RS, Heffner HE: Hearing range of the domestic cat, *Hearing Res* 19:85–88, 1985.

125. Hein A, Held R, Gower EC: Development and segmentation of visually controlled movement by selective exposure during rearing, *J Comp Physiol Psychol* 73(2):181–187, 1970.

126. Hein A, Vital-Durand F, Salinger W, Diamond R: Eye movements initiate visual-motor development in the cat, *Science* 204:1321–1322, Jun 22, 1979.

127. Herbert JM, Harsh CM: Observational learning by cats, *J Comp Psychol* 37:81–95, 1944.

128. Holy TE, Dulac C, Meister M: Responses of vomeronasal neurons to natural stimuli, *Science* 289:1569–1572, Sep 1, 2000.

129. Houpt K, Drewer E, Eickwort A, Sappington B: A cat (or dog) of a different color: the influence of coat color and breed on behavior problems. Paper presented at American Veterinary Society of Animal Behavior meeting, Baltimore, July 27, 1998.

130. Houpt KA: Companion animal behavior: a review of dog and cat behavior in the field the laboratory and the clinic, *Cornell Vet* 75:248–261, 1985.

131. Houpt KA: Cognitive dysfunction in geriatric cats. In August JR, editor: *Consultations in feline internal medicine,* vol 4, Philadelphia, 2001, WB Saunders.

132. Houpt KA, Wolski TR: Domestic animal behavior for veterinarians and animal scientists, Ames, 1982, Iowa State University Press.

133. Hubel DH: The visual cortex of the brain. In Held R, Richards W, editors: *Perception: mechanisms and models,* San Francisco, 1972, Scientific American.

134. Hubel DH, Wiesel TN: Receptive fields of single neurons in the cat's striate cortex, *J Physiol* 148:547–591, 1959.

135. Hubel DH, Wiesel TN: Receptive fields binocular interaction and functional architecture in the cat's visual cortex, *J Physiol* 160:106–154, Jan 1962.

136. Hubel DH, Wiesel TN: The period of susceptibility to the physiological effects of unilateral eye closure in kittens, *J Physiol* 206:419–436, 1970.

137. Hubel DH, Wiesel TN: Aberrant visual projections in the Siamese cat, *J Physiol* 218:33–62, 1971.

138. Hughes A: Vergence in the cat, *Vision Res* 12:1961–1994, Dec 1972.

139. Hughes A: Observing accommodation in the cat, *Vision Res* 13:481–482, Feb 1973.

140. Hughes CP, Chi DY: Visual function in the ventral lateral geniculate nucleus of the cat, *Exp Neurol* 79:611–621, March 1983.

141. Jacobs GH: *Comparative color vision,* New York, 1981, Academic Press.

142. Jacobson SG, Franklin KBJ, McDonald WI: Visual acuity of the cat, *Vision Res* 16:1141–1143, 1976.

143. Jane JA, Masterton RB, Diamond IT: The function of the tectum for attention to auditory stimuli in the cat, *J Comp Neurol* 125:165–192, 1965.

144. Jenkins TW: *Functional mammalian neuroanatomy,* Philadelphia, 1972, Lea & Febiger.

145. Jewett DL: Volume-conducted potentials in response to auditory stimuli as detected by averaging in the cat, *Electroencephalogr Clin Neurophysiol* 28:609–618, 1970.

146. Jewett DL, Romano MN: Neonatal development of auditory system potentials averaged from the scalp of rat and cat, *Brain Res* 36:101–115, 1972.

147. Johnson SB: The "dark side" of catnip, *AVSAB Newsletter* 10(1):6, 1987.

148. Joshua JO: Abnormal behavior in cats. In Fox MW, editor: *Abnormal behavior in animals,* Philadelphia, 1968, WB Saunders.

149. Kaas JH, Krubitzer LA, Chino YM: Reorganization of retinotopic cortical maps in adult mammals after lesions of the retina, *Science* 248:229–231, 1990.

150. Kakolewski JW: Psychopharmacology: clinical and experimental aspects. In Fox MW, editor: *Abnormal behavior in animals,* Philadelphia, 1968, WB Saunders.

151. Kasprzak H, Tapper DN, Craig PH: Functional development of the tactile pad receptor system, *Exp Neurol* 26:439–446, March 1970.

152. Kemp IR, Kaada BR: The relation of hippocampal theta activity to arousal attentive behaviour and somato-motor movements in unrestrained cats, *Brain Res* 95:323–342, Sep 23, 1975.

153. Kennedy JL, Smith KU: Visual thresholds of real movement in the cat, *J Gen Psychol* 46:470–476, 1935.

154. Kenshalo DR: The temperature sensitivity of furred skin of cats, *J Physiol* 172:439–448, Aug 1964.

155. Kenshalo DR: Cutaneous temperature sensitivity. In Dawson WW, Enoch JM, editors: *Foundations of sensory science,* New York, 1984, Springer-Verlag.

156. Kenshalo DR, Duncan DG, Weymark C: Thresholds for thermal stimulation of the inner thigh footpad and face of cats, *J Comp Physiol Psychol* 63:133–138, Feb 1967.

157. Kenshalo DR, Hensel H, Graziadei P, Fruhstorfer H: On the anatomy, physiology and psychophysics of the cat's temperature-sensing system. In Dubner R, Kawamura Y, editors: *Oral-facial sensory and motor mechanisms,* New York, 1971, Appleton-Century-Crofts.

158. Keverne EB: The vomeronasal organ, *Science* 286:716–720, Oct 22, 1999.

159. Klinke R, Kral A, Heid S, et al: Recruitment of the auditory cortex in congenitally deaf cats by long-term cochlear electrostimulation, *Science* 285(5434):1729–1733, 1999.

160. Kolb B, Nonneman AJ: The development of social responsiveness in kittens, *Anim Behav* 23:368–374, May 1975.

161. Konrad KW, Bagshaw M: Effect of novel stimuli on cats reared in a restricted environment, *J Comp Physiol Psychol* 70:157–164, Jan 1970.

162. Kruger S, Boudreau JC: Responses of cat geniculate ganglion tongue units to some salts and physiological buffer solutions, *Brain Res* 47:127–145, Nov 27, 1972.

163. Landsberg G: Behavior problems in the geriatric dog and cat, Friskies PetCare Symposium. *Small Anim Behav Proc* pp 37–42, Oct 4, 1998.

164. Landsberg GM: Behavior problems of older cats, *Proc Am Vet Med Assoc* pp 317–320, 1998.

165. Leventhal AG, Vitek DJ, Creel DJ: Abnormal visual pathways in normally pigmented cats that are heterozygous for albinism, *Science* 229:1395–1397, Sep 27, 1985.

166. Levine MS, Hull CD, Buchwald NA, Villablanca JR: Effects of caudate nuclei or frontal cortical ablations in kittens: motor activity and visual discrimination performance in neonatal and juvenile kittens, *Exp Neurol* 62(3):555–569, 1978.

167. Loop MS, Millican CL, Thomas SR: Photopic spectral sensitivity of the cat, *J Physiol* 382:537–553, 1987.

168. Lott D, Hart BL, Verosub KL, Howell MW: Is unusual animal behavior observed before earthquakes? Yes and no, *DVM* 11(3):65–69, 1980.

169. Lubar JF, Numan R: Behavioral and physiological studies of septal function and related medial cortical structures, *Behav Biol* 8:1–25, Jan 1973.

170. Martin P, Bateson P: The ontogeny of locomotory play behaviour in the domestic cat, *Anim Behav* 33:502–510, May 1985.

171. Martin P, Bateson P: The influence of experimentally manipulating a component of weaning on the development of play in domestic cats, *Anim Behav* 33:511–518, May 1985.

172. Martin P, Bateson P: Behavioural development in the cat. In Turner DC, Bateson PPG, editors: *The domestic cat: the biology of its behaviour,* Cambridge, 1988, Cambridge University Press.

173. Marzi CA, Stefano M: Role of Siamese cat's crossed and uncrossed retinal fibres in pattern discrimination and interocular transfer, *Arch Ital Biol* 116:330–337, Sep 1978.

174. Masterton B, Thompson GC, Bechtold JK, RoBards MJ: Neuroanatomical basis of binaural phase-difference analysis for sound localization: a comparative study, *J Comp Physiol Psychol* 89:379–386, July 1975.

175. Mead LC: Visual brightness discrimination in the cat as a function of illumination, *J Genet Psychol* 60:223–257, 1942.

176. Mendelson JR, Cynader MS: Sensitivity of cat primary auditory cortex (AI) neurons to the direction and rate of frequency modulation, *Brain Res* 327:331–335, 1985.

177. Mendl M: The effects of litter-size variation on the development of play behaviour in the domestic cat litters of one and two, *Anim Behav* 36:20–34, Feb 1988.

178. Middlebrooks JC, Knudsen EI: Changes in external ear position modify the spatial tuning of auditory units in the cat's superior colliculus, *J Neurophysiol* 57(3):672–686, March 1987.

179. Miles RC: Learning in kittens with manipulatory exploratory and food incentives, *J Comp Physiol Psychol* 51:39–42, Feb 1958.

180. Mitchell DE, Giffin F, Wilkinson F, et al: Visual resolution in young kittens, *Vision Res* 16:363–366, 1976.

181. Moore CN, Casseday JH, Neff WD: Sound localization: the role of the commissural pathways of the auditory system of the cat, *Brain Res* 82:13–26, Dec 20, 1974.

182. Morgenson GJ, Huang YH: The neurobiology of motivated behavior, *Prog Neurobiol* 1(1):55–83, 1973.

183. Mosier JE: Common medical and behavioral problems in cats, *Mod Vet Pract* 56:699–703, Oct 1975.

184. Movshon JA: Reversal of the physiological effects of monocular deprivation in the kitten's visual cortex, *J Physiol* 261:125–174, Sep 1976.

185. Muir DW, Mitchell DE: Visual resolution and experience: acuity deficits in cats following early selective visual deprivation, *Science* 180:420–422, April 27, 1973.

186. Muir WW: Hallucinations caused by xylazine-ketamine, *Mod Vet Pract* 58:654, Aug 1977.

187. Nagaki J, Yamashita S, Sato M: Neural response of cat to taste stimuli of varying temperatures, *Jpn J Physiol* 14:67–89, 1964.

188. Neer TM: Complex partial seizures (behavioral epilepsy). Paper presented at Texas Veterinary Medical Association Summer Seminar, Corpus Christi, Tex, Aug 6, 1995.

189. Neff WD: Discriminatory capacity of different divisions of the auditory system. In Brazier MAB, editor: *Brain and behavior,* vol 1, Washington, DC, 1961, American Institute of Biological Science.

190. Neff WD, Diamond IT: The neural basis of auditory discrimination. In Harlow HF, Woolsey CN, editors: *Biological and biochemical bases of behavior,* Madison, 1958, University of Wisconsin Press.

191. Nelson PG, Erulkar SD: Synaptic mechanisms of excitation and inhibition in the central auditory pathway, *J Neurophysiol* 26:908–923, Nov 1963.

192. Nilsson BY: Structure and function of the tactile hair receptors on the cat's foreleg, *Acta Physiol Scand* 77:396–416, Dec 1969.

193. Nilsson BY, Skoglund CR: The tactile hairs on the cat's foreleg, *Acta Physiol Scand* 65:364–369, Dec 1965.

194. Nonneman AJ, Kolb BE: Lesions of hippocampus or prefrontal cortex alter species-typical behaviors of the cat, *Behav Biol* 12:41–54, Sep 1974.

195. Norton TT: Receptive-field properties of superior colliculus cells and development of visual behavior in kittens, *J Neurophysiol* 37(4):674–690, 1974.

196. Olmstead ChE, Villablanca JR: Development of behavioral audition in the kitten, *Physiol Behav* 24:705–712, 1980.

197. Overall KL: Preventing behavior problems: early prevention and recognition in puppies and kittens, *Behav Probl Small Anim Purina Specialty Review* pp 13–29, 1992.

198. Overall KL: Animal models for human psychiatric illness. Paper presented at American Veterinary Medical Association meeting, San Francisco, July 10, 1994.

199. Passanisi WC, Macdonald DW: Group discrimination on the basis of urine in a farm cat colony. In Macdonald DW, Müller-Schwarze D, Natynczwk SE, editors: *Chemical signals in vertebrates,* ed 5, New York, 1990, Oxford University Press.

200. Payne BR, Berman N: Functional organization of neurons in cat striate cortex: variations in preferred orientation and orientation selectivity with receptive-field type ocular dominance and location in visual-field map, *J Neurophysiol* 49(4):1051–1072, 1983.

201. Peters G, Wozencraft WC: Acoustic communication in fissiped carnivores. In Gittleman JL, editor: *Carnivore behavior ecology and evolution,* Ithaca, NY, 1989, Cornell University Press.

202. Peterson EA, Heaton WC, Wruble SD: Levels of auditory response in fissiped carnivores, *J Mammal* 50(3):566–578, Aug 1969.

203. Pfaffmann C: Differential responses of the new-born cat to gustatory stimuli, *J Genet Psychol* 49:61–67, 1936.

204. Pfaffman C: Gustatory afferent impulses, *J Cell Comp Physiol* 17:243–258, 1941.

205. Pickles JO: *An introduction to the physiology of hearing,* ed 2, New York, 1988, Academic Press.

206. Pinchoff BS, Winterkorn JMS: Deficits in luminous flux discrimination by cats with lesions of the superior colliculus-pretectum, *Brain Res* 173(2):217–224, 1979.

207. Prince JH: *Comparative anatomy of the eye,* Springfield, Ill, 1956, Charles C Thomas Publisher.

208. Prince JH, Diesem CD, Eglitis I, Ruskell GL: *Anatomy and histology of the eye and orbit in domestic animals,* Springfield, Ill, 1960, Charles C Thomas Publisher.

209. Rauschecker JP, Singer W: The effects of early visual experience on the cat's visual cortex and their possible explanation by Hebb synapses, *J Physiol* 310:215–239, 1981.

210. Rhine JB, Feather SR: The study of cases of "psi-trailing" in animals, *J Parapsychol* 26:1–22, March 1962.

211. Romanes GJ: *Mental evolution in animals,* New York, 1969, AMS Press.

212. Rose GH, Lindsley DB: Development of visually evoked potentials in kittens: specific and nonspecific responses, *J Neurophysiol* 31:607–623, July 1968.

213. Rose JE, Gross NB, Geisler CD, Hind JE: Some neural mechanisms in the inferior colliculus of the cat which may be relevant to localization of a sound source, *J Neurophysiol* 29:288–314, March 1966.

214. Rosenblatt JS: Suckling and home orientation in the kitten: a comparative development study. In Tobach E, Aronson LR, Shaw E, editors: *The biopsychology of development,* New York, 1971, Academic Press.

215. Rosenblatt JS: Learning in newborn kittens, *Sci Am* 227:18–25, 1972.

216. Rosenblatt JS, Turkewitz G, Schneirla TC: Development of home orientation in newly born kittens, *Trans N Y Acad Sci* 31:231–250, 1969.

217. Rosenzweig MR, Bennett EL: *Neural mechanisms of learning and memory,* Cambridge, Mass, 1976, MIT Press.

218. Sales G, Pye D: *Ultrasonic communication by animals,* New York, 1974, John Wiley and Sons.

219. Scheibel M, Scheibel A: Some structural and functional substrates of development in young cats, *Prog Brain Res* 9:6–25, 1964.

220. Schiffman HR: Evidence for sensory dominance: reactions to apparent depth in rabbits cats and rodents, *J Comp Physiol Psychol* 71:38–41, April 1970.

221. Schilder MBH: The (in)effectiveness of anti-cat repellents and motivational factors, *Appl Anim Behav Sci* 32(2–3):227–236, 1991.

222. Schmidt JP: Psychosomatics in veterinary medicine. In Fox MW, editor: *Abnormal behavior in animals,* Philadelphia, 1968, WB Saunders.

223. Schweikert GE III, Treichler FR: Visual probability learning and reversal in the cat, *J Comp Physiol Psychol* 67:269–272, Feb 1969.

224. Seitz PFD: Infantile experience and adult behavior in animal subjects, *Psychosom Med* 21:353–378, 1959.

225. Shansky MS, Chino YM, Hamasaki DI: Response properties of retinal ganglion cells in Siamese cats. In Cool SJ, Smith EL, editors: *Frontiers in visual science,* New York, 1977, Springer-Verlag.

226. Shapley R, Victor J: Hyperacuity in cat retinal ganglion cells, *Science* 231:999–1002, Feb 28, 1986.

227. Shell L: Feline ischemic encephalopathy (cerebral infarct), *Virginia Vet Notes* 35:3, Sep/Oct 1988.

228. Sherman SM: Development of interocular alignment in cats, *Brain Res* 37:187–203, 1972.

229. Sherman SM: Visual field defects in monocularly and binocularly deprived cats, *Brain Res* 49:25–45, Jan 15, 1973.

230. Sherman SM: Permanence of visual perimetry deficits in monocularly and binocularly deprived cats, *Brain Res* 73:491–501, 1974.

231. Sherman SM, Guillery RW, Kaas JH, Sanderson KJ: Behavioral electrophysiological and morphological studies of binocular competition in the development of the geniculo-cortical pathways of cats, *J Comp Neurol* 158:1–18, 1974.

232. Sherman SM, Wilson JR: Behavioral and morphological evidence for binocular competition in the postnatal development of the dog's visual system, *J Comp Neurol* 161:183–195, 1975.

233. Short CE: Fundamentals of pain perception in animals, *Appl Anim Behav Sci* 59(1–3):125–133, 1998.

234. Simoni A, Sprague JM: Perimetric analysis of binocular and monocular visual fields in Siamese cats, *Brain Res* 111:189–196, July 23, 1976.

235. Sireteanu R: The development of visual acuity in very young kittens: a study with forced-choice preferential looking, *Vision Res* 25(6):781–788, 1985.

236. Smith BA, Jansen GR: Behavior and brain composition of offspring of underfed cats, *Federal Proceedings* 36:1108, 1977.

237. Smith KU: Visual discrimination in the cat. III. The relative effect of paired and unpaired stimuli in the discriminative behavior of the cat, *J Genet Psychol* 48:29–57, 1936.

238. Smith KU: Visual discrimination in the cat. IV. The visual acuity of the cat in relation to stimulus distance, *J Genet Psychol* 49:297–313, 1936.

239. Smith KU: The relation between visual acuity and the optic projection centers in the brain *Science* 86:564–565, Dec 17, 1937.

240. Smith RC: *The complete cat book,* New York, 1963, Walker & Company.

241. Snyder A, Shapley R: Deficits in the visual evoked potentials of cats as a result of visual deprivation, *Exp Brain Res* 37(1):73–86, 1979.

242. Spear PD: Role of binocular interactions in visual system development in the cat. In Cool SJ, Smith EL, editors: *Frontiers in visual science,* New York, 1977, Springer-Verlag.

243. Starr A: Suppression of single unit activity in cochlear nucleus of the cat following sound stimulation, *J Neurophysiol* 28:850–862, Sep 1965.

244. Steigerwald ES, Sarter M, March P, Podell M: Effects of feline immunodeficiency virus on cognition and behavioral function in cats, *J Acquir Immune Defic Syndr* 20(5):411–419, 1999.

245. Stone J: The number and distribution of ganglion cells in the cat's retina, *J Comp Neurol* 180:753–772, 1978.

246. Stone J, Campion JE: Estimate of the number of myelinated axons in the cat's optic nerve, *J Comp Neurol* 180:799–806, 1978.

247. Suehsdorf A: The cats in our lives, *National Geographic* 125:508–541, April 1964.

248. Sutherland NS, Mackintosh NJ: *Mechanisms of animal discrimination learning,* New York, 1971, Academic Press.

249. Tamura T, Nakatani K, Yau K-W: Light adaptation in cat retinal rods, *Science* 245:755–758, Aug 18, 1989.

250. Thompson RF, Johnson RH, Hoopes JJ: Organization of auditory somatic sensory and visual projection to association fields of cerebral cortex in the cat, *J Neurophysiol* 26:343–364, May 1963.

251. Thorn F, Gollender M, Erikson P: The development of the kitten's visual optics, *Vision Res* 16:1145–1149, 1976.

252. Thorpe WH: *Learning and instinct in animals,* Cambridge, Mass, 1963, Harvard University Press.

253. Tieman SB: Effects of monocular deprivation on geniculocortical synapses in the cat, *J Comp Neurol* 222(2):166–176, 1984.

254. Tilney F, Casamajor L: Myelinogeny as applied to the study of behavior, *Arch Neurol Psychiatry* 12:1–66, July 1924.

255. Trachtenberg JT, Trepel C, Stryker MP: Rapid extragranular plasticity in the absence of thalamocortical plasticity in the developing primary visual cortex, *Science* 287:2029–2032, March 17, 2000.

256. Tretter F, Cynader M, Singer W: Modification of direction selectivity of neurons in the visual cortex of kittens, *Brain Res* 84:143–149, 1975.

257. Tritsch MF: Color choice behavior in cats and the effect of changes in the color of the illuminant, *Naturwissenschaften* 80(6):287–288, 1993.

258. Tucker AO, Tucker SS: Catnip and the catnip response, *Econ Botany* 42:214–231, April/June 1988.

259. Turner D, Appleby D, Magnus E: The Association of Pet Behaviour Counsellors: annual review of cases, 2000. Available at www.apbc.org.uk/2000/report.htm.

260. Vakkur GJ, Bishop PO: The schematic eye in the cat, *Vision Res* 3:357–381, 1963.

261. Villablanca JR, Olmstead CE: Neurological development of kittens, *Dev Psychobiol* 12:101–127, 1979.

262. Voith VL: Personal communication, 1978.

263. Volokhov AA: The ontogenetic development of higher nervous activity in animals. In Himwich WA, editor: *Developmental neurobiology,* Springfield, Ill, 1970, Charles C Thomas Publisher.

264. von Grünau MW: The role of maturation and visual experience in the development of eye alignment in cats, *Exp Brain Res* 37(1):41–47, 1979.

265. Wallach MB, Gershon S: The induction and antagonism of central nervous system stimulant-induced stereotyped behavior in the cat, *Eur J Pharmacol* 18:22–26, April 1972.

266. Walls GL: *The vertebrate eye and its adaptive radiation,* New York, 1967, Hafner Publishing.

267. Warden CJ: Animal intelligence, *Sci Am* 184:64–68, 1951.

268. Warkentin J, Smith KU: The development of visual acuity in the cat, *J Genet Psychol* 50:371–399, 1937.

269. Warren JM: Oddity learning set in a cat, *J Comp Physiol Psychol* 53:433–434, Oct 1960.

270. Warren JM: Overtraining extinction and reversal learning by kittens, *Anim Learn Behav* 3:340–342, Nov 1975.

271. Warren JM: Irrelevant cues and shape discrimination learning by cats, *Anim Learn Behav* 4:22–24, Feb 1976.

272. Warren JM, Baron A: The formation of learning sets by cats, *J Comp Physiol Psychol* 49:227–231, June 1956.

273. Washburn MF: *The animal mind,* ed 3, New York, 1976, Macmillan.

274. Wassle H: Optical quality of the cat eye, *Vision Res* 11:995–1006, Sep 1971.

275. Weigel I: Small cats and clouded leopards. In Grzimek HCB, editor: *Grzimek's animal life encyclopedia,* vol 12, New York, 1975, Van Nostrand Reinhold.

276. West CD: The relationship of the spiral turns of the cochlea and the length of the basilar membrane to the range of audible frequencies in ground dwelling mammals, *J Acoust Soc Am* 77(3):1091–1101, 1985.

277. West M: Social play in the domestic cat, *Am Zool* 14:427–436, Winter 1974.

278. Wever EG, Vernon JA, Rahm WE, Strother WF: Cochlear potentials in the cat in response to high-frequency sounds, *Proc Natl Acad Sci U S A* 44:1087–1090, 1958.

279. Widdowson EM: Food growth and development in the suckling period. In Graham-Jones O, editor: *Canine and feline nutritional requirements,* New York, 1965, Pergamon Press.

280. Wienrich M, Zrenner E: Colour-opponent mechanisms in cat retinal ganglion cells. In Mollon J, Sharpe LT, editors: *Colour vision: physiology and psychophysics,* New York, 1983, Academic Press.

281. Wiesel TN, Hubel DH: Effects of visual deprivation on morphology and physiology of cells in the cat's lateral geniculate body, *J Neurophysiol* 26:978–993, Nov 1963.

282. Wilson M, Warren JM, Abbott L: Infantile stimulation activity and learning by cats, *Child Dev* 36:843–853, Dec 1965.

283. Windle WF: Normal behavioral reactions of kittens correlated with the postnatal development of nerve-fiber density in the spinal gray matter, *J Comp Neurol* 50:479–503, 1930.

284. Windle WF, Griffin AM: Observations on embryonic and fetal movements of the cat, *J Comp Neurol* 52:149–188, Feb 15, 1931.

285. Wolski TR, Riter R, Houpt KA: The effectiveness of animal repellents on dogs and cats in the laboratory and field, *Appl Anim Behav Sci* 12(1–2):131–144, 1984.

286. Worden AN: Abnormal behaviour in the dog and cat, *Vet Rec* 71:966–978, Dec 26, 1959.

Additional Readings

Ables M, Goldstein MH: Functional architecture in cat primary auditory cortex: columnar organization and organization according to depth, *J Neurophysiol* 33:172–187, 1970.

Ables M, Goldesin MH Jr: Responses of single units in the primary auditory cortex of the cat to tones and to tone pairs, *Brain Res* 42:337–352, 1972.

Achor LJ, Starr A: Auditory brain stem response in the cat. I. Intracranial and extracranial recordings, *Electroencephalogr Clin Neurophysiol* 48:155–173, 1980.

Achor LJ, Starr A: Auditory brain stem response in the cat. II. Effects of lesions, *Electroencephalogr Clin Neurophysiol* 48:174–190, 1980.

Adamec R: Behavioral and epileptic determinants of predatory attack behavior in the cat, *Can J Neurol Sci* 2:457–466, Nov 1975.

Adamec RE: Hypothalamic and extrahypothalamic substrates of predatory attack: suppression and the influence of hunger, *Brain Res* 106:57–69, April 16, 1976.

Albus K: The detection of movement direction and effects of contrast reversal in the cat's striate cortex, *Vision Res* 20:289–293, 1980.

Algers B: TV apparatus upsets cats, *Friskies Res Dig* 13:14, Fall 1977.

Allikmets LH: Cholinergic mechanisms in aggressive behaviour, *Med Biol* 52:19–30, Feb 1974.

Andersen RA, Snyder RL, Merzenich MM: The topographic organization of corticocollicular projections from physiologically defines loci in AI AII and anterior cortical auditory fields of the cat, *J Comp Neurol* 191:479–494, 1980.

Anderson HT: Problems of taste specificity. In Wolstenholme GEW, Knight J, editors: *Taste and smell in vertebrates,* London, 1970, Churchill Livingstone.

Animal vision research focuses on seeing colors, *DVM* 17(3):84–85, 1986.

Appelle S: Perception and discrimination as a function of stimulus orientation: the "oblique effect" in man and animals, *Psychol Bull* 78:266–278, Oct 1972.

Baccelli G, Albertini R, Mancia G, Zanchetti A: Interactions between sino-aortic reflexes and cardiovascular effects of sleep and emotional behavior in the cat, *Circ Res* 38(suppl 1):30, 34, 1976.

Barinaga M: Listening in on the brain, *Science* 280:376–378, April 17, 1998.

Basbaum AI, Fields HL: The origin of descending pathways in the dorsolateral funiculus of the spinal cord of the cat and rat: further studies on the anatomy of pain modulation, *J Comp Neurol* 187(3):513–523, 1979.

Bateson P: The development of play in cats, *Appl Anim Ethol* 4:290, Sep 1978.

Baumgartner G, Brown JL, Schulz A: Responses of single units of the cat visual system to rectangular stimulus patterns, *J Neurophysiol* 28:1–18, Jan 1965.

Beach FA: Current concepts of play in animals, *Am Nat* 79:523–541, Nov/Dec 1945.

Bergsma DR, Brown KS: White fur blue eyes and deafness in the domestic cat, *J Hered* 62:171–185, May/June 1971.

Berkley KJ, Parmer R: Somatosensory cortical involvement in responses to noxious stimulation in the cat, *Exp Brain Res* 20:363–374, July 31, 1974.

Berkley MA: A system for behavioral evaluation of the visual capacities of cats, *Behav Res Methods Instrumentation* 11:545–548, 1979.

Berkson G: Maturation defects in kittens, *Am J Ment Defic* 72:757–777, 1959.

Berman AL: Interaction of cortical responses to somatic and auditory stimuli in anterior ectosylvian gyrus of cat, *J Neurophysiol* 24:608–620, Nov 1961.

Berman AL: Overlap of somatic and auditory cortical response fields in anterior ectosylvian gyrus of cat, *J Neurophysiol* 24:595–607, Nov 1961.

Berntson GG: Blockage and release of hypothalamically and naturally elicited aggressive behaviors in cats following midbrain lesions, *J Comp Physiol Psychol* 81(3):541–554, 1972.

Berntson GG, Hughes HC, Beattie MS: A comparison of hypothalamically induced biting attack with natural predatory behavior in the cat, *J Comp Physiol Psychol* 90:167–178, Feb 1976.

Berntson GG, Leibowitz SF: Biting attack in cats: evidence for central muscarinic mediation *Brain Res* 51:366–370, 1973.

Bjursten LM, Norrsell K, Norrsell U: Behavioral repertory of cats without cerebral cortex from infancy, *Exp Brain Res* 25:115–130, May 28, 1976.

Blake R, DiGianfilippo A: Spatial vision in cats with selective neural deficits, *J Neurophysiol* 43:1197–1205, May 1980.

Bland KP: Tom-cat odor and other pheromones in feline reproduction, *Vet Sci Comm* 3:125–136, 1979.

Bogen JE, Suzuki M, Campbell B: Paw contact placing in the hypothalamic cat given caffeine, *J Neurobiol* 6:125–127, Jan 1975.

Bosher SK, Hallpike CS: Observations on histological features development and pathogenesis of the inner ear degeneration of the deaf white cat, *Proc R Soc Lond Biol* 162:147–170, Apr 13, 1965.

Bradley NS, Smith JL, Villablanca JR: Absence of hind limb tactile placing in spinal cats and kittens, *Exp Neurol* 82(1):73–88, Oct 1983.

Brito GNO, Webster WG: Electrophysiological indicant of asymmetric hemispheric involvement in discrimination performance by cats, *Brain Res* 175(1):150–154, 1979.

Brogden WJ, Girden E, Mettler FA, Culler E: Acoustic value of the several components of the auditory system in cats, *Am J Physiol* 116:252–261, 1936.

Brooks C: Teaching tricks to your cat, *Pet News* 3:40–41, Sep/Oct 1977.

Brooks VB, Rudomin P, Slayman CL: Sensory activation of neurons in the cat's cerebral cortex, *J Neurophysiol* 24:286–301, March 1961.

Brunner F: The application of behavior studies in small animal practice. In Fox MW, editor: *Abnormal behavior in animals,* Philadelphia, 1968, WB Saunders.

Buchwald JS, Hinman C, Normal RJ, et al: Middle- and long-latency auditory evolved responses recorded from the vertex of normal and chronically lesioned cats, *Brain Res* 205(1):91–109, 1981.

Buizza A, Schmid R: New experimental data on cat's optokinetic responses: is there need to revise previous models of the optokinetic reflex? *Biol Cybern* 51(5):301–304, 1985.

Buser P, Bignall KE: Nonprimary sensory projections on the cat neocortex, *Int Rev Neurobiol* 10:111–165, 1967.

Cain DP: The role of the olfactory bulb in limbic mechanisms, *Psychol Bull* 81:654–671, Oct 1974.

Caird D, Klinke R: Processing of binaural stimuli by cat superior olivary complex neurons, *Exp Brain Res* 52:385–399, 1983.

Camuti LJ: Can cats be trained? *Feline Pract* 4(4):50, 1974.

Camuti LJ: Cats are not dumb, *Feline Pract* 4(6):52, 1974.

Caro TM: Effects of the mother object play and adult experience on predation in cats, *Behav Neural Biol* 29:29–51, 1980.

Carpenter JA: Species differences in taste preferences, *J Comp Physiol Psychol* 49:139–141, April 1959.

Carreras M, Andersson SA: Functional properties of neurons of the anterior ectosylvian gyrus of the cat, *J Neurophysiol* 26:100–126, Jan 1963.

Celesia GG: Segmental organization of cortical afferent areas in the cat, *J Neurophysiol* 26:193–206, March 1963.

Chi CC, Bandler RJ, Flynn JP: Neuroanatomic projections related to biting attack elicited from ventral midbrain in cats, *Brain Behav Evol* 13:91–110, 1976.

Chow KL, Stewart DL: Reversal of structural and functional effects of long-term visual deprivation in cats, *Exp Neurol* 34:409–433, March 1972.

Clemente CD, Chase MH: Neurological substrates of aggressive behavior, *Annu Rev Physiol* 35:329–356, 1973.

Cohen DH, Obrist PA: Interactions between behavior and the cardiovascular system, *Circ Res* 37:693–706, Dec 1975.

Coile DC, O'Keefe LP: Schematic eyes for domestic animals, *Opthalmic Physiol Opt* 8:125–220, 1988.

Colavita FB: Auditory cortical lesions and visual pattern discrimination in the cat, *Brain Res* 39:437–447, 1972.

Colpaert FC: The ventromedial hypothalamus and the control of avoidance behavior and aggression: fear hypothesis versus response-suppression theory of limbic system function, *Behav Biol* 15:27–44, Sep 1975.

Comis SD, Davies WE: Acetylcholine as a transmitter in the cat auditory system, *J Neurochem* 16:423–429, 1969.

Cornwell AC: Electroretinographic responses following monocular visual deprivation in kittens *Vision Res* 14:1223–1227, Nov 1974.

Cornwell P, Overman W, Levitsky C, et al: Performance on the visual cliff by cats with marginal gyrus lesions, *J Comp Physiol Psychol* 90:996–1010, Oct 1976.

Cornwell P, Overman W, Ross C: Extent of recovery from neonatal damage to the cortical visual system in cats, *J Comp Physiol Psychol* 92(2):255–270, 1978.

Costalupes JA: Representation of tones in noise in the responses of auditory fibers in cats. I. Comparison with detection thresholds, *J Neurosci* 5(12):3261–3269, 1985.

Costalupes JA, Yound ED, Gibson DJ: Effects of continuous noise backgrounds on rate response of auditory nerve fibers in cats, *J Neurophysiol* 51:1326–1344, 1984.

Cragg BG: The development of synapses in kitten visual cortex during visual deprivation, *Exp Neurol* 46:445–451, March 1975.

Cranford JL: Role of neocortex in binaural hearing in the cat. I. Contralateral masking, *Brain Res* 100:395–406, 1975.

Cranford JL: Detection versus discrimination of brief tones by cats with auditory cortex lesions, *J Acoust Soc Am* 65(6):1573–1575, 1979.

Cranford JL, Igarashi M, Stramler JH: Effect of auditory neocortex ablation on pitch perception in the cat, *J Neurophysiol* 39:143–152, 1976.

Crowley JC, Katz LC: Early development of ocular dominance columns, *Science* 290:1321–1324, Nov 17, 2000.

Cynader M: Strengthening visual connections, *Science* 287:1943–1944, March 17, 2000.

Daves WF, Boostrom E: Object properties mediating visual object discrimination in the cat *Percept Mot Skills* 19:343–350, Oct 1964.

DeLanerolle NC, Lang FF: Functional neural pathways for vocalization in the domestic cat. In Newman JD, editor: *Physiological control of mammalian vocalization,* New York, 1988, Plenum Publishing.

DeMolina AF, Hunsperger RW: Organization of subcortical systems governing defense and flight reactions in the cat, *J Physiol* 160:200–213, Feb 1962.

Derdzinski D, Warren JM: Perimeter complexity and form discrimination learning by cats, *J Comp Physiol Psychol* 68:407–411, July 1969.

Dews PB, Wiesel TN: Consequences of monocular deprivation on visual behaviour in kittens, *J Physiol* 206:437–455, Feb 1970.

Dewson JH: Speech sound discrimination by cats, *Science* 144:555–556, May 1, 1964.

Diamond IT, Neff WD: Ablation of temporal cortex and discrimination of auditory patterns, *J Neurophysiol* 20:300–315, May 1957.

Divac I: Delayed response in blind cats before and after prefrontal ablation, *Physiol Behav* 4(5):795–799, 1969.

Dursteler MR, Garey LJ, Movshon JA: Reversal of the morphological effects of monocular deprivation in the kitten's lateral geniculate nucleus, *J Physiol* 261:189–210, Sep 1976.

Dworkin S: Conditioned motor reflexes in cats, *Am J Physiol* 109:31, 1934.

Ehret G: Categorical perception of mouse-pup ultrasounds in the temporal domain, *Anim Behav* 43(3):409–416, March 1992.

Eleftheriou BE, Scott JP: *The physiology of aggression and defeat,* New York, 1971, Plenum Publishing.

Evans EF, Whitfield IC: Classification of unit responses in the auditory cortex of the unanaesthetised cat, *J Physiol* 171:476–493, 1964.

Ewer RF: *Ethology of mammals,* London, 1968, Paul Elek Ltd.

Ezure K, Wilson VJ: Interaction of tonic neck and vestibular reflexes in the forelimb of the decerebrate cat, *Exp Brain Res* 54(2):289–292, 1984.

Feaver J, Mendle M, Bateson P: A method for rating the individual distinctiveness of domestic cats, *Anim Behav* 34:1016–1025, 1986.

Fox MW: Natural environment: theoretical and practical aspects for breeding and rearing laboratory animals, *Lab Anim Care* 16:316–321, Aug 1966.

Fox MW: Psychomotor disturbances. In Fox MW, editor: *Abnormal behavior in animals,* Philadelphia, 1968, WB Saunders.

Fox MW: Psychopathology in man and lower animals, *J Am Vet Med Assoc* 159:66–77, July 1, 1971.

Fox MW: *Understanding your cat,* New York, 1974, Coward McCann & Geoghegan.

Fraser AF: Behavior disorders in domestic animals. In Fox MW, editor: *Abnormal behavior in animals,* Philadelphia, 1968, WB Saunders.

Frégnac Y, Imbert M: Development of neuronal selectivity in primary visual cortex of the cat, *Phys Rev* 64(1):325–434, 1984.

Fried PA: Septum and behavior: a review, *Psychol Bull* 78:292–310, Oct 1972.

Fukada Y: Receptive field organization of cat optic nerve fibers with special reference to conduction velocity, *Vision Res* 11:209–226, March 1971.

Ganz L, Hirsch HVB, Tieman SB: The nature of perceptual deficits in visually deprived cats, *Brain Res* 11:547–568, Sep 29, 1972.

Gerken GM: Central denervation hypersensitivity in the auditory system of the cat, *J Acoust Soc Am* 66(3):721–727, 1979.

Gerken GM: Temporal summation of pulsate brain stimulation in normal and deafened cats, *J Acoust Soc Am* 66(3):728–734, 1979.

Gerken GM, Sandlin D: Auditory reaction time and absolute threshold in the cat, *J Acoust Soc Am* 61(2):602–607, 1988.

Gibbs EL, Gibbs FA: A purring center in the brain of the cat, *J Comp Neurol* 64:209–211, 1936.

Gibson EJ, Walk RD: The visual cliff, *Sci Am* 202:64–71, 1960.

Glassman RB: Cutaneous discrimination and motor control following somatosensory cortical ablation, *Physiol Behav* 5:1009–1019, Sep 1970.

Glusman M: The hypothalamic "savage" syndrome, *Res Publ Assoc Nerv Ment Dis* 52:52–90, 1974.

Goldberg JM, Neff WD: Frequency discrimination after bilateral ablation of cortical auditory areas, *J Neurophysiol* 24:119–128, March 1961.

Gorham ME, Mitchell R: Classifying the catnip response: the low-down on feline highs, *DVM* 10:32–33, Jan 1979.

Guillery RW: Binocular competition in the control of geniculate cell growth, *J Comp Neurol* 144:117–127, 1972.

Grbović L, Radmanović B: Prostaglandins E_2 and $F_{2\alpha}$ and gross behavioural effects of cholinomimetic substances injected into the cerebral ventricles of unanesthetized cats, *Neuropharmacology* 18(8–9):667–671, 1979.

Gruber SH: Mechanisms of color vision: an ethologist's primer. In Burtt EH Jr, editor: *The behavioral significance of color,* New York, 1979, Garland Publishing.

Gunter R: The absolute threshold for vision in the cat, *J Physiol* 114:8–15, June 29, 1951.

Guthrie ER, Horton GP: Behavior in the puzzle box. In Henderson RW, editor: *Learning in animals,* Stroudsburg, Pa, 1982, Hutchinson Ross Publishing.

Guthrie ER, Horton GP: Interpretation of results. In Hendersen RW, editor: *Learning in animals,* Stroudsburg, Pa, 1982, Hutchinson Ross Publishing.

Hamilton LW: Active avoidance impairment following septal lesions in cats, *J Comp Physiol Psychol* 69:420–431, Nov 1979.

Hara K, Cornwell PR, Warren JM, Webster IH: Posterior extramarginal cortex and visual learning by cats, *J Comp Physiol Psychol* 87:884–904, Nov 1974.

Harris LR: Contrast sensitivity and acuity of a conscious cat measured by the occipital evoked potential, *Vision Res* 18:175–178, 1978.

Hart BL: Disease processes and behavior, *Feline Pract* 3(6):6–7, 1973.

Hart BL: A quiz on feline behavior, *Feline Pract* 5(3):12, 14, 1975.

Hart BL: Quiz on feline behavior, *Feline Pract* 7(3):20–21, 1977.

Hekmatpanah J: Organization of tactile dermatomes C1 through L4 in cat, *J Neurophysiol* 24:129–140, March 1961.

Hemmer H: Gestation period and postnatal development in felids. In Eaton RL, editor: *The world's cats,* vol 3, Seattle, 1976, Carnivore Research Institute.

Hendersen RW: *Learning in animals,* Stroudsburg, Pa, 1982, Hutchinson Ross Publishing.

Henry GH, Harvey AR, Lund JS: The afferent connections and laminar distribution of cells in the cat striate cortex, *J Comp Neurol* 187(4):725–744, 1979.

Henry JP: Mechanisms of psychosomatic disease in animals, *Adv Vet Sci Comp Med* 20:115–145, 1976.

Hirsch HVB, Spinelli DN: Visual experience modifies distribution of horizontally and vertically oriented receptive fields in cats, *Science* 168:869–871, May 15, 1970.

Hoffman KP, Sherman SM: Effects of early monocular deprivation on visual input to the cat superior colliculus, *J Neurophysiol* 37:1276–1286, 1974.

Horn G, Wiesenfeld Z: Attention in the cat: electrophysiological and behavioural studies, *Exp Brain Res* 21:67–82, 1974.

Houpt KA: Animal behavior as a subject for veterinary students, *Cornell Vet* 66:73–81, Jan 1976.

Houpt KA: *Domestic animal behavior for veterinarians and animal scientists,* ed 2, Ames, 1991, Iowa State University Press.

Hubel DH, Wiesel TN: Receptive fields of cells in striate cortex of very young visually inexperienced kittens, *J Neurophysiol* 26:994–1002, Nov 1963.

Hubel DH, Wiesel TN: Receptive fields and functional architecture in two nonstriate visual areas (18 and 19) of the cat, *J Neurophysiol* 28:229–289, March 1965.

Hubel DH, Wiesel TN: Binocular interaction in striate cortex of kittens reared with artificial squint, *J Neurophysiol* 28:1041–1051, Nov 1965.

Hutchinson RR, Ulrich RE, Azrim NH: Effects of age and related factors on the pain-aggression reaction, *J Comp Physiol Psychol* 59(3):365–369, 1965.

Jackson B, Reed A: Catnip and the alteration of consciousness, *JAMA* 207:1349–1350, Feb 17, 1969.

Jacobs BL, Trulson ME, Stern WC: An animal behavior model for studying the actions of LSD and related hallucinogens, *Science* 194:741–743, Nov 12, 1976.

Jenkins WM, Merzenich MM: Role of cat primary auditory cortex for sound-localization behavior, *J Neurophysiol* 52(5):819–847, 1984.

Johansson GG, Kalimo R, Niskanen H, Ruusunen S: Effects of stimulation parameters on behavior elicited by stimulation of the hypothalamic defense area, *J Comp Physiol Psychol* 87:1100–1108, Dec 1974.

John ER, Chesler P, Bartlett F, Victor I: Observation learning in cats, *Science* 159:1489–1491, March 29, 1968.

Kaelber WW: Escape from and avoidance of nociception elicited by intracranial stimulation of the cat subthalamus, *Exp Neurol* 73(3):397–420, 1981.

Kaelber WW, Mitchel CL: Alteration in escape responding in the cat, *Brain Behav Evol* 12:137–150, 1975.

Kare MR, Halpern BP: *Physiological and behavioral aspects of taste,* Chicago, 1961, University of Chicago Press.

Karmel BZ, Miller PN, Dettweiler L, Anderson G: Texture density and normal development of visual depth avoidance, *Dev Psychobiol* 3:73–90, 1970.

Keidel WD: The sensory detection of vibrations. In Dawson WW, Enoch JM, editors: *Foundations of sensory science,* New York, 1984, Springer-Verlag.

Kiang NYS, Sachs MB, Peake WT: Shapes of tuning curves for single auditory-nerve fibers, *J Acoust Soc Am* 42(6):1341–1342, 1967.

Kim EHJ, Woody CD, Berthier NE: Rapid acquisition of conditioned eye blink responses in cats following pairing of an auditory CS with glabella tap US and hypothalamic stimulation, *J Neurophysiol* 49(3):767–779, 1983.

Kling A, Kovach JK, Tucker TJ: The behaviour of cat. In Hafez ESE, editor: *The behaviour of domestic animals,* ed 2, Baltimore, 1969, Williams & Wilkins.

Kling A, Orbach J, Schwartz NB, Towne JC: Injury to the limbic system and associated structures in cats, *Arch Gen Psychiatry* 3:391–420, 1960.

Koepke JE, Pribram KH: Effect of milk on the maintenance of sucking behavior in kittens from birth to six months, *J Comp Physiol* 75:363–377, June 1971.

Krettek JE, Price JL: Amygdaloid projections to subcortical structures within the basal forebrain and brainstem in the rat and cat, *J Comp Neurol* 178:225–254, 1978.

Krettek JE, Prince JL: A description of the amygdaloid complex in the rat and cat with observations on intra-amygdaloid connections, *J Comp Neurol* 178:255–280, 1978.

Kuffler SW, Fitzhugh R, Barlow HB: Maintained activity in the cat's retina in light and darkness, *J Gen Physiol* 40:683–702, May 20, 1957.

Kuhn RA: Organization of tactile dermatomes in cat and monkey, *J Neurophysiol* 16:169–182, March 1953.

Kurtsin IT: Pavlov's concept of experimental neurosis and abnormal behavior in animals. In Fox MW, editor: *Abnormal behavior in animals,* Philadelphia, 1968, WB Saunders.

Kurtsin IT: Physiological mechanisms of behavior disturbances and corticovisceral interrelations in animals. In Fox MW, editor: *Abnormal behavior in animals,* Philadelphia, 1968, WB Saunders.

Kuwada S, Yin TCT, Wickesberg RE: Response of cat inferior colliculus neurons to binaural beat stimuli: possible mechanisms for sound localization, *Science* 206(4418):586–588, 1979.

Langworthy OR: Behavioral disturbances related to the decomposition of reflex activity caused by cerebral injury: an experimental study of the cat, *J Neuropathol Exp Neurol* 3:87–100, 1944.

Layton BS, Toga AW, Horestein S, Davenport DG: Temporal pattern discrimination serves simultaneous bilateral ablation of suprasylvian cortex but not sequential bilateral ablation of insular-temporal cortex in the cat, *Brain Res* 173(2):337–340, 1979.

Levinson BM: Man and his feline pet, *Mod Vet Pract* 53:35–39, Nov 1972.

Levinson PK, Flynn JP: The objects attacked by cats during stimulation of the hypothalamus, *Anim Behav* 13:217–220, April/July 1965.

Liberman MC: Auditory-nerve response from cats raised in a low-noise environment, *J Acoust Soc Am* 63(2):442–455, 1978.

Liberman MC, Kiang NYS: Acoustic trauma in cats, *Acta Otolaryngol Supp* 358:1–63, 1978.

Loop MS, Bruce LL, Petuchowski S: Cat color vision: the effect of stimulus size shape and viewing distance, *Vision Res* 19:507–513, 1979.

Lorenz K, Leyhausen P: *Motivation of human and animal behavior,* New York, 1973, Van Nostrand Reinhold.

MacDonnell MF, Flynn JP: Control of sensory fields by stimulation of hypothalamus, *Science* 152:1406–1408, June 3, 1966.

Macleod AJ: Chemistry of odours. In Stoddart DM, editor: *Olfaction in mammals,* London, 1980, Academic Press.

Mancia G, Baccelli G, Zanchetti A: Regulation of renal circulation during behavioral changes in the cat, *Am J Physiol* 227:536–542, Sep 1972.

Margoshes A: Angle sense in cats and ants, *J Genet Psychol* 110(1):41–43, 1967.

Marler P, Vandenbergh JG: *Handbook of behavioral neurobiology,* vol 3, *Social behavior and communication,* New York, 1979, Plenum Publishing.

Martin P: The energy cost of play: definition and estimation, *Anim Behav* 30(1):294–295, 1982.

Martin P: The (four) whys and wherefores of play in cats: a review of functional evolutionary developmental and casual issues. In Smith PK, editor: *Play in animals and humans,* Oxford, 1984, Basil Blackwell.

Maruyama N, Kanno Y: Experimental study on functional compensation after bilateral removal of auditory cortex in cats, *J Neurophysiol* 24:193–202, March 1961.

Masterton RB: Adaptation for sound localization in the ear and brainstem of mammals, *Federal Proceedings* 33:1904–1910, Aug 1974.

Masterton RB, Jane JA, Diamond IT: Role of brain-stem auditory structures in sound localization. II. Inferior colliculus and its brachium, *J Neurophysiol* 31:96–108, Jan 1968.

Mayers KS, Robertson RT, Rubel EW, Thompson RF: Development of polysensory responses in association cortex of kitten, *Science* 171:1038–1040 March 12, 1971.

McAllister WG, Berman HD: Visual form discrimination in the domestic cat, *J Comp Psychol* 12:207–241, 1931.

McClung AW, Hart BL: Olfactory loss affecting behavior? *Feline Pract* 8:17, May 1978.

McFarland CA, Hart BL: Aggressive behavior, *Feline Pract* 8:13, July 1978.

Meaney MJ, Stewart J, Beatty WW: Sex differences in social play: the socialization of sex roles, *Adv Study Behav* 15:1–58, 1985.

Mello NK, Peterson NJ: Behavioral evidence for color discrimination in cat, *J Neurophysiol* 27:323–333, 1964.

Melzceck R, Stotler WA, Livingston WK: Effects of discrete brainstem lesions in cats on perception of noxious stimulation, *J Neurophysiol* 21:353–367, 1958.

Meyer DR, Anderson RA: Colour discrimination in cats. In de Reuck AVS, Knight J, editors: *Colour vision,* London, 1965, Churchill Livingstone.

Middlebrooks JC, Dykes RW, Merzenich MM: Binaural response-specific bands in primary auditory cortex (A1) of the cat: topographical organization orthogonal to isofrequency contours, *Brain Res* 181:31–48, 1980.

Mignard M, Malpeli JG: Paths of information flow through visual cortex, *Science* 251:1249–1251, March 8, 1991.

Miller JD, Watson CS, Covell WP: Deafening effects of noise on the cat, *Acta Otolaryngol Stockholm* 176(suppl):2–81, 1963.

Morgane PJ, Kosman AJ: Alterations in feline behavior following bilateral amygdalectomy, *Nature* 180:598–600, Sep 21, 1957.

Motles E, Gonzalez M, Infante C: Rotational behavior in the cat induced by electrical stimulation of the pulvinar-lateralis posterior nucleus complex: role of the cholinergic system, *Exp Neurol* 82(1):43–54, 1983.

Movshon JA: Reversal of the behavioural effects of monocular deprivation in the kitten, *J Physiol* 261:175–187, Sep 1976.

Muir DW, Mitchell DE: Behavioral deficits in cats following early selected visual exposure to contours of a single orientation, *Brain Res* 85:459–477, March 7, 1975.

Munk MHJ, Roelfsema PR, König P, et al: Role of reticular activation in the modulation of intracortical synchronization, *Science* 272(5259):271–274, 1996.

Murakami DM, Wilson PD: The effect of monocular deprivation on cells in the C-laminae of the cat lateral geniculate nucleus, *Dev Brain Res* 9:353–359, 1983.

Murata K, Cramer H, Bach-y-Rita P: Neuronal convergence of noxious acoustic and visual stimuli in the visual cortex of the cat, *J Neurophysiol* 28:1223–1239, Nov 1965.

Murphy EH, Berman N: The rabbit and the cat: a comparison of some features of response properties of single cells in the primary visual cortex, *J Comp Neurol* 188(3):401–427, 1979.

Neff WD, Fisher JF, Diamond IT, Yela M: Role of auditory cortex in discrimination requiring localization of sound in space, *J Neurophysiol* 19:500–512, Nov 1956.

Neff WD, Hind JE: Auditory thresholds of the cat, *J Acoust Soc Am* 27:480–483, May 1955.

Negus VE: The organ of Jacobson, *J Anat* 90:515–519, Oct 1956.

Oliver J: Determinants of experimental neurosis in cats, *J Clin Psychol* 31:594–600, Oct 1975.

Oswaldo-Cruz E, Kidd C: Functional properties of neurons in the lateral cervical nucleus of the cat, *J Neurophysiol* 27:1–14, Jan 1964.

Overall KL: Recognition diagnosis and management of obsessive-compulsive disorders. Part 1. A rational approach, *Canine Pract* 17(2):40–44, 1992.

Overall KL: Recognition diagnosis and management of obsessive-compulsive disorders. Part 2. A rational approach, *Canine Pract* 17(3):25–27, 1992.

Overall KL: Rational behavior pharmacology. *The Friskies Symposium on Behavior* pp 18–28, 1996.

Paden GF, Goddard GV: Catnip and oestrous behaviour in the cat, *Anim Behav* 14:372–377, 1966.

Pasternal T, Merigan WH: The luminance dependence on spatial vision in the cat, *Vision Res* 21:1333–1339, 1981.

Peck CK, Blakemore C: Modification of single neurons in kitten's visual cortex after brief periods of monocular visual experience, *Exp Brain Res* 22:57–68, 1975.

Plantz RG, Williston JS, Jewett DL: Spatio-temporal distribution of auditory-evoked far field potentials in the rat and cat, *Brain Res* 68(1):55–71, 1974.

Quilliam TA: Non-auditory vibration receptors, *Int Audiol* 7:311–321, 1968.

Ratliff F: Form and function: linear and nonlinear analyses of neural networks in the visual system. In McFadden D, editor: *Neural mechanisms in behavior: a Texas symposium,* New York, 1980, Springer-Verlag.

Reale RA, Kettner RE: Topography of binaural organization in primary auditory cortex of the cat: effects of changing interaural intensity, *J Neurophysiol* 56(3):663–682, 1986.

Reis DJ: Central neurotransmitters in aggression, *Res Publ Assoc Nerv Ment Dis* 52:119–147, 1974.

Rheingold HL, Eckerman CO: Familiar social and nonsocial stimuli and the kitten's response to a strange environment, *Dev Psychobiol* 4:71–89, 1971.

Rizzolatti G, Tradardi V: Pattern discrimination in monocularly reared cats, *Exp Neurol* 33:81–94, 1971.

Roberts WW, Bergquist EH: Attack elicited by hypothalamic stimulation in cats raised in social isolation, *J Comp Physiol Psychol* 66:590–595, Dec 1968.

Roberts WW, Keiss HO: Motivational properties of hypothalamic aggression in cats, *J Comp Physiol Psychol* 58:187–193, Oct 1964.

Robertson RT: Patterns of habituation to electrical stimulation of cerebral cortex in the awake cat, *Brain Res* 173(3):557–561, 1979.

Robinson FR, Cohen JL, May J, et al: Cerebellar targets of visual pontine cells in the cat, *J Comp Neurol* 223(4):471–482, 1984.

Robinson JS, Voneida J: Central cross-integration of visual inputs presented simultaneously to the separate eyes, *J Comp Physiol Psychol* 57:22, Feb 1964.

Rodieck RW, Stone J: Response of cat retinal ganglion cells to moving visual patterns, *J Neurophysiol* 28:819–832, Sep 1965.

Roldan E, Alvarez-Pelaez R, de Molina AF: Electrographic study of the amygdaloid defense response, *Physiol Behav* 13:779–787, Dec 1974.

Rose JE, Woolsey CN: Cortical connections and functional organization of the thalamic auditory system of the cat. In Harlow HF, Woolsey CN, editors: *Biological and biochemical bases of behavior,* Madison, 1958, University of Wisconsin Press.

Rosenkilde CE, Divac I: Time-discrimination performance in cats with lesions in prefrontal cortex and caudate nucleus, *J Comp Physiol Psychol* 90:343–352, April 1976.

Rosenzweig M: Discrimination of auditory intensities in the cat, *Am J Psychol* 59:127–136, Jan 1946.

Rothfield L, Harman PJ: On the relation of the hippocampal-fornix system to the control of rage responses in cats, *J Comp Neurol* 101:265–282, Oct 1954.

Rubel EW: A comparison of somatotopic organization in sensory neocortex of newborn kittens and adult cats, *J Comp Neurol* 143:447–480, Dec 1971.

Scharlock DP, Neff WD, Strominger NL: Discrimination of tone duration after bilateral ablation of cortical auditory areas, *J Neurophysiol* 28:673–681, July 1965.

Scharlock DP, Tucker TJ, Strominger NL: Auditory discrimination by the cat after neonatal ablation of temporal cortex, *Science* 141:1197–1198, Sep 20, 1963.

Schilder P: Loss of a brightness discrimination in the cat following removal of the striate area, *J Neurophysiol* 29:888–897, 1966.

Schmied A, Bénita M, Condé H, Dormont JF: Activity of ventrolateral thalamic neurons in relation to a simple reaction time task in the cat, *Exp Brain Res* 36(2):285–300, 1979.

Schwartz AS, Whalen RE: Amygdala activity during sexual behavior in the male cat, *Life Sci* 4:1359–1366, July 1965.

Scott JP: *Aggression,* ed 2, Chicago, 1975, University of Chicago Press.

Sechzer JA, Brown JL: Color discrimination in the cat, *Science* 144:427–429, April 24, 1964.

Segundo JP: A hypothesis concerning the sharp pitch discrimination observed in the sleeping cat, *Experientia* 20(7):415–416, 1964.

Seksel K, Linderman MJ: Use of clomipramine in the treatment of anxiety-related and obsessive-compulsive disorders in cats, *Aust Vet J* 76(5):317–321, 1998.

Semple MN, Aitkin LM: Representation of sound frequency and laterality by units in the central nucleus of cat inferior colliculus, *J Neurophysiol* 42(6):1626–1639, 1979.

Seward JP, Humphrey GL: Changes in heart rate during avoidance training and extinction in the cat, *J Comp Physiol Psychol* 66:764–768, Dec 1968.

Shapley R, Victor JD: The contrast gain control of the cat retina, *Vision Res* 19:431–434, 1979.

Sherman SM: Visual development in cats, *Invest Ophthalmol* 11:394–401, May 1972.

Sherman SM, Hoffman KP, Stone J: Loss of a specific cell type from the dorsal lateral geniculate nucleus in visually deprived cats, *J Neurophysiol* 35:532–541, 1972.

Sherman SM, Wilson JR: Permanence of lateral geniculate abnormalities in visually deprived cats, *Anat Rec* 181:478, 1975 (abstract).

Shipley C, Buchwald JS, Norman R, Guthrie D: Brain stem auditory evoked response development in the kitten, *Brain Res* 182:313–326, 1980.

Siegel A, Edinger H, Dotto M: Effects of electrical stimulation of the lateral aspect of the prefrontal cortex upon attack behavior in cats, *Brain Res* 93:473–484, Aug 15, 1975.

Skultety FM: The behavioral effects of destructive lesions of the periaqueductal grey matter in adult cats, *J Comp Neurol* 110:337–365, 1958.

Smith BA, Jansen GR: Early undernutrition and subsequent behavior patterns in cat, *J Nutr* 103:19, July 1973.

Smith KU: Visual discrimination in the cat. I. The capacity of the cat for visual figure discrimination, *J Genet Psychol* 44:301–320, 1934.

Smith KU: Visual discrimination in the cat. II. A further study of the capacity of the cat for visual figure discrimination, *J Genet Psychol* 45:336–357, 1934.

Solijarvi ARA, Hyvärinen J: Auditory cortical neurons in the cat sensitive to the direction of sound source movement, *Brain Res* 73:455–471, 1974.

Spear PD, Baumann TP: Effects of visual cortex removal on receptive-field properties of neurons in lateral suprasylvian visual area of the cat, *J Neurophysiol* 41(suppl 1, pt 1):31–56, 1979.

Spear PD, Baumann TP: Neurophysiological mechanisms of recovery from visual cortex damage in cats: properties of lateral suprasylvian visual area neurons following behavioral recovery, *Exp Brain Res* 35(1):177–192, 1979.

Spinelli DN: Neural correlates of visual experience in single units of cat's visual and somatosensory cortex. In Cool SJ, Smith EL, editors: *Frontiers in visual science,* New York, 1977, Springer-Verlag.

Sprague JM, Chambers WW, Stellar E: Attentive affective and adaptive behavior in the cat, *Science* 133(3447):165–173, 1961.

Squires RD, Jacobson FH, Bergey GE: Hypothermia in cats during physical restraint, *Nat Tech Info Service* AD-735:883, 1971.

Stevenson JC: Dido—an impression from the past, *VMSAC* 74(2):161, 1979.

Straschill M, Hoffmann KP: Functional aspects of localization in the cat's tectum optium, *Brain Res* 13:274–283, 1969.

Sutin J, Rose J, Van Atta L, Thalmann R: Electrophysiological studies in an animal model of aggressive behavior, *Res Publ Assoc Res Nerv Ment Dis* 52:93–118, 1974.

Thomas GJ, Fry WJ, Fry FJ, et al: Behavioral effects of mammillothalamic tractotomy in cats, *J Neurophysiol* 26:857–876, Nov 1963.

Thompson RF: Function of auditory cortex of cat in frequency discrimination, *J Neurophysiol* 23:321–334, 1960.

Thompson RF, Smith HE, Bliss D: Auditory, somatic sensory, and visual response interactions and interrelations in association and primary cortical fields of the cat, *J Neurophysiol* 26:365–378, May 1963.

Thorn F: Detection of luminance differences by the cat, *J Comp Physiol Psychol* 70:326–334, Feb 1970.

Thorndike EL: *Animal intelligence,* New York, 1970, Hafner Publishing.

Tieman DG, McCall MA, Hirsch HVB: Physiological effects of unequal alternating monocular exposure, *J Neurophysiol* 49(3):804–818, 1983.

Trianna E, Pasnak R: Object permanence in cats and dogs, *Anim Learn Behav* 9(1):135–139, 1981.

Trotter Y, Fregnac Y, Buisseret P: Synergy between vision and extraocular proprioception in gaining functional plasticity of the kitten's primary visual cortex, *C R Acad Sc Paris* (III), 296(14):665–668, 1983.

Tucker T, Kling A: Differential effects of early vs. late brain damage on visual duration discrimination in cat, *Federal Proceedings* 25:207, March/April 1966.

Ursin H, Divac I: Emotional behavior in feral cats with ablations of prefrontal cortex and subsequent lesions in amygdala, *J Comp Physiol Psychol* 88(1):36–39, 1975.

Van Hof-Van Duin J: Development of visuomotor behavior in normal and dark-reared cats, *Brain Res* 104:233–241, March 12, 1976.

Verberne G: Beobachtungen und versuche uber das flehmen katzenartiger raubtiere, *Z Tierpsychol* 27:807–827, Oct 1970.

Verberne G: Chemocommunication among domestic cats mediated by the olfactory and vomeronasal senses. II. The relation between the function of Jacobson's organ (vomeronasal organ) and flehmen behaviour, *Z Tierpsychol* 42:113–128, Oct 1976.

Verberne G, DeBoer J: Chemocommunication among domestic cats mediated by the olfactory and vomeronasal senses. I. Chemocommunication, *Z Tierpsychol* 42:86–109, Sep 1976.

Vital-Durand F, Jeannerod M: Eye movement related activity in the visual cortex of dark-reared kittens, *Electroencephalogr Clin Neurophysiol* 38:295–301, March 1975.

Wada JA, Sato M: Directedness of defensive emotional behavior and motivation for aversive learning, *Exp Neurol* 40:445–456, Aug 1973.

Walk RD: The study of visual depth and distance perception in animals. In Lehrman DS, Hinde RA, Shaw E, editors: *Advances in the study of behavior,* vol 1, New York, 1965, Academic Press.

Walker AD: Taste preferences in the domestic dog and cat, *Gaines Dog Res Prog* Summer 1975.

Waller GR, Price GH, Mitchell ED: Feline attractant cis trans-nepetalactone: metabolism in the domestic cat, *Science* 164:1281–1282, June 13, 1969.

Ward DG, Ward JH: Control of water intake: evidence for the role of a hemodynamic pontine pathway, *Brain Res* 262(2):314–318, 1983.

Warkentin J, Carmichael L: A study of the development of the air-righting reflex in cats and rabbits, *J Genet Psychol* 55:67–80, 1939.

Warren JM: Discrimination of mirror images by cats, *J Comp Physiol Psychol* 69:9–11, Sep 1969.

Warren JM: Transfer of responses to open and closed shapes in discrimination by cats, *Perc Psychophys* 12:449–452, 1972.

Warren JM, McGonigle BO: Perimeter complexity and generalization of a form discrimination by cats, *Psychon Sci* 17:16–17, 1969.

Warren JM, Warren HB, Akert K: Orbitofrontal cortical lesions and learning in cats, *J Comp Neurol* 118:17–41, Feb 1962.

Watson CS: Masking of tones by noise for the cat, *J Acoust Soc Am* 35:167–172, 1963.

Wemmer C, Scow R: Communication in the Felidae with emphasis on scent marking and contact patterns. In Sebeok TA, editor: *How animals communicate,* Bloomington, 1977, Indiana University Press.

Wenzel BM: Tactile stimulation as reinforcement for cats and its relation to early feeding experience, *Psychol Rep* 5:297–300, 1959.

West CD, Harrison CD: Transneuronal cell atrophy in the congenitally deaf white cat, *J Comp Neurol* 151:377–398, Sep/Oct 1973.

West MJ: Exploration and play with objects in domestic kittens, *Dev Psychobiol* 10(1):53–57, 1977.

Wickelgren I: Heretical view of visual development, *Science* 290:1271, 1273, Nov 17, 2000.

Wickelgren WO: Effects of walking and flash stimulation on click-evoked responses in cats, *J Neurophysiol* 31:769–776, Sep 1968.

Wiesel TN, Gilbert CD: Morphological basis of visual cortical function, *Q J Exp Physiol* 68:525–543, 1983.

Wiesel TN, Hubel DH: Single-cell responses in striate of kittens deprived of vision in one eye, *J Neurophysiol* 26:1003–1017, 1963.

Wiesel TN, Hubel DH: Comparison of the effects of unilateral and bilateral eye closure on cortical unit responses in kittens, *J Neurophysiol* 28:1029–1040, Nov 1965.

Wiesel TN, Hubel DH: Extent of recovery from the effects of visual deprivation in kittens, *J Neurophysiol* 28:1060–1072, Nov 1965.

Wikmark RGE: Maturation of spatial delayed responses to auditory cues in kittens, *J Comp Physiol Psychol* 86(2):322–327, 1974.

Wilkinson F, Dodwel PC: Young kittens can learn complex visual pattern discriminations, *Nature* 284(5753):258–259, 1980.

Williams RW, Bastiani MJ, Lia B: Growth cones dying axons and developmental fluctuations in the fiber population of the cat's optic nerve, *J Comp Neurol* pp 246–269, 1986.

Williams RW, Cavada C, Reinoso-Suàrez F: Rapid evolution of the visual system: a cellular assay of the retina and distal lateral geniculate nucleus of the Spanish wildcat and the domestic cat, *J Neurosci* 13:208–228, 1993.

Winans SS: Visual form discrimination after removal of the visual cortex in cats, *Science* 158:944–946, Nov 17, 1967.

Würbel H, Freire R, Nicol CJ: Prevention of stereotypic wire-gnawing in laboratory mice: effects on behaviour and implications for stereotypy as a coping response, *Behav Process* 42:61–72, 1998.

Yehuda S, Chorover SL, Carasso RL: Habituation and transfer during sleep in cats, *Int J Neurosci* 9(4):225–227, 1979.

Yen HCY, Krop S, Mendez HJC, Katz MH: Effects of some psychoactive drugs in experimental neurotic (conflict induced) behavior in cats, *Pharmacology* 3:32–40, 1970.

Zagrodzka J, Hedberg CE, Mann GL, Morrison AR: Contrasting expressions of aggressive behavior released by lesions of the central nucleus of the amygdala during wakefulness and rapid eye, *Behav Neurosci* 112(3):589–602, 1998.

Zetterstrom B: The effect of light on the appearance and development of the electroretinogram in newborn kittens, *Acta Physiol Scand* 35:272–279, 1956.

Zvartau EE, Patkina NA: Motivational properties of hypothalamic stimulation in cats, *Bull Exp Biol Med* 75:233–235, March 1973.

3

Feline Communicative Behavior

Intraspecies communication takes three major forms: vocal expression, body postures, and visual or olfactory marks. For most animals, body language is the primary messenger, not vocalizations. Chemical communications are often underappreciated by humans. Interspecies communication is more complicated than intraspecies communication because animals of different species generally are not considered to have the innate ability to understand the communications of each other. However, because humans can learn many feline signals, understanding and communication between people and cats is possible.

VOCAL COMMUNICATION

Vocal communications are used to transmit general messages and are not associated with the complexities typically found in human communication. Both vocalizations and marking behaviors, which are discussed later in this chapter, are important tools for the relatively asocial cat; these methods of communication enable an individual to determine if there are any other cats nearby and can thus help prevent direct confrontations. Distance-reducing vocal patterns in response to humans generally do not occur if the distance between the cat and the human is greater than 8 feet.[66] The variations of tonal elements during specific-goal emotional states result from changes in the laryngopharynx due to touch reception and tension variations rather than from oral position variations typical in human speech.[66,83] Phonetically distinct sounds have been carefully differentiated and placed into one of three groups, depending on how the sound is produced (see Appendix A). Spectrogram analysis recognized 23 patterns that could be divided into two major types of cat vocalizations. Pure calls are homogeneous, whereas complex ones have major changes in frequency ranges, harmonic structures, or pulse modulations.[20] Postural communication might also be important in modulating vocal signals.[20] These could include such things as position of the ears or piloerection. Although kittens can recognize familiar voices by 4 weeks of age, they usually do not take specific notice of one another's vocal communication patterns until their ninth week.[66]

Murmur Patterns

Murmur vocalizations involve sounds a cat produces while its mouth is closed.[66]

Acknowledgment

The cat that is very bonded to its owner may use a single short murmur of "acknowledgment" when it visualizes something it is about to receive.[66] This trill vocalization implies a friendly approach. More than 90% of the time it occurs as the cat is moving, and more than half of the time this is when the cat is changing elevation.[12] The acknowledgment sound does not start until sometime after the twelfth week of age.

Call

The feline "call" sound is used primarily to draw someone or something toward the cat; it is also the female's signal that she is ready to mate.[27,28,66] Variations include the coaxing sounds used by a tomcat to notify females that he is ready to mate, to invite young males out to fight, and to announce his presence to other males. This advertising sound is not used by all South American domestic cats, indicating that a learning component may be present in vocalization.[79]

Grunt

The "grunt" sound, present at birth, generally disappears at maturity, but an occasional adult will voice a grunt when particularly baffled by a difficult obstacle.[66]

Purr

The "purr" has been described in a number of ways, from *mhrn*, the most common, to *brrp* and *chirp*.[16] By 2 days of age the purr is present and is produced by both nursing kittens and the queen. The queen uses the purr initially when approaching her kittens.[16] It then serves as a form of communication between them (vocal for the queen and tactile for the kittens). The young kittens will stop the purr only for swallowing.[66] The frequency of its use increases as the queen adopts a lactation position, as the kittens nuzzle her fur, or if the queen shifts position while nursing her young.[43]

As the kitten matures the purr can develop several other inflections and meanings. A "greeting" or request vocalization is an expanded form of a single inhalation segment of the purr. In the kitten this purring vocalization increases in intensity until it reaches the greeting level by about the third week of life, when it may alert other kittens as the first reaches the queen to nurse.[25,66,67] This sound, although usually short, can be prolonged sequences of individual purr segments, as when a cat approaches from a distance. The "request" purr for food or attention develops after the twelfth week[66] and becomes adultlike by 20 weeks.[67]

A cat may purr in almost any situation, including just before death following a chronic disease. This may reflect a state of euphoria, perhaps resulting from an endorphin release. A similar sensation has been experienced by terminally ill humans. Experiences that are interpreted to be either pleasurable or distressing may also be accompanied by purring vocalizations. The purr has been equated with the human smile. This may be fairly accurate, although anthropomorphic. Just as people smile when they are happy, are fearful, or want something, cats too are most likely to purr in these situations. Studies show that it is very common for the cat to produce an inaudible purr in the presence of humans.[77]

There have been many descriptions of how the purr is generated. Theories include fremitus caused by blood passing through kinetic angulation in major vessels and soft palate vibrations. Electromyographic studies, however, show that the purr results from activation of the intrinsic laryngeal muscles, which results in partial glottal closure and increased transglottal pressure for 20- to 30-ms bursts.[77,89] That in turn is controlled by the neural infundibulum.[30] The diaphragm is alternately activated to produce the more or less continuous sound.[77,89] Inhalation is often the louder, longer, and lower-pitched component of the purr, although there is considerable individual variation. In some cats the exhalation portion of the purr may be the major component. The purring interval is variable and depends on the cat's intensity of interest.

Vowel Patterns

The five types of sounds produced when the mouth is first opened and then gradually closed are called *vowel patterns*.[66]

Anger wail

A common form of vocalization for the young kitten has been termed the *anger wail*.[66] This distress vocalization can be heard as early as the first day of life and seems to be related to the absence of the smell of the mother, littermates, or both. The anger wail is even more common in cold environments and during physical restraint.[43] During the first few days, the mean number of distress cries is one or two during a 3-minute period, but this number increases rapidly during the first 5 days of life. It reaches a peak soon after the 2-week-old period, which is the most vocal period of the kitten's life.[78,81] Although the anger wail is first associated with competition during nursing, it later becomes individualized and associated with rough forms of play, fights, and protests.[27,66,78]

Bewilderment

"Bewilderment" is a minor vowel pattern that first occurs after 79 days of age and has a prolonged or more intense terminal sound. The initial portion of this sound can also indicate high expectations or a lack of confidence if the cat is stressed.[66]

Complaint

Vocalizations of "complaint" also begin sometime after 79 days of age.[22,66] Some cats that express a vocal complaint are apparently satisfied with a human's verbal sympathy.[66]

Demand

"Demand," like several other patterns, is often the intermediate form of a series of vocalizations that increase in intensity with time. Kittens do not acquire this pattern until after 79 days of age.[66] Variations by means of voice inflections allow the cat to indicate different moods. In tense situations more stress is given to the initial sound, and the opposite occurs in situations of hopelessness.[66] A coaxing variation is soft and begins with a closed mouth. The "whisper" occurs when the cat is aware that it is not advisable to make noise but is unable to suppress the demand.[66] That results in a mouthing movement with little or no noise (a "silent meow"). A chirping variation of demand, accompanied by intense tail flicking, is commonly expressed when the cat is highly aroused by the sight of prey. Queens use another form of demand to call their kittens over to observe prey.[3] A slower, more drawn-out vocalization is expressed when the cat is absorbed in a goal pursuit. The demand then becomes a "begging demand."[66]

Mating cry

The cat can express mild forms of the "mating cry" by gradually closing an open mouth.[66] It is a characteristic two-syllable call used by an estrous female.[49]

Siamese vocalizations

Most of the unusual, excessive, and loud vocalizations associated with the Siamese cat are classified as vowel patterns. The distinctive qualities of these sounds are apparently associated with the same recessive gene that carries their typical pigmentation.[93]

Ultrasonic variations

Around 6 weeks of age, kittens will use a pure ultrasonic call, and the components are separated by low-intensity, low-frequency sounds within the human hearing range.[16] The queen responds with a similar call, although the meaning of this communication remains unclear.[16]

Strained-Intensity Patterns

Sounds that express an intense emotional state are produced with the mouth held open.[66]

Growl

The warning "growl" occurs during a slow, steady exhalation. The queen uses this vocalization to scatter her kittens and warn them to seek immediate shelter; if necessary, she reinforces the warning with a bat from her paw. When the queen is particularly alarmed, this vocalization takes on a dog-bark quality.[27,28] Young kittens can produce this sound and usually first do so when they have matured enough to escape with pieces of food.[66] During a fight, the growl is 400 to 800 Hz in frequency.[49]

Hiss

"Hiss" and its more intense variation "spit" are involuntary reactions to surprise by an enemy. The sound is produced as air is forced through a small oral opening while the cat is changing positions to view the approacher.[66] These vocalizations can occur even before the eyes open in the kitten and are controlled, along with other forms of defensive behavior, by the amygdala and the hypothalamus.

Mating cry

The "mating cry" of the tomcat is an intense form of vocalization, which is probably a highly modified form of demand. Often accompanying this caterwauling cry are the parasympathetic reactions of drooling, increased swallowing, and licking.[66]

Refusal

"Refusal," a minor sound that is low and rasping, is generally associated with occasions when a cat draws back from something forced on it.[66]

Scream

As copulation ends, the female cat vocalizes a form of "scream." This sudden loud pattern, also termed *pain shriek,* probably represents a very intense variation of the complaint vocal pattern.[66,77] Vaginal stimulation by the penile spines is normally the initiating factor.

Snarl

Active fighting, especially between males, is accompanied by a "snarl." Following a noisy inhalation the vocalization is expressed and abruptly stopped.[66] The amount of noise is intense but generally is quite out of proportion to the amount of actual physical damage.

Neural Regulation

Several areas of the brain are associated with vocalization, but the periaqueductal gray is the most important site.[20,86,87] The lateral tegmentum is associated with the growl, the ventral nucleus III with the scream, the tegmentum and medial lemniscus with the meow,[20] the cerebral aqueduct with the purr,[2] and the amygdala and hypothalamus with growling and hissing.[21]

Dopamine and acetylcholine are the two primary neurotransmitters associated with vocal communication. When dopamine is released and reuptake is prevented (D-amphetamine), the cat hisses, spits, and meows.[20] Blocking dopamine receptors (bulbocapnine) results in a cat that will vocalize easily and loudly at little disturbances.[20] Activation of muscarinic cholinergic receptors in the hypothalamus results in a vocal response.[20]

POSTURAL COMMUNICATION

The cat uses various body postures as its primary methods of communication, but these postures are probably less significant for the cat than for other animals, because maintaining harmony within a social group is less significant. Nevertheless, a cat generally uses certain patterns to indicate whether another individual may approach.

Distance-Reducing Postures
Submissive postures

Submissive postures are of minimal significance and, if present, are less highly developed than those of other species. Submission involves postures that serve mainly to inhibit an attack if flight is not possible. The ears may be flattened back against the cat's head. This posture is commonly shown by a nonterritorial male or female when approached by the territorial male, which may then use the mounting postures associated with mating on the lower-ranking individual. The mounted individual tolerates mounting only until it can escape. Crouching may also be an invitation to approach, as with a female in heat.[28]

Active approaches

When one cat is actively approaching another, the tail is held vertically.[54] When a cat approaches a generally friendly being, or when a kitten approaches the queen, the vertical tail position is particularly obvious (Figure 3-1). This tail position may have been derived from the queen's licking of the anogenital area of the kittens,[27,28] but more likely it evolved to make the message of benevolence very obvious. Cats often rub against each other or a friendly person. This usually begins with the head and corner of the lips and progresses along the shoulder and rest of the body. It may then be repeated using the other side of the cat's body.[67] At the same time the vertical tail is rubbed against the other cat along its cheek, side, or back.[13,53] Eventually the two cats end up with the rear end of one cat near the face of the other and with the tail of the first tilting toward the other cat.

When petted, a friendly cat responds by pushing the petted part of its body closer to the person for contact (Figure 3-2). Thus the cat will extend its pelvic limbs when the base of the tail is rubbed or flex its forelimbs and turn its head for a neck massage.

Play postures

Play postures, described in Chapter 2, are distance reducing, as are play-soliciting postures, such as rolling over to expose the abdominal area. In the dog, that is a submissive posture, but it is seen in the cat only in play solicitation, courtship, and extreme defense.[27,28]

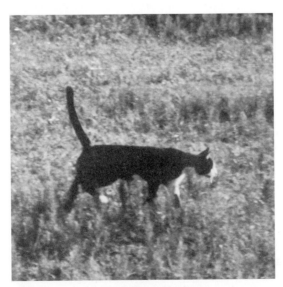

Figure 3-1 The vertical tail posture of a friendly approach.

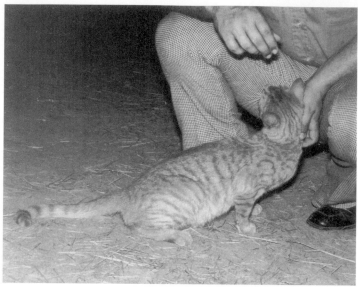

Figure 3-2 A cat responds to petting by pushing the petted area closer.

Rolling

Cats that roll onto their side or back expose the most vulnerable portion of their body, the abdomen, to potential attack. Thus it has been suggested that this is a submissive or greeting posture.[14,26,67] The behavior is commonly displayed to adult tomcats. In 795 of the cats studied, the cat rapidly approaches another cat and immediately rolls before the other cat can respond.[26] The paws are flexed and the legs are splayed.[26] Rolling is also used as an invitation to play by kittens.[26]

Other postures

Many facial expressions and tail postures without piloerection have a "come-closer" meaning. Arching of the tail over the cat's back indicates a high arousal, as in play (Figure 3-3). An inverted U shape to the tail is most significant in the play chase (Figure 3-4). Extreme excitement, as when watching a bird, can result in a twitching tail movement often accompanied by a chirping vocalization. Facial expressions involving half-closed eyes, protrusion of the third eyelid, or both are most often associated with the performance of a natural body function, such as eating, defecating, social grooming, or copulating.[28,82] The play face usually includes dilated pupils and forward-pointing ears (Figure 3-5). Rapid head shaking from side to side has been associated with the response to acute stress.[90]

Distance-Increasing Postures

Interactions between cats often involve patterns of silent communication that indicate when the cat prefers minimal social contact. Thus many body signs are used to convey a "distance-increasing" message. The cat usually gives adequate warning before an attack. Unfortunately, humans and other species do not always interpret the threat postures accurately.

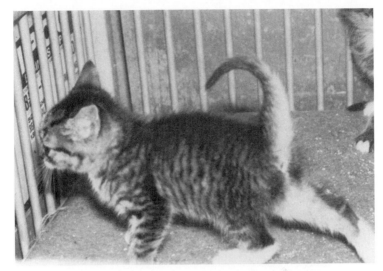

Figure 3-3 Arching of the tail over the back is a distance-reducing posture.

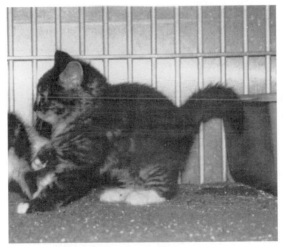

Figure 3-4 The inverted-U tail posture associated with distance-reducing behavior.

Offensive threat

In the offensive threat, direct eye contact with constricted pupils, forward-directed whiskers, and a straight-forward body position indicate an intention to attack (Figure 3-6).[3,27,55,70] It also permits the cat to block all movements by the other cat.[70] This stare technique is used to regulate social distances. A more subtle, deliberate back-and-forth flagging of the tail, particularly the tail tip, expresses the cat's disturbance with the situation and its agitation.[54] Threat postures as part of the conditioned defensive reflex can appear before the kitten's eyes have opened, and they will stabilize by 35 days. Even at this young age, the threat usually involves the optical effect of a rapid approach

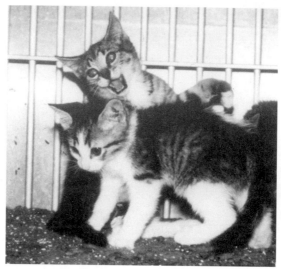

Figure 3-5 An intense-play facial expression.

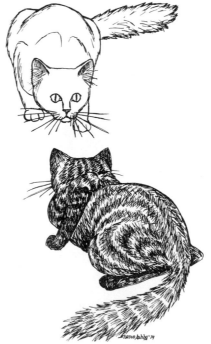

Figure 3-6 Offensive threat posture.

created by a sudden, apparent increase in size resulting from piloerection. Tomcats use another variation of this threat.[13,14,60] The cat stiffens his rear limbs and straightens his back to "slope downhill." Piloerection starts in the thoracolumbar region and increases caudally. The tail comes straight caudally for a short distance and then makes an abrupt bend downward. It too is bristled. The head may move slowly side to side.

Defensive threat

The typical "Halloween cat" posture is associated with the defensive threat (Figure 3-7). The cat presents to the aggressor an arched, lateral display with piloerection, instead of the straight-forward view, to appear larger in overall size and thus more of a threat. The ears are flattened against the back of its head, the corners of the mouth are pulled back to bare its teeth, the whiskers are drawn against the side of its head, and the nose is wrinkled. In wild species, males use this posture only in play.[92]

Pariah threat

The lowest ranking cat of a group of cats, the pariah, may show a crouched posture whenever approached by the territorial male (Figure 3-8). This behavior is accompanied with flattened ears, and the cat will often bare its teeth. Because the cat is in a crouched posture, the act is often compared with the submissive behavior shown by dogs, and controversy remains about the true nature of the position.[14,15] It is listed here as a distance-increasing behavior because the crouched posture is rarely seen without some elements of defensive threat.[15] This posture can also be shown to a person, so providing a description of the posture becomes important when cat aggression is a problem. It represents a time for the approaching person to back off to lessen the threat.

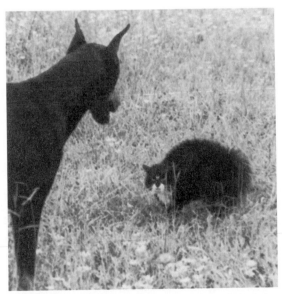

Figure 3-7 The lateral display of defensive threat.

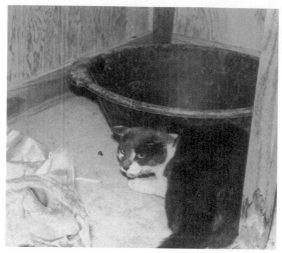

Figure 3-8 The crouched display of the pariah threat.

Other postures

Tail postures can send messages. For distance-increasing signals, tail lashing indicates general irritation in an aggressive situation and is particularly characteristic of defensive aggression or escape.[8,54] Piloerection of the tail is associated with a threat posture. When the tail is vertical with piloerection, a moderately intense offensive threat is indicated (Figure 3-9). This signal is commonly used when the resident cat chases away an intruder. In defensive threats the tail can be arched over the back with hair erect (Figure 3-10), whereas a tail curved into an inverted "U" with the hair standing is associated with postures that are intermediate between offensive and defensive threats (Figure 3-11).[27,28] This inverted-U tail posture is also used during defensive withdrawals.[95] During an immobile confrontation the tail posture is similar, but the ears are back, the pupils are dilated, and, except for head movement to closely watch the threatening individual, the cat is motionless.[95] The tail can also be between the legs, as when defensive or escape behaviors are attempted.[8] These tail positions are far more common during play behaviors than they are in defensive or offensive ones.

Fighting between male cats is very ritualized and is usually far more noisy than injurious. With pupils dilated and claws protruding, the tomcat directs his biting and clawing at the cheeks, neck, and shoulders (Figure 3-12). That is probably the evolutionary reason for the regional thickening of the skin in these areas as a secondary sex characteristic. Initially the ears, head, and piloerect tail are raised, but they are lowered as the attack becomes serious. Weight is shifted backward and one forelimb is raised with claws unsheathed. As one cat bites for the other's nape, the other cat responds by suddenly throwing itself on its back, biting, holding the opponent with the foreclaws, and lashing out with rear claws.[60] Soon both cats are rolling on the ground. They will suddenly leap apart and start the encounter again. Usually cats avoid direct confrontations or fights if at all possible. When attacking a dog that has come within its critical distance, the cat will direct its blows to the eyes and nose but will flee if given the opportunity.

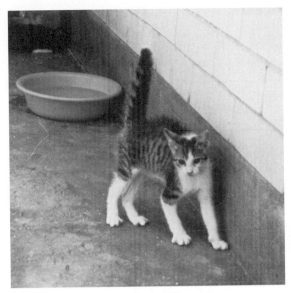

Figure 3-9 A vertical tail posture of threat includes piloerection.

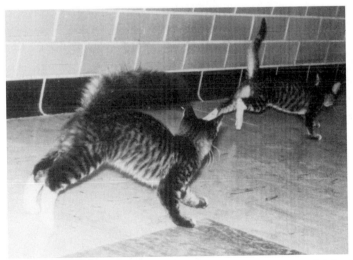

Figure 3-10 The tail is arched over the back with the hair standing in play and defensive threats.

If a severe challenge continues, the cat may roll onto its back so that all four feet can be used as weapons (Figure 3-13). There is very little biting, because the cat needs to protect its face.[24,92] There is a lack of ritualized submissive or appeasement gestures following tomcat aggression toward another tomcat.[18] The loser backs away very slowly after its ears move back and the stare is broken.[13]

Fear can be associated with forms of distance-increasing silent communication. In addition to the arched back and piloerection of the other threat postures, the fearful

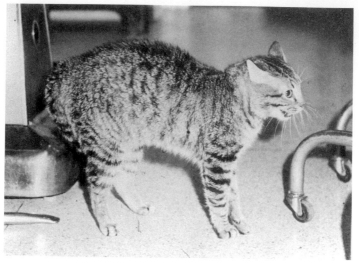

Figure 3-11 Piloerection of an inverted U-shaped tail as part of an immobile confrontation.

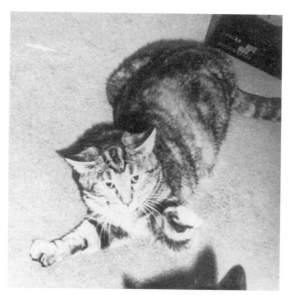

Figure 3-12 Clawing is directed toward the head of another.

threat includes signs of apprehension such as salivation, extreme mydriasis, sweating of the foot pads, flattened ears, and panting.[27,52] The body may be lowered into a crouched position similar to that of the pariah threat; the head is down, and the tail is down or tucked between the rear limbs.[13] These fearful cats are best approached from overhead.[52] If the fear stimulus is great enough, the cat may go from the fearful threat reaction into a cataleptic shock syndrome.

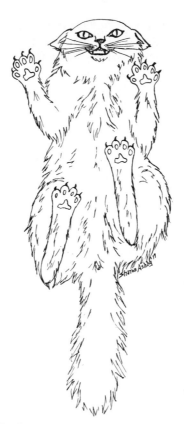

Figure 3-13 The extreme defensive posture.

Neural regulation

Distance-increasing behavior is controlled from within the central nervous system. Electrical stimulation of the ventromedial hypothalamus in kittens as young as 12 days produces behaviors typically observed in threat situations.[28] Behavioral alerting, mydriasis, ear retraction, piloerection, hissing, and claw protrusion are some of the general displays. Extreme ragelike displays include opening the mouth and baring the teeth, curving the tongue, and blowing air.[29] The prefrontal cortex and thalamus apparently play a role in moderating these reactions.[85,95] In addition, the lateral septal nuclei with their connections into this area are evidently important in overriding the formation of conditioned emotional responses such as fear.[62] A defensive cat personality appears between 30 and 50 days of age and correlates positively with readiness to adapt defensive immobility and negatively with olfactory exploration and purring during human contact.[1]

Ambivalent Postures

Although most of the cat's body communications are ambivalent to some degree because of conflicting situations, each attitude usually has one overriding posture, on the basis of which it is classified. Occasionally, however, the cat truly alternates between distance-increasing and distance-reducing behaviors. For example, when approaching an older kitten, the queen may react with maternal grooming when presented with a caudal view and with a clawing attack when presented with a cranial view.[24] The "Halloween cat" posture of the defensive threat has been classified as ambivalent with the thought that the front half of the cat tries to leave while the rear end stands its ground. Because the lateral threat is common in other species, such as cattle, and is used to give a larger appearance during a threat, it is reasonable to expect that in small-sized animals it probably represents a defensive threat posture, rather than a true mental conflict.[28]

MARKING COMMUNICATION

Marking is a more permanent form of communication than either postures or vocalizations. It allows the cat to leave olfactory and visual messages that remain long after the communicator has gone. Thus individuals can space themselves to prevent meetings, recognize territorial owners by smell, and control reproduction. Marking provides information regarding the individual and sexual identity, the amount of time spent at the location, and the reproduction cycle stage of the marker—all without threat.[6,32,61]

Rubbing Behavior

The cat has greatly enlarged sebaceous glands around the mouth, on the chin, in the ear canals, in the perianal area, and at the cranial portion of the base of the tail; these are areas that the cat specifically likes to rub or to have rubbed. This rubbing (or bunting)[49] behavior is directed toward certain individuals, perhaps suggesting a social relationship.[53] When rubbing humans, the cat may be using a greeting form of distance-reducing behavior, rather than a true marking behavior.[24] Rubbing is also directed toward familiar or novel objects. A protruding object or hand is often rubbed first by the very rostral portion of the cat's nose, then by its cheek from the commissure of the mouth toward the lateral commissure of the eye. Cats will often show facial rubbing on objects and follow that behavior with flehmen, particularly if the emotion is intense. The cat may rub a higher object with the dorsal aspect of its head while standing on its hind feet. It may rub its dorsum and tail along an object such as a chair. Low-lying objects are usually rubbed by a stroke from the chin to the laryngeal area. The sebaceous scent is probably thus transferred to the rubbed object. Although intact adult males do not rub any more frequently than females, their glands are particularly active.[80,91]

Cheek rubbing can also be seen in agonistic and sexual contexts, although neither situation is oriented toward a scent. After aggressive interactions, a cat may rub its head on the nearest protruding objects.[76] Estrous behavior is also associated with cheek rubbing. In both cases the behaviors are ritualized and probably function as visual or appeasement displays.[76] Urine will elicit an investigative response for up to 3 days.[49] Cats will occasionally spray urine after rubbing a place, but they do not rub their faces in sprayed urine and then rub another place.[72] When petted, the cat may also profusely salivate and then rub the corner of its mouth against the individual doing the petting. The saliva transferred may provide another form of olfactory mark.[93]

Scent rubbing is the transfer of scents from the environment onto the animal's body.[76] Although this behavior is generally common in carnivores, it is not common in cats. When it does occur, it usually takes a specific and powerful scent like catnip; even then, a cat is as likely to show cheek rubbing as a scent-rubbing response. Other possible responses to an odor include flehmen and earth raking.[76]

Secretions from the glands of the anal sac may have an olfactory marking function. In carnivores the secretions contain a number of volatile carboxylic acids, including acetic, butyric, isobutyric, isocaproic, isovaleric, propionic, and valeric.[31] However, the exact role of these secretions in cats is questioned, because the anal sacs are expressed primarily during traumatic experiences and because the anogenital approach is not of major social significance.[91,93]

Pheromones are associated with rubbing behaviors in cats and have been recently introduced commercially. Each pheromone is species specific in context. For example, one may serve as a label for self, indicate a social status or reproductive state, or mark a territory.[88] They control estrus and mating behaviors and guide blind neonates to a nipple.[88] The F_3 fraction of the cat's facial pheromone has been produced commercially for its calming effect. It has been shown to be of some benefit to cats undergoing intravenous catheterization[56]; to increase interest in face rubbing, grooming, and food[33]; and to reduce urine spraying.[71]

Wood Scratching

Wood scratching is a second major type of marking behavior, one that uses visual cues. The cat may use either a horizontally or a vertically oriented piece of soft wood or bark and grips the object with both extended forelimbs (Figures 3-14 and 3-15). The body

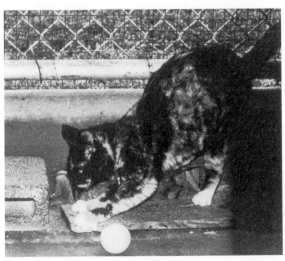

Figure 3-14 Scratching a horizontal piece of wood.

may be positioned so that the thorax is lower than the hindquarters if the object is near the ground, or the cat may reach upward. On alternating paws the cat extends and withdraws its claws. These jerky motions vary in length and speed and may serve two purposes: to create a visual marker and to condition the claw by removing any thin loose pieces of sheaths (Figure 3-16).[41,42,59,64] Outer parts of the rear claws are removed by the teeth. Sweat glands in the skin of the foot have been said to leave a secondary olfactory cue,[40,59] but these locations are not investigated by other cats, so the olfactory function is probably insignificant in territorial marking. Instead, the odor may provide reassurance to the resident cat.[6,42] New objects and old favorites are scratching sites, and the longer the object serves as a scratching medium, the greater the significance it is likely to have to the individual. Cats are most likely to scratch shortly after awakening and may use the behavior as a form of stretching.[9,34,37,59]

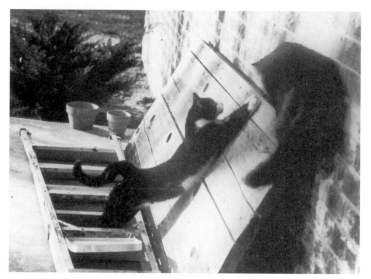

Figure 3-15 Scratching a vertically directed object.

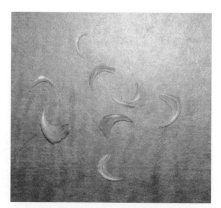

Figure 3-16 Nail fragments left after using a scratching post.

Newborn kittens are unable to completely withdraw their claws until they are about 4 weeks of age (see Appendix D). Scratching is an inborn behavior that can be performed by 5 weeks of age. The behavior is common in older cats, such that a farm cat will show this behavior one to six times (average 3.5 times) in a 24-hour period.[46,72] The motions are so instinctive that they can be observed even if the animal was declawed shortly after birth.[34]

Scratching loose soil leaves a disruption that serves as both a visual marker and a possible olfactory one.[23,93]

Excrement Marking

Because of the territorial, sexual, or agonistic connotation in which it occurs, urine marking is used for communication, or scent marking, particularly by intact male cats. By spraying the urine, a cat covers a large area at a height convenient for sniffing. Males spend a great deal of time marking their home range, particularly near pathways, crossings, and boundaries.[23,36] The typical marking posture is with the cat standing (Figure 3-17). There is an erratic twitching motion of the vertical tail and urine pulses backward. This motion has been described as either neurologically initiated automatic behavior or as a voluntary behavior cued for a visual signal.[92,93]

Visual signals are apparently important to draw a cat's attention to an olfactory cue, so the wet mark of freshly sprayed urine is particularly attractive.[17] The freshest urine (up to 4 hours) is explored first, and the intensity of the response generally decreases as the urine gets older.[17,73] This complements the theory that the age of a urine mark may

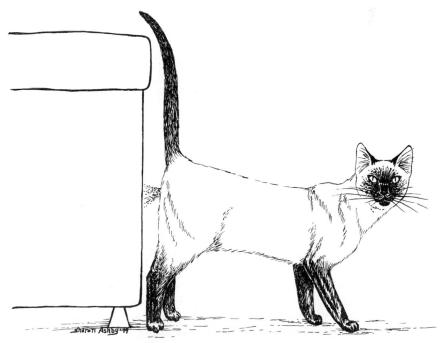

Figure 3-17 The marking posture usually used for urine spraying.

help direct traffic in an area to minimize chance encounters between tomcats—a feline version of "time sharing."[10,17,31]

Cats use urine spraying to leave their own scent, not to cover odors from other cats. Although a cat will smell the urine mark of another, no responses of fear or intimidation are evoked and the animal makes no obvious attempt to cover the odor with his own.[35,91] A number of chemicals have been identified in carnivore urine, including isopent-3-enyl methyl sulfide, 2-phenylethyl methyl sulfide, 4-heptanone, 6-methylhept-5-en-2-one, benzaldehyde, acetophenone, and 2-methylquinoline.[31] Cat urine also has felinine, isovalthine, and cysteine-S-isopentanol.[31,45] Adult males spend more time investigating urine than adult females, although both show considerably more interest in sprayed urine than urine voided in a normal squatting posture.[10,73] Urine from unknown cats is also sniffed longer than that from familiar cats.[31,73] Both sexes spray urine, but males do it at a much higher rate than females—62.6 times per hour compared with a female's 6.0 times.[53] Estrus increases the frequency of a queen's spraying, however. Other reports indicate that solitary males spray every 33 minutes.[53] In farm cats 61.5% of the spraying bouts are associated with hunting.[72] Although cats average one spray bout every 22.2 minutes of hunting time, they often go for longer periods without marking.[72] The number of sprays in 24 hours when primarily associated with hunting is up to 42 (mean 11.1).[72] Most sprays are not accompanied by the prior sniffing of the location, suggesting that odors are not significant to the individual eliciting them.[72]

Besides indicating movement and identity, sprayed urine serves to bring the male and female together during mating season by attracting the female and to acclimate an individual cat with a particular area. The latter function is commonly served when a tomcat is placed in a new area. Not only does the odor of his own distinct scent provide relief from anxiety and aggression, but it also allows him to establish his own small breeding territory.[35,36,38]

Feces are rarely used by the cat as a scent marker, although situations have been described in which defecation on raised areas served such a purpose.[10,31,92,93] Territorially dominant cats in an untamed population leave feces uncovered in conspicuous places, particularly along trails of good hunting areas.[53,63]

More is discussed about spraying as a normal and problem behavior in Chapter 8.

Communicative Behavior Problems

Although the inability to understand feline communication can be hazardous for humans, the real problem behaviors are associated with marking.

Clawing of Furniture and Household Items

Clawing represents an expression of a normal behavior in an atypical environment, but it represents approximately 15% of feline behavior complaints.[44] Cats that are confined indoors will use household items for clawing if there is nothing else to scratch. Prominent objects and areas are favored, including soft furniture (30%), carpet (25%), logs or wood (11%), wicker furniture (6%), and hard furniture (6%).[12]

Once scratching on an object is started, the chosen object continues to be used,[40] with cats going back to favorites whenever possible.[64] Discouragement of scratching a particular object is not successful without providing an acceptable substitute. Direct attempts at punishment usually teach the cat to run from the owner and do not stop the scratching.

The physical characteristics of a scratching post or board can affect its suitability. In addition to being stable, the object should be tall enough (at least 12 inches and preferably $2\frac{1}{2}$ to 3 feet) for the cat to rest on its hind limbs and reach out to claw. The texture of the scratching post is of some significance, with the preferred primary orientation of the fabric weave being longitudinal to provide the cat with the most efficient conditioning of each claw.[34,40,42] An outdoor cat that is coming indoors may prefer a post of the same wood as its preferred tree. Another option is a sisal scratching post, which many cats prefer to carpet posts.[47] Horizontal scratching surfaces are favored by some cats, so carpets are used. Alternatives like soft wood pieces and catnip-impregnated cardboard can be substituted for these cats.[47]

When raising a kitten, the owner can best prevent the development of furniture scratching by providing a scratching post in a prominent location, preferably near the kitten's sleeping area, and by keeping other potential targets hidden.[9,34,65] Post usage can be encouraged by placing a favorite toy on top; by leaving the kitten in a room where the post is the only furniture; or by having an older, post-trained cat to provide a source for observational learning.[9,40] Because cats have the tendency to develop preferences for specific scratching objects, once the kitten has started using the post, it is best to keep the same one. In play a kitten will occasionally use its claws to climb, and if confined indoors the substitute trees can be a scratching post, curtains, furniture, and even the owner's leg. The behavior should consistently be discouraged so that it does not continue into adulthood, but it is unrealistic to expect that it can be totally prevented.

If the owner has been unable to prevent furniture damage, behavior modification can be used to retrain the cat. Access to the scratched furniture should be controlled. Every time the cat scratches areas other than the post, "no" should be followed by placing the cat on the post and manipulating its legs as if it were scratching the post.[4,52] The cat can also be startled immediately upon starting the behavior.[69] The alternative is that the object scratched should be removed or moved and covered, preferably with plastic, and replaced with an acceptable scratching object.[9,40] If the cat is scratching the carpet, the owner should place the scratching post horizontally over the clawed carpet. Every successful effort to scratch the old object reinforces the unacceptable location, so physical barriers and consistent retraining efforts are important. Remote punishment, in which the location is associated with the punishment, can be effective in behavior modification. This method has the advantage of punishing each occurrence and eliminating the necessity for the owner to physically contact the animal.[39,51] Using two-sided sticky tape or activating a fan or hair dryer by placing a motion-detecting device near the undesirable scratching location are examples of remote punishment. The advantage to remote punishment is that the cat is less likely to develop an aversion to the owner. Olfactory cues rather than physical ones can also be used for negative reinforcement. Smell aversion makes the cat fearful of the particular odor associated with that event. With the cat out of the room, the scratched object should be sprayed well and the mist allowed to settle before the cat returns to the area. A suitable object to be scratched must still be provided. When the cat must be left alone, it should be placed in a room where scratching has not been a problem.

Other ways to minimize the scratching problem include clipping the cat's claws or using plastic claw covers. Although there is no correlation between the clipping of claws or using the claw covers and the frequency of scratching, less damage is done.[9] The synthetic feline facial pheromone has been reported to reduce the incidence of furniture clawing by 96% after 28 days when sprayed on each scratch site.[50]

Other owners prefer to prevent furniture scratching or human injuries by having the cat declawed. Studies indicate between 24.4% and 52.3% of cats have had this surgery.[74] In the general population, owners report about 20% of the cat population scratches furniture and 4% scratch people.[74] For veterinarians, about 86% of the cats are presented for this surgery because of household damage. Twenty-nine percent are presented to prevent human injuries.[58] The outcome can be particularly satisfactory for indoor cats. Between 59% and 78% of declawed cats will continue to go through the motions associated with claw sharpening.[94] Outdoor cats can relearn defense, hunting, and climbing, particularly if the rear claws remain.[41,69] Care should be taken, however, because cats that depend on their claws as weapons or for climbing can become traumatized if they must suddenly discover their lack of claws. A gradual introduction to the outdoor environment is appropriate.

Without the declawing surgery, veterinarians estimate that about half of the owners would have chosen to get rid of the cat.[41,58,59] With it, 70% to 90% of declawed cat owners report an improvement in the cat-owner relationship.[41,58,59] Even though studies have shown no evidence of long-term physical or behavioral problems as a result of this procedure, there remains a moral controversy about the surgery. There is a perception that the cat will develop other problems, such as biting and jumping on counters or tables.[*] This must be tempered by the reminder that for some cats, declawing truly is a life-saving procedure.

Excessive Vocalization

In one study, 2 of 23 cats that were presented for problem behaviors other than house-soiling or aggression were diagnosed as being excessively vocal.[5] Although this problem is often associated with Siamese or estrous females, excessive vocalizations are not restricted to such cats. Excessive vocalization is common after a move or dramatic change in the cat's schedule. It can also occur in outdoor cats that have become indoor ones. For those cats, allowing them the time to adjust to the change and providing them with a strict new schedule is helpful. A window perch or noise in the house might also provide distractions.[47] Antianxiety drug therapy can be added if the cat's stress levels indicate such treatment.[84]

Learned vocalizations can become a problem and may actually be encouraged by an owner. A cat may learn to meow as a signal to go outside or to get food. Some cats have a tendency to start meowing about 4 o'clock in the morning, and because most owners have a very low threshold for this noise, they get up and feed the cat. When an

[*]References 7, 19, 57, 58, 65, 68, 74, 75.

owner ignores the behavior, the cat vocalizes longer and eventually is rewarded with what it wants. Because this does not take much energy, the cat can usually successfully outlast the owner.[47]

Excessive vocalization and the reversal of daytime and nighttime behaviors have been described as the two primary behaviors associated with what has been called "feline cognitive dysfunction."[11,48]

REFERENCES

1. Adamec RE, Stark-Adamec C, Livingston KC: The expression of an early developmentally emergent defensive bias in the adult cat *(Felis catus)* in non-predatory situations, *Appl Anim Ethol* 10:89–108, March 1983.
2. Adametz J, O'Leary JL: Experimental mutism resulting from periaqueductal lesions in cats, *Neurology* 9:636–642, 1959.
3. Beadle M: *The cat: history, biology, and behavior,* New York, 1977, Simon & Schuster.
4. Beaver BVG: Feline behavioral problems, *Vet Clin North Am* 6:333–340, Aug 1976.
5. Beaver BV: Feline behavioral problems other than housesoiling, *J Am Anim Hosp Assoc* 25:465–469, July/Aug 1989.
6. Beaver BV: Disorders of behavior. In Sherding RG, editor: *The cat: diseases and clinical management,* New York, 1989, Churchill Livingstone.
7. Bennett M, Houpt KA, Erb HN: Effects of declawing on feline behavior, *Companion Anim Pract* 2:7–9, 12, 1988.
8. Bernstein P, Strack M: Home ranges, favored spots, time-sharing patterns, and tail usage by 14 cats in the home, *Animal Behavior Consultant Newsletter* 10(3):1–3, 1993.
9. Bryant D: *The care and handling of cats,* New York, 1944, Ives Washburn.
10. Cooper LL: Feline inappropriate elimination, *Vet Clin North Am Small Anim Pract* 27(3):569–600, 1997.
11. Cooper LL: Personal communication, July 23, 2000.
12. Crowell-Davis SL: Social behavior and gender in domestic cats. Paper presented at American Veterinary Medical Association meeting, Reno, Nev, July 22, 1997.
13. Crowell-Davis SL: Social behavior in cats. Paper presented at Western Veterinary Conference, Las Vegas, February 22, 2000.
14. Crowell-Davis SL, Barry K, Wolfe R: Social behavior and aggressive problems of cats, *Vet Clin North Am Small Anim Pract* 27(3):549–568, 1997.
15. Dards JL: The behavior of dockyard cats: interactions of adult males, *Appl Anim Ethol* 10:133–153, 1983.
16. Deag JM, Manning A, Lawrence CE: Factors in influencing the mother-kitten relationship. In Turner DC, Bateson PPG, editors: *The domestic cat: the biology of its behavior,* Cambridge, 1988, Cambridge University Press.
17. DeBoer JN: The age of olfactory cues functioning in chemocommunication among male domestic cats, *Behav Process* 2:209–225, 1977.
18. DeBoer JN: Dominance relations in pairs of domestic cats, *Behav Process* 2:227–242, 1977.
19. Declawing not related to behavior problems, *DVM* 22(1):8, 1991.
20. deLanerolle NC, Lang FF: Functional neural pathways for vocalization in the domestic cat. In Newman JD, editor: *Physiological control of mammalian vocalization,* New York, 1988, Plenum Publishing.
21. deMolina AF, Hunsperger RW: Organization of the subcortical system governing defense and flight reactions in the cat, *J Physiol* 160:200–213, 1962.

22. Dhume RA, Gogate MG, deMascarenhas JF, Sharma KN: Functional dissociation within hippocampus: correlates of visceral and behavioral patterns induced on stimulation of ventral hippocampus in cats, *Indian J Med Res* 64:33–40, Jan 1976.

23. Eaton RL: The evolution of sociality in the Felidae. In Eaton RL, editor: *The world's cats,* vol 3, Seattle, 1976, Carnivore Research Institute.

24. Ewer RF: *Ethology of mammals,* London, 1968, Paul Elek.

25. Ewer RF: *The carnivores,* Ithaca, NY, 1973, Cornell University Press.

26. Feldman HN: Domestic cats and passive submission, *Anim Behav* 47:457–459, 1994.

27. Fox MW: *Understanding your cat,* New York, 1974, Coward, McCann & Geoghegan.

28. Fox MW: The behavior of cats. In Hafez ESE, editor: *The behavior of domestic animals,* ed 3, Baltimore, 1975, Williams & Wilkins.

29. Giammanco S, Paderni MA, Carollo A: The effect of thermic stress on the somatic reaction of rage and on rapid circling turns, in the cat, *Arch Int Physiol Biochem* 84:787–799, Oct 1976.

30. Gibbs EL, Gibbs FA: A purring center in the brain of the cat, *J Comp Neurol* 64:6–8, 1936.

31. Gorman ML, Trowbridge BJ: The role of odor in the social lives of carnivores. In Gittleman JL, editor: *Carnivore behavior, ecology and evolution,* Ithaca, NY, 1989, Cornell University Press.

32. Gosling LM: A reassessment of the function of scent marking in territories, *Z Tierpsychol* 60:89–118, 1982.

33. Griffith CA, Steigerwald ES, Buffington CAT: Effects of a synthetic facial pheromone on behavior of cats, *J Am Vet Med Assoc* 217(8):1154–1156, 2000.

34. Hart BL: Behavioral aspects of scratching in cats, *Feline Pract* 2(2):6–8, 1972.

35. Hart BL: Normal behavior and behavioral problems associated with sexual function, urination, and defecation, *Vet Clin North Am* 4:589–606, Aug 1974.

36. Hart BL: Behavioral patterns related to territoriality and social communication, *Feline Pract* 5(1):12–14, 1975.

37. Hart BL: Behavioral aspects of raising kittens, *Feline Pract* 6(6):8, 10, 20, 1976.

38. Hart BL: Olfaction and feline behavior, *Feline Pract* 7(5):8–10, 1977.

39. Hart BL: Water sprayer therapy, *Feline Pract* 8(6):13, 15–16, 1978.

40. Hart BL: Starting from scratch: a new perspective on cat scratching, *Feline Pract* 10(4):8, 10, 12, 1980.

41. Hart BL: *Feline behavior problems, Friskies Symposium on Behavior,* p 28–39, 1994.

42. Hart BL, Hart LA: *Canine and feline behavioral therapy,* Philadelphia, 1985, Lea & Febiger.

43. Haskins R: A causal analysis of kitten vocalizations: an observational and experimental study, *Anim Behav* 27(3):726–736, 1979.

44. Heidenberger E: Housing conditions and behavioral problems of indoor cats as assessed by their owners, *Appl Anim Behav Sci* 52(3,4):345–364, April 1997.

45. Hendricks WH, Moughan PJ, Tarttelin MF, Woolhouse AD: Felinine: a urinary amino acid of Felidae, *Comp Biochem Physiol* 112B(4):581–588, 1995.

46. Houpt KA: Companion animal behavior: a review of dog and cat behavior in the field, the laboratory and the clinic, *Cornell Vet* 75:248–261, 1985.

47. Houpt KA: Transforming an outdoor cat into an indoor cat, *Vet Med* 95(11):830, 2000.

48. Houpt KA: Cognitive dysfunction in geriatric cats. In August JR, editor: *Consultations in feline internal medicine,* vol 4, Philadelphia, 2001, WB Saunders.

49. Houpt KA, Wolski TR: *Domestic animal behavior for veterinarians and animal scientists,* Ames, 1982, Iowa State University Press.

50. Hunthausen W: For scratching. Available at http://msnhomepages.talkcity.com/Terminus/wwah/feliway.htm.

51. Jacobs DL: Behavior modification technique, *Feline Pract* 8(2):6, 1978.
52. Joshua JO: Abnormal behavior in cats. In Fox MW, editor: *Abnormal behavior in animals,* Philadelphia, 1968, WB Saunders.
53. Kerby G, Macdonald DW: Cat society and the consequences of colony size. In Turner DC, Bateson PPG, editors: *The domestic cat: the biology of its behavior,* Cambridge, 1988, Cambridge University Press.
54. Kiley-Worthington M: The tail movements of ungulates, canids and felids with particular reference to their causation and function as displays, *Behaviour* 56(1–2):69–115, 1975.
55. Kleiman DG, Eisenberg JF: Comparisons of canid and felid social systems from an evolutionary perspective, *Anim Behav* 21:637–659, Nov 1973.
56. Kronen PW, Ludders JW, Erb HN, et al: The F_3-fraction of feline facial pheromones calms cats prior to intravenous catheterization. Paper presented at the Seventh World Congress of Veterinary Anaesthesia, Berne, Switzerland, Sep 20–24, 2000.
57. Landsberg G: Personal communication, 1989.
58. Landsberg G: Declawing revisited: controversy over consequences, *Vet Forum* 94–95, Sep 1994.
59. Landsberg G: Feline behavior and welfare, *J Am Vet Med Assoc* 208(4):502–505, 1996.
60. Leyhausen P: *Cat behavior: the predatory and social behavior of domestic and wild cats,* New York, 1978, Garland STPM Press.
61. Liberg O: Spacing patterns in a population of rural free roaming domestic cats, *Oikos* 35(3):336–349, 1980.
62. Lubar JF, Numan R: Behavioral and physiological studies of septal function and related medial cortical structures, *Behav Biol* 8(1):1–25, 1973.
63. MacDonald DW: Patterns of scent marking with urine and faeces amongst carnivore communities, *Symp Zool Soc Lond* 45:107–139, 1980.
64. Marder A: Managing behavioral problems in puppies and kittens, *Small Anim Behav Friskies PetCare* 15–24, 1997.
65. McKeown D, Luescher A, Machum M: The problem of destructive scratching by cats, *Can Vet J* 29:1017, Dec 1988.
66. Moelk M: Vocalizing in the house cat: a phonetic and functional study, *Am J Psychol* 57:184–205, 1944.
67. Moelk M: The development of friendly approach behavior in the cat: a study of kitten-mother relations and the cognitive development of the kitten from birth to eight weeks, *Adv Study Behav* 10:163–224, 1979.
68. Morgan M, Houpt KA: Personal communication, 1989.
69. Overall KL: Management related problems in feline behavior, *Feline Pract* 22(1):13–15, 1994.
70. Overall KL: Behavioral knowledge can help smooth introduction of new pet to household, *DVM Newsmagazine* 26(11):6S, 12S, 13S, 1995.
71. Pageat P: Experimental evaluation of the efficacy of a synthetic analogue of cats' facial pheromones (Feliway) in inhibiting urine marking of sexual origin in adult tom-cats, *J Vet Pharmacol Ther* 20(suppl 1):169, 1997.
72. Panaman R: Behavior and ecology of free-ranging female farm cats (*Felis catus* L), *Z Tierpsychol* 56:59–73, 1981.
73. Passanisi WC, Macdonald DW: Group discrimination on the basis of urine in a farm cat colony. In Macdonald DW, Müller-Schwarze D, Natynczwk SE, editors: *Chemical signals in vertebrates,* ed 5, New York, 1990, Oxford University Press.
74. Patronek GJ: Assessment of claims of short- and long-term complications associated with onychectomy in cats, *J Am Vet Med Assoc* 219(8):932–937, 2001.

75. Patronek GJ, Glickman LT, Beck AM, et al: Risk factors for relinquishment of cats to an animal shelter, *J Am Vet Med Assoc* 209(3):582–588, 1996.

76. Reiger I: Scent rubbing in carnivores, *Carnivore* 2(1/2):17–25, 1979.

77. Remmers JE, Gautier H: Neural and mechanical mechanisms of feline purring, *Respir Physiol* 16:351–361, 1972.

78. Rheingold HL, Eckerman CO: Familiar social and nonsocial stimuli and the kitten's response to a strange environment, *Dev Psychobiol* 4(1):71–89, 1971.

79. Romanes GJ: *Mental evolution in animals,* New York, 1969, AMS Press.

80. Rose CE, Doering GG: "Stud tail" in cats, *Feline Pract* 6(5):28, 1976.

81. Rosenblatt JS: Learning in newborn kittens, *Sci Am* 227:18–25, 1972.

82. Rosenblueth A, Bard P: The innervation and functions of the nictitating membrane in the cat, *Am J Physiol* 100(3):537–544, 1932.

83. Sampson S, Eyzaguirre C: Some functional characteristics of mechanoreceptors in the larynx of the cat, *J Neurophysiol* 27(3):464–480, 1964.

84. Seksel K, Lindeman MJ: Use of clomipramine in the treatment of anxiety-related and obsessive-compulsive disorders in cats, *Aust Vet J* 76(5):317–321, 1998.

85. Siegel A, Edinger H, Dotto M: Effects of electrical stimulation of the lateral aspect of the prefrontal cortex upon attack behavior in cats, *Brain Res* 93:473–484, Aug 15, 1975.

86. Skultety FM: The behavioral effects of destructive lesions of the periaqueductal gray matter in adult cats, *J Comp Neurol* 110:337–365, 1958.

87. Skultety FM: Mutism in cats with rostral midbrain lesions. Part 1, *Arch Neurol* 12:211–225, Feb 1965.

88. Sommerville BA, Broom DM: Olfactory awareness, *Appl Anim Behav Sci* 57(3–4):269–286, 1998.

89. Stogdale L, Delack JB: Feline purring, *Compend Contin Educ* 7(7):551–553, 1985.

90. van den Bos R: Post-conflict stress-response in confined group-living cats *(Felis silvestris catus), Appl Anim Behav Sci* 59(4):323–330, 1998.

91. Verberne G, DeBoer J: Chemocommunication among domestic cats, mediated by the olfactory and vomeronasal senses. I. Chemocommunication, *Z Tierpsychol* 42:86–109, Sep 1976.

92. Weigel I: Small cats and clouded leopards. In Grzimek HCB, editor: *Grzimek's animal life encyclopedia,* vol 12, New York, 1975, Van Nostrand Reinhold.

93. Wemmer C, Scow K: Communication in the Felidae with emphasis on scent marking and contact patterns. In Sebeok TA, editor: *How animals communicate,* Bloomington, 1977, Indiana University Press.

94. Yeon SC, Flanders JA, Scarlett JM, et al: Attitudes of owners regarding tendonectomy and onychectomy in cats, *J Am Vet Med Assoc* 218(1):43–47, 2001.

95. Zanchetti A, Baccelli G, Mancia G: Fighting, emotions, and exercise: cardiovascular effects in the cat. In Onesti G, Fernandes M, Kim KE, editors: *Regulation of blood pressure by the central nervous system,* New York, 1976, Grune & Stratton.

Additional Readings

Blacklock GA: A cat's purr...on purpose? *Cat Fancy* 16:20–22, Aug 1973.

Borchelt PL: Cat elimination behavior problems, *Vet Clin North Am Small Anim Pract* 21(2):257–264, 1991.

Boudreau JC, Tsuchitani C: *Sensory neurophysiology,* New York, 1973, Van Nostrand Reinhold.

Brown KA, Buchwald JS, Johnson JR, Mikolich DJ: Vocalization in the cat and kitten, *Dev Psychobiol* 11(6):559–570, 1978.

Cannon WB: *Bodily changes in pain, hunger, fear and rage,* ed 2, Boston, 1953, Charles T Branford.

Darwin CR: *The expression of the emotions in man and animals,* New York, 1969, Greenwood Press.

De Molina AF, Hunsperger RW: Organization of subcortical systems governing defense and flight reactions in the cat, *J Physiol* 160(2):200–213, 1962.

Dewson JH: Speech sound discrimination by cats, *Science* 144:555–556, May 1, 1964.

Eisenberg JF, Kleiman DG: Olfactory communication in mammals, *Annu Rev Ecol Syst* 3:1–32, 1972.

Eleftheriou BE, Scott JP: *The physiology of aggression and defeat,* New York, 1971, Plenum Publishing.

Franks JN, Boothe HW, Taylor L, et al: Evaluation of transdermal fentanyl patches for analgesia in cats undergoing onychectomy, *J Am Vet Med Assoc* 217(7):1013–1018, 2000.

Fried PA: The septum and hyper-reactivity: a review, *Br J Psychol* 64(2):267–275, 1973.

Hart BL: Gonadal androgen and sociosexual behavior of male mammals: a comparative analysis, *Psychol Bull* 81(7):383–400, 1971.

Hart BL: Social interactions between cats and their owners, *Feline Pract* 6(1):6, 8, 1976.

Hart BL: Behavioral aspects of selecting a new cat, *Feline Pract* 6(5):8, 10, 14, 1976.

Houpt KA: Animal behavior as a subject for veterinary students, *Cornell Vet* 66(1):73–81, 1976.

Houpt KA: *Domestic animal behavior for veterinarians and animal scientists,* Ames, 1991, Iowa State University Press.

Houpt KA, Honig SU, Reisner IR: Breaking the human-companion animal bond, *J Am Vet Med Assoc* 208(10):1653–1659, 1996.

Jenkins TW: *Functional mammalian neuroanatomy,* Philadelphia, 1972, Lea & Febiger.

Johansson GG, Kalimo R, Niskanen H, Ruusunen S: Effects of stimulation parameters on behavior elicited by stimulation of the hypothalamic defense area, *J Comp Physiol Psychol* 87:1100–1108, Dec 1974.

Kahn B: Out of the frying pan—into the litter pan, *Cat Fancy* 15:18–21, Nov/Dec 1972.

Knol BW, Egberink-Alink ST: Treatment of problem behavior in dogs and cats by castration and progestogen administration: a review, *Vet Q* 11(2):102–107, 1989.

Langworthy OR: Behavioral disturbances related to the decomposition of reflex activity caused by cerebral injury: an experimental study of the cat, *J Neuropathol Exp Neurol* 3:87–100, 1944.

Levinson BM: Forecast for the year 2000. In Anderson RS, editor: *Pet animals and society,* London, 1974, Baillière Tindall.

Leyhausen P: *Cat behavior: the predatory and social behavior of domestic and wild cats,* New York, 1978, Garland STPM Press.

Mattina MJI, Pignatello JJ, Swihart RK: Identification of volatile components of bobcat *(Lynx rufus)* urine, *J Chem Ecol* 17(2):451–462, 1991.

McCuistiom WK: Feline purring and its dynamics, *Vet Med Small Anim Clin* 61:562–566, June 1966.

McFarland C, Niebuhr BR, Beaver B, et al: Excessive vocalization, *Feline Pract* 15(3):8–9, 1985.

McKeown DB, Luescher UA, Halip J: Stereotypies in companion animals and obsessive-compulsive disorder, behavior problems in small animals, *Purina Specialty Review* pp 30–35, 1992.

Mykytowycz R: Reproduction of mammals in relation to environmental odors, *J Reprod Fertil* 19(suppl):433–446, 1973.

Science probing why cats purr, *Friskies Research Digest* 10:16, Spring 1974.

Suehsdorf A: The cats in our lives, *National Geographic* 125:508–541, April 1964.

Ursin H: Flight and defense behavior in cats, *J Comp Physiol Psychol* 58(2):180–186, 1964.

Verberne G: Chemocommunications among domestic cats, mediated by the olfactory and vomeronasal senses. II. The relation between the function of Jacobson's organ (vomeronasal organ) and flehmen behavior, *Z Tierpsychol* 42:113–128, Oct 1976.

Verberne G, Leyhausen P: Marking behavior of some viverridae and Felidae: time-interval analysis of the marking pattern, *Behaviour* 58(3–4):192–253, 1977.

Volokhov AA: The ontogenetic development of higher nervous activity in animals. In Himwich WA, editor: *Developmental neurobiology,* Springfield, Ill, 1970, Charles C Thomas Publisher.

Wada JA, Sato M: Directedness of defensive emotional behavior and motivation for aversive learning, *Exp Neurol* 40(2):445–456, 1973.

Worden AN: Abnormal behavior in the dog and cat, *Vet Rec* 71:966–978, Dec 26, 1959.

Wynne-Edwards VC: *Animal dispersion in relation to social behavior,* Edinburgh, 1962, Oliver & Boyd.

4

Feline Social Behavior

The social behavior patterns of animals are complex. Nine major social patterns can combine in 45 ways during the interaction of two or more cats.[171] Investigative, ingestive, eliminative, and sexual behaviors have some social adaptations but are considered in other appropriate sections.

The social behavior of a species is of evolutionary importance in the survival of that species, and most behaviors are a direct reflection of social organization.

SOCIAL ORGANIZATION

Domestication involves selective breeding for several generations, but until recently cat breeding has generally been uncontrolled. Cats that received food from humans tended to breed to each other, but with little selective criteria. As a result, today's cats are organized socially much like their early ancestors, although these social patterns are often interspersed with patterns introduced by selective breeding.[182] Social maturity probably does not occur until 2 to 4 years of age,[150] so this too must be considered when studying individuals at any location.

Social groups are made up of animals of the same species that are organized in a cooperative manner.[37,38,197] There is a relatively stable, long-term membership in the group, and the animals live in family groups or groups larger than the nuclear family.[37,38] In contrast, solitary species do not form enduring social relationships and live most of their lives alone.[37,38] It is also important to differentiate asocial from antisocial. An asocial species is primarily solitary, coming together for reproduction and when raising young. In contrast, antisocial animals are aggressive toward each other even during reproduction, and young have a very short time of maternal dependency.

Intraspecies Relationships

The ancient Egyptians used a cat symbol to denote a false or deceitful friendship.[110] Because cats are not seen in consistently sized groups, their exact social behaviors are difficult to study and are only beginning to be appreciated for their complexity. Speculation often replaces fact. The cat social system is flexible, allowing cats to live alone or in groups of varying size. Cats tend to exist in four very different lifestyles. At one extreme is the feral, independent wildlife, which are totally self-sufficient.[108,132] Another lifestyle is the feral, interdependent, free-roaming/unowned cats, which tend to have a colony type of interaction.[132] The domesticated, interdependent, free-roaming/ loosely owned cats are exemplified by barn cats and those fed by caring strangers.[132] Domesticated household cats are almost dependent on their owners.[132]

Feline social behavior is characterized by an avoidance of interactions,[73] or "living apart together."[42] Cats use an active spacing pattern and so are not randomly distributed within a space. Regular, if not actually rigid, schedules of daily activity help maintain spacing between individuals.[199] Communication, both by visual contact and by marking behaviors, also helps minimize the amount of close contact between individuals. The cat is able to differentiate conspecifics by urine odors.[155] Studies suggest that most cats living without human intervention are solitary.[100] Whether any animal tends to be solitary or highly social depends mostly on its primary type of food.[104] As a hunter, a cat typically hunts mice, one of which is a single meal for the hunter without any to share. But when cats do live in groups, they are more concentrated near food and shelter.[139] Variation in the number of associating individuals is based largely on the local abundance of food and relatedness of individuals.[39] Even those living in a group often spend much of their time alone.[3,42] Farm cat groups vary from 2 to 11 adult females (mode 4.5), with at least some being related.[100] There tends to be an alpha male, but there does not seem to be a typical linear hierarchy, because other parameters typical of such a social order are not present.[140]

Cats do make social contacts, and the primary one is between a female and her young. Specific epimeletic (caregiving) behavior is covered with maternal behavior, but the social development of the young can be significantly affected by this early experience. Early contact with the queen is obviously significant to the kittens, because when placed in a strange environment, they immediately display ectepimeletic (care-seeking) behavior.[163,173] Kittens raised with other kittens tend to become more stressed in loner situations than single-raised kittens.[129] Particularly at 2 and 4 weeks of age, contact between littermates is important to calm them in strange surroundings.[163,166] Social and play behavior are affected by social contacts with both the mother and the littermates. Deprivation of interaction with littermates results in kittens that do not learn social communication skills, and they have hyperresponses to play objects and in social play.[64,125] Kittens who are raised without the mother cat or whose mothers were on low-protein diets during the month either side of parturition have retarded or hyper-gregarious social behaviors.[64,125] Normal social relationships are most readily formed during the first 2 months of age, although there can be a lot of individual variation even within a litter.[125]

Feline social relationships are often nonenduring: The queen weans her young and the sexual partners do not form bonds. Kittens are social, depending on the interactions of littermates and the queen to develop the skills and knowledge they will later need for a solitary existence. The young males will disperse between 6 and 36 months.[39,115,190,200] Males that disperse usually move farther away than do females that leave, and they settle in areas where there is no dominant male.[115] Females usually do not go much farther than 650 yards from their birthplace.[115] Cats tend to live around other cats, particularly when food is plentiful, and to be solitary hunters. Most of the cats' time is spent out of each other's sight, with 35% of the time spent within 10 feet of another cat.[5] Even house cats tend to divide the house into individual zones, so the addition or removal of one member can be disruptive as cats redistribute the space.[199,200] Males are more likely to be closer than 3 feet.[3,5] The rolling behavior often seen may help inhibit overt aggression.[52] Female outdoor cats are more likely than males to show affiliative behavior, including social grooming, toward both males and females.[5] Cats also are more likely to approach the opposite gender.[198] Some cats simply tolerate each other, whereas others can become very devoted and protective toward one or two social partners.

Female cats are more likely to remain in one place their whole life, living alone or in groups of up to eight.[115] Usually group members are closely related. When trapped and neutered, the original group remains relatively constant, retaining approximately 75% of the original membership over a 3-year period.[202] Group membership does not necessarily mean the cats will spend long periods together, however.[100] Although the cats may be near the core area, they are usually alone when in the fields.

The longer these individual cats are together, the stronger their bond becomes, particularly if the relationship started when both cats were young. Littermates that stay together will spend more time in close social behaviors than will happen between unrelated cats.[22] Unrelated cats tend to eat one at a time or at well-separated bowls compared with the littermates that often share a food bowl.[22] Such a close relationship is characterized by mutual grooming, hunting close to each other (about 50 yards apart), running together (about 6 feet apart), and sleeping together.[6,49,59,112,197] The relationships between these cats can be highly structured, with approximately 65% of the interactions involving licking and 28% involving rubbing.[100] Feline groups are resistant to the introduction of new cats. New males tend to attack kittens, and new females would initiate a new gene line rather than promote the existing one.[37] Because cats have a tendency to be matrilineal, it is best to keep females and their offspring together with only a few males.[159] Acceptance of a new cat into a feral colony is a slow process, beginning with life on the periphery.[37] Loss of one partner can produce some interesting behavior changes in the other, including anorexia and excessive vocalization.[87] In some cases, a previously unassertive cat can show a dramatic personality change that is totally different than the previous one. The time lived together is negatively correlated with the amount of aggression observed.[4,5,36,178] Just as close bonds can form,[196] it is now known that some cats may actively avoid particular individuals.[84,197,198]

A very high percentage of cats that live in outdoor colonies are fed by people nearby or have access to food in waste bins. Food is often the common thread that keeps several cats in a specific area. Approximately 45% of the groups have fewer than 10 cat members, as is typical, and 11% have more than 50 members.[53,116] Three fourths of the British colonies are older than 5 years and have been altered by human interactions in the past. Barn cats that are mainly self-sufficient almost always live in a population density of less than 100 cats/km^2 and usually less than 25 cats/km^2.[199] Urban densities can reach more than 2000 cats/km^2.[88,100,199] Social densities of 2.5 to 3.3 cats/km^2 or fewer have been reported,[96,100,116,192] but such spaces tend to repel cats.[88] Distribution data for areas where cats must survive solely on natural prey are not available.

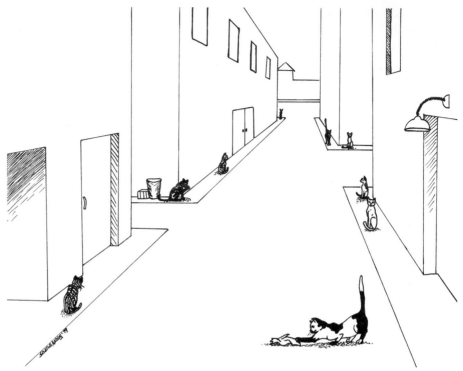

Figure 4-1 Social gatherings of neighborhood cats are one form of social contact between cats.

A modification of this semisocial relationship is the neighborhood meeting. In a neutral area in the early evening, local cats of both sexes may gather and sit in a loosely formed circle, usually within 5 yards of each other (Figure 4-1). This quiet social gathering often lasts several hours before the participants depart for their own home areas.[6,41,50,59]

Cat-Human Relationships

Cats have had a variety of relationships with people over the centuries. Even today the tendency is to love them or hate them. They have a number of traits that make them desirable pets.[78] Their small size is the first. That they will eliminate in a litterbox rather than requiring special trips outdoors is particularly nice for high-rise apartment living. In addition, they adapt well to being the only pet and to staying alone for long periods. As the human demographics began changing to more urban living, the popularity of cats soared.

The role of nature versus nurture has been questioned regarding the relationship of cats to humans. Genetics, particularly the sire's contribution, has been reported to be more significant in the amount of a cat's friendliness toward humans than how it was handled or socialized as a kitten.[162,184] However, friendlier mothers do not tend to have friendlier kittens.[184] This genetics research has since been reinterpreted to suggest that the parameter being evaluated as friendliness was actually boldness.[127] Cats socialized to people and those from friendly sires are not only friendlier to unfamiliar people, but they also show fewer signs of distress when approached and handled by strangers.[127] Socialization to humans is different from and independent of socialization to other cats.[130] For those cats that do interact with people, their behavior toward people tends to be relatively constant after socialization.[184] Kittens that are not socialized to people take longer to approach and have fewer interactions.[98] When they are socialized to people but encounter unfamiliar people, cats will show more direct contacts with them than with familiar people, with most of the attention behaviors shown to people of both groups on the first day.[158] Availability, sex, and age of the person with whom the cat interacts affect the relationship.[130] In general, the strongest relationships tend to occur with women and the weakest occur with juveniles,[130] although this might be related to the human's activity and vocal patterns.[131]

The cat-human relationship may be more like an ectepimeletic, kitten-mother relationship than an adult conspecific one. Behaviors such as rubbing against a person's leg, lying down to be petted, and kneading while being held, all behaviors for which cats have been selectively bred, illustrate this infant-mother relationship.[70,74] Vertical tail approaches to humans suggest a kitten approaching its queen rather than its littermates. Conversely, a cat licking a human is mimicking mutual grooming of contemporaries.

While the cat population was increasing because of the cat's desirability as a pet, those who did not like cats continued to express their views. Approximately 10 million cats are surrendered to shelters each year, with around 70% of those having to be euthanized.[88] Some of these cats have to be trapped to get them, and they are poor candidates for pets because most can be tamed only after a great deal of time and patience.[132] Few people are willing to put in that amount of effort. The feral cat programs may have another impact that is not well recognized. Those cats that are not trapped and thus not neutered may increase the genetic selection for wildness.[23]

The cat's reactions to environmental happenings reflect its lack of strong social bonds. When trapped in a dangerous situation, such as a house fire, the cat's instinct for self-preservation dictates escape. Only if escape is blocked will the cat recruit assistance from a human and coincidentally save the human's life. Cats are most often honored with hero awards when using this behavior in a burning building. Occasionally cats have been reported to serve as seeing-eye cats or hearing-ear cats, to fight off snakes endangering a child, and to call attention to a trapped cat or person.[156,164]

Social Distances

Several distances and areas have social significance to the cat. The area traveled during normal activities is called the *home range,* and although it is generally considered circular, the shape is actually quite variable (Figure 4-2). A home range will have enough food to sustain the individual and perhaps others, and it is not uniformly used by the individual.[93] The size of area is highly correlated to metabolic needs and amount of meat needed in the diet.[62] The central, or core, area, where a cat spends 80% of its time, is approximately 0.5 acre, or 20,000 m^2.[154] In addition to the core, the cats may use the range evenly or have radiating paths leading to secondary home sites for special purposes, such as hunting, elimination, or resting.* As size of the home range increases,

*References 72, 84, 113, 121, 181, 186.

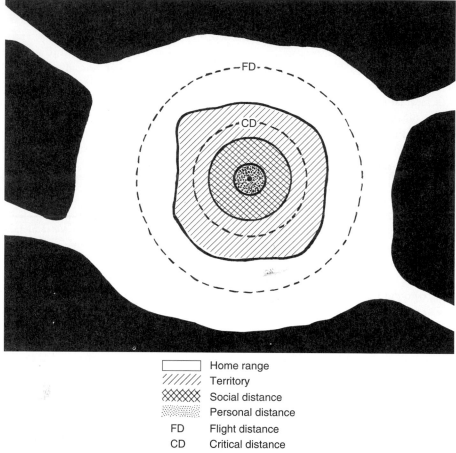

Home range
///// Territory
XXXXX Social distance
:::::: Personal distance
FD   Flight distance
CD   Critical distance

Figure 4-2 The social distances of cats.

the percentage of the area visited daily drops from 38% to as low as 5% without apparent consequences.[186] Paths to commonly used locations are chosen for length and direction.[160] Both the paths and the special areas may be part of the home range of several individuals.[72,165,186] Usage of the paths is not based on dominance but on a passive first-come, first-served basis. Scheduling can be very important in a cat's routine, with feeding times or travel schedules determining when a cat is in a certain location. Cats arriving at an intersection at the same time will sometimes sit for long periods, each waiting for the other to take the initiative[59,113] (Figure 4-3).

The size of a home range varies considerably, depending on food availability and sex of the cat. The size for males averages 3.5 times larger than for females in the same general area,[117] and cats are reported to travel 230 to 2770 feet daily.[154,185] The size of the home range varies from 0.2 acre for females and 2.1 acres for males where cats are well fed, up to 667 acres for females and 1038 acres for males in the Australian bush.[*]

[*]References 6, 50, 88, 96, 100, 114–117, 120, 192.

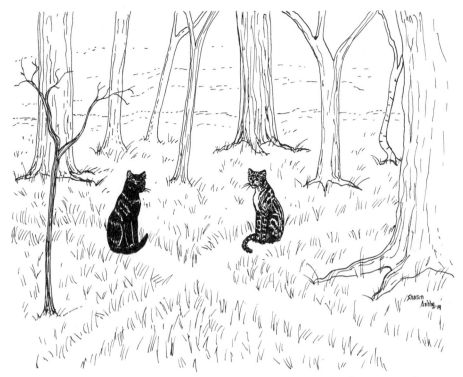

Figure 4-3 Cats meeting at an intersection of paths may wait for each other to proceed.

The mean for free-roaming females is 42 acres, and that for males is 153 acres.[100] The home ranges of solitary cats overlap more than expected by chance.[100] Home ranges of females do not overlap between groups but are shared by females of that specific group, sometimes with their male.[40,115] Female cats from the same farm have a 55.1% overlap of each other's home ranges compared with a 3.5% overlap with nonresident female cats.[39] Males from the same farm have a 56.5% overlap with each other and a 14.4% overlap with the home range of males from other locations.[39] Specifics are more inconsistent in free-ranging male cats because their home ranges may not have a specific outer boundary.[112] Inside a house the average cat uses 40 square yards of living space.[80] Adult males use more rooms in the home (average 5.4) than adult females (average 3.9) as part of their home range.[12,13] Most cats have favorite spots where they can be predictably found, with different spots used at different times of the day.[13] Generally there will be individuals moving to empty or recently vacated spots rather than groups lying together.[13]

Juveniles tend to appropriate parts of their dam's home range in the spring, and if they do not stay in the group, they will use a distinct range in the summer.[200] When juvenile males emigrate, they may establish their home range next to that of their sire.[200] If a tom is removed, immigration of another tom will occur within a few days; however, immigration of females into an established area is uncommon.[200]

A *territory* is an area that is actively defended against strangers of the same species (see Figure 4-2), and such an aggressive encounter should be won almost exclusively by the territory's owner.[39] Generally a territory is smaller than a home range, but in the case of the house cat, territory and home range may be identical. The difficulty in obtaining more precise information about social distances is related to the cat's solitary nature, its agility, and its nocturnal patterns. In roaming cats, the minimal territorial size is estimated to be 0.1 square mile.[6,113,181] Males are more territorial and form larger, more rigid, and more permanent territories.[181,193] These areas are small enough to be observed by the resident male cat in toto and are regularly patrolled and marked by him.[113] Although tomcats may eat at a common source and sleep in close proximity, their territories seldom overlap, they avoid each other on common pathways, and their territories are not contiguous with those of other males.[6,88,115,181] When population permits, cats spread out and make maximal use of the available space.[112]

Some males will allow females into their territory but not in the immediate proximity of their home site. In fact, the amount of aggression directed toward an intruder is inversely proportional to the distance from the core area.[140,181]

When approached by a stranger of an unfamiliar species, a cat will flee when the stranger reaches a certain distance. That distance is called the *flight distance* (see Figure 4-2). A cat that cannot flee or that is unaware of the intruder will defend itself at a second, closer distance, known as the *critical distance* (see Figure 4-2). Unfortunately, flight and critical distances have been used interchangeably, which causes some confusion to the reader. The flight distance for the cat is approximately 6 feet and probably somewhat longer for the kitten.[25,135] Females with young have a greater critical distance than other cats, and some will aggressively meet an intruder from quite a distance.[193]

When the cat is approached by individuals of a species that it does not fear, two other distances become important. Special well-accepted individuals are allowed an intimate approach, including physical contact, and thus may enter the cat's *personal distance* (see Figure 4-2). Other acquaintances will not be attacked but are not allowed within the personal distance. Their accepted space is called the *social distance* (see Figure 4-2). Threat displays often serve to inhibit further approach by a violator of the personal distance.

As for all species, social distances are important to the cat. In fact, most cats form a stronger bond with home range and territory than with any social being.

Social Orders

The significance and display of social ranking between individual animals has undergone a lot of reflection in recent years. For a long time, it was thought that social animal species have fairly well-defined dominance rankings to minimize agonistic behavior between individuals. A threat display by the dominant animal leads to a submissive display by the subordinate. This is still generally true. Exceptions, however, are easy to point out. There are times when a higher ranking individual might not find a resource particularly important and chooses to defer to an otherwise lower ranking animal. This in essence creates two hierarchies within the same group. At other times, peaceful coexistence seems to occur without strong evidence of a well-defined social rank. That is apparently the case for cats living together. Instead of a linear ranking, there tends to be three general positions. One male assumes relative dominance based on territorial ownership.[116,120,190] These dominant cats tend to be larger and older than other males.[129] For several days this despot walks stiff legged with raised back and tail, seizing each of the other cats, pushing their backs down with his hindquarters, and mounting

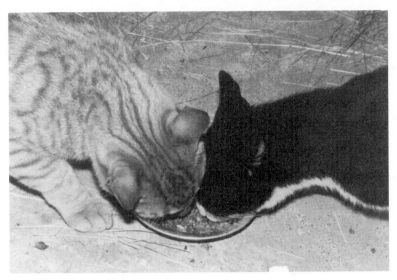

Figure 4-4 Two male cats sharing a meal.

each as if for copulation.[195] This mounting behavior is a sign of dominance in several other species, also without sexual connotations. The subordinate animal, male or female, responds with much vocalization and struggling and dashes away as soon as possible.[195] Aside from this dominant male, the female cats apparently do not differ in rank.* The tendency to rub the face of another is a poor but clear single indicator of which individual might rank lower.[121] There may also be one or more pariahs.[6,112,190] These are the lowest ranking cats that display an almost constant growl and lowered body posture in the presence of the top cat and occasionally for the group as a whole. Both social outcasts and progestin-treated females, because they are frequently attacked by members of the group and become chronically wary of other cats, temporarily lose social position.[94] Cats may even choose a specific human to treat as a pariah, attacking frequently.

A differentiated and fairly linear dominance order has been described in cats.[2] Variations occur between individuals and between groups. Stability of the hierarchies also varies.[2]

Lack of a complete hierarchy between cats makes it difficult to predict the outcome of a confrontation. For social animals, size, weight, and sex factors can alter this agonistic behavior; however, for the cat, location, time of day, presence of food, past history, and the number of cats present are more significant.† For example, if two cats meet on a path, the one arriving last or at a different time than is usual often yields to the other cat. One cat does not take food away from another as a dominant would do from a subordinate in a rigid social hierarchy. Instead, each cat waits its turn or shares if possible (Figure 4-4). The addition of neutered animals to cat populations further complicates these relationships because of behavior changes resulting from changes in hormones.

*References 12, 13, 41, 108, 140, 195.
†References 6, 31, 50, 59, 110, 201.

Social Approaches

Two cats approaching each other use species-specific behaviors and investigate scent gland locations. In 7% of approaches, aggression is shown. For the other approaches, 28% involve sniffing, more than 12% use a trill vocal greeting sound, and 7% show mutual grooming.[35] The territorial cat smells the nose first and then the anal area of the intruder, who continues a slow exploration of the strange environment.[193,201] The facial approach, followed by the anogenital approach, is generally used by cats that already know each other and have no reason for hostility (Figure 4-5).[6] The facial approach is the most commonly used and involves smelling the mouth and temporal regions, touching noses and areas of tactile hairs, and rubbing heads. The facial approach is also commonly used by a cat approaching a human and even in this situation is followed by the anogenital posture as the cat presents its hindquarters to the human. The odor associated with the anogenital approach apparently has social significance to the cat because the scent of an anestrous female may actually have a repelling effect on a sexually mature male.[49,194] Approaching cats will usually align themselves in one of four ways, depending on the position of the cat being approached. Body to body contact, including that between nursing kittens, occurs in 79% of the contacts; body to head-neck contact, 9%; head-neck to head-neck contacts, 6%; and head-neck to body contact, including the greeting sniff, 5%.[194]

When confronted with its image in a mirror, a cat usually approaches with interest and often tries to locate the image behind the mirror. This indicates no self-identification.[65] If a threat reaction is initiated, it usually intensifies because of the continually increasing threat display by the image.

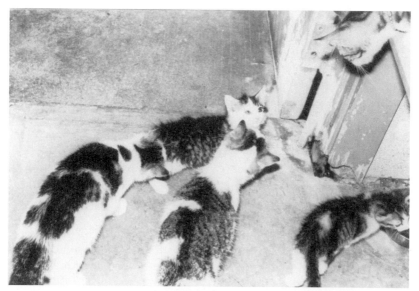

Figure 4-5 Adult cats showing a facial approach and an anogenital approach to a newly introduced kitten.

SOCIALIZATION

Although every age is important in the normal development of a kitten, four periods are unique and particularly critical in behavioral development.[58,167] The infantile or neonatal period is characterized by neonatal ingestive and sleep patterns. The transitional or intermediate period begins during the second week with the appearance of adult patterns of eating and locomotion and of immature forms of social behavior. The socialization period is the time when all primary social bonds are formed and constitutes the single most important period during the cat's life. During this phase, striking behavioral changes also occur because of growth and experience. The fourth period of kitten development, the adolescent or juvenile period, is primarily a time for maturation of motor skills.

Socialization is a process by which an individual forms an attachment to the other species it contacts during a limited time (see Appendix D). The socialization period is a developmentally sensitive time during which the individual is the most responsive to social stimuli.[144] If the kitten is not exposed to appropriate stimuli, it may never develop appropriate responses. Early environments and social relationships are definitely important in socialization. The socialization process can occur between a kitten and humans or between a kitten and its "natural enemies," such as dogs, rats, mice, or birds (Figure 4-6). These attachments result in the "unusual" yet perfectly normal pictures so often seen in newspapers (Figure 4-7). Only after a great deal of training might a grown cat accept or tolerate a species with which it was not acquainted during its socialization phase.

The long process of domestication generally produces animals with a naturally reduced tendency to flee from humans. By working with a young animal, domesticated or not, one can reduce the flight distance to zero and thus environmentally effect a psychologic change in an individual, which is called *taming*. Kittens handled after 2 weeks of age become more responsive to people than those not handled or those not handled

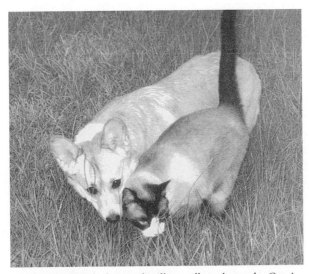

Figure 4-6 This cat was raised with dogs and will actually seek out the Corgi.

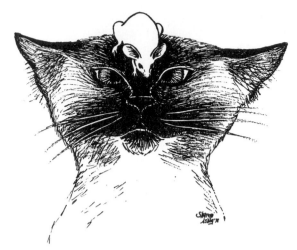

Figure 4-7 Kittens socialized to certain species accept that species as a normal part of their adult environment.

until at least 7 weeks of age.[97,98,119] Handling before 2 weeks makes no difference. Handling by multiple people makes kittens much less fearful of people compared with those with single-person handlers.[32] The downside is that the kittens exposed to multiple people show less social and play behaviors.[32,98] Without this environmental contact the kitten naturally tends to avoid humans, as often is the case with cats raised in a woodpile or hayloft. Even when carefully raised in association with humans, kittens have a normal period of human avoidance, which gradually appears between 40 and 50 days of age, is strongly obvious shortly thereafter, and if socialization to humans has occurred, ends sometime after the seventieth day.

The kitten that generalizes taming to all members of a species is said to be *socialized* to that species. Because eyesight is still developing in the kitten, visual recognition is probably somewhat limited, as in the dog. Forms of young children do not look the same as those of adults to a kitten, so exposing it to both types of humans might be important to ensure proper socialization. Rough play and handling during socialization result in the cat's becoming either wild and aggressive or timid and nervous with people.[26] Similar results occur if the kitten has little or no human contact during this early stage or if it is separated from its littermates and mother at 2 weeks of age.[23,65,67,188]

Species identification also occurs during the socialization period. Not only does this permit the cat to recognize other felines so that future matings are not a problem, but it also teaches the animal to tolerate if not fully accept other cats in social situations. Cats raised with members of other species in addition to their own will accept both but form stronger attachments with their own species. If raised only with other species during socialization, the cat forms attachments only to the adopted species.[98,105] Future mate selection can then be a serious problem because the cat fails to identify with its own species.

The exact amount of time necessary for socialization of the cat is not known. In other species, socialization begins with the appearance of behavioral mechanisms that maintain or prevent social contacts, and perhaps for the kitten, socialization starts with the development of emotional reactions.[172] The critical period ends with development of a fear response,[97] which is probably associated with a particular stimulus causing the young to leave the vicinity.[172] The socialization period must then include the ages of 5 to 7 weeks and probably ranges from 2 to 9 weeks of age. Careful handling of the kitten may extend this period for a few more weeks, and prolonged social exposure to certain individuals may even result in some form of attachment.[54,59,172]

The socialization process is faster if the kitten encounters stress; has a strong emotional experience such as hunger, pain, or loneliness[172]; or is handled intensively.[98,144] This experience encourages rapid species identification. Once the socialization period passes, however, it becomes extremely difficult to acquaint the cat with other species except to occasional individuals. Hand-reared kittens are slower to develop normal responses.[144]

The young kitten is imprinted to its mother within the first few days of life, as evidenced by its reaction to separation, and olfaction plays an important role in the formation of the bond. Early approach behaviors also ensure early socialization to cats. The end of this species identification period is signaled by an increased tendency to avoid the unfamiliar,[57] and the 3- to 6-week age seems the most important in intraspecies socialization.[144] Secondary social relationships can then be developed by means of socialization. About 15% of cats will be resistant to socialization.[107]

AGGRESSION

Agonistic behavior is a competitive interaction between two or more individuals that involves body postures and displays related to flight, defensive attack, and offensive attack. Aggression and the associated escape and passive postures are relatively common in the feline species. Neutering may not dramatically decrease the amount of aggression between cats, except in forms of aggression that are testosterone dependent. Neutering does, however, result in an increase in "friendly" interactions in both males and females.[39,141]

Much of the confusion in the literature regarding aggression has resulted because there are several different kinds of aggression displayed by the cat. This fact has often been neglected, so studies of cats attacking rats are equated with cats protecting themselves, showing fear, and being involved in other aggressive situations. It has made reviewing the literature very difficult. Classification of aggression can be done in several ways—by target, active or passive defense reflexes, learning, or function.[20] Classification by function is practical in a clinical setting, resulting in approximately 15 different categories.[11]

In certain situations, aggressive behavior is considered perfectly normal; however, cat owners generally consider it to be a problem behavior. Because it is difficult to differentiate normal from problem aggression, most forms are discussed here. Aggression is a commonly reported behavior problem for cats, representing 17% of the problems in geriatric cats[27] and up to 35% of the regular behavior cases.* Because the claws and teeth of a cat are such formidable weapons, aggression by the cat can become a significant problem. Although figures vary, somewhere between 6% and 20% of the reported bites that animals inflict on humans are caused by cats, and most of those bitten are children.[63,83,95,187]

*References 9, 15, 16, 21, 39, 80, 124, 183.

Affective Aggression

Affective and nonaffective aggression are broad categories defined by the presence of an intensive, patterned autonomic activation, which especially involves sympathoadrenal interactions. Cats that hiss and show aggressive body postures are displaying affective aggression. Eight types of aggressive behavior can be classified as affective aggression, but several behavioral characteristics appear in all types.[161] Although menacing vocalizations and threat postures may be only displays, they may progress to a full-rage attack with teeth and claws that is directed toward the provoking or threatening object, to escape flight, or to tonic immobility.[47,56,188] These threats range from low intensity, in which the cat crouches and holds its ears slightly back; to middle intensity, in which the cat flattens its ears and hisses; to high intensity, in which these displays are combined with arched back, piloerection, inverted-U tail position, and lowered head. Submission is generally not considered a major part of a cat's behavioral repertoire, because it retreats instead. Unlike the social species, a fleeing cat does not induce flight behavior in other cats. There is no "sympathetic induction of mood."[118]

Because it is not related to sexual or food-gathering behaviors, various types of affective aggression are often not goal directed but are usually initiated by either a somatic or an external stimulus that lowers the irritability threshold for the aggression.[161] Genetic factors are related to these behaviors. Some cats that are basically aggressive toward humans, other cats, or both have produced offspring showing these same behaviors regardless of how they were raised. Visual and olfactory stimuli can elicit adultlike agonistic behavior patterns as early as 6 weeks of age.[102]

A cat that stands firm during an attack of affective aggression from another cat, rather than running away or submitting, has about a 65% chance of inhibiting or avoiding the attack.[138]

Intermale aggression

Fighting between tomcats is a common form of feline aggression. The presence of testosterone in the prenatal and neonatal kitten masculinizes the young brain. Later production of testosterone potentiates the earlier presence of the hormone and produces male behaviors, including fighting. Castration usually eliminates this later facilitation of male aggression, so castrated cats do not commonly fight.[76] Testosterone plays a significant role in intermale aggressive behavior in the cat, because it is selectively taken up by the portions of the brain that control aggressive behavior. In addition, it is responsible for the loose attachment and dermal thickness of the neck skin. Intermale aggression increases during periods of overcrowding and the mating season, but an estrous female need not be present. The increased frequency during mating season results from a greater number of encounters with young wandering males, called *floaters,* as they emigrate from their birthplace rather than from cyclic hormone changes.[45,140] Differential diagnoses for intermale aggression include competitive, territorial, and sexual aggression.

Area males establish a "brotherhood" or "fraternity" by aggressive interactions. When a young male reaches puberty, one or two of the local tomcats begin to call in a soft vocalization similar to that of a tomcat calling an estrous female. When the young male approaches, severe fighting ensues.[41,112,114] These encounters continue for about a year, and if the younger cat is still alive and has not become totally fearful, he is accepted into the group.[59,112] Unlike other social groupings, the brotherhood has an absolute ranking order that holds regardless of whenever or wherever members meet.[112] The cats are of almost equal strength, so even a threat display rivalry can change the narrowly separated ranking positions.[59,112,113]

Any initial meeting between two males arriving in a new territory simultaneously results in a similar behavior. An intense fight allowed to go to completion is followed by a situation in which threat displays adequately prevent further interactions.[6,112]

Because intermale aggression is related to testosterone, castration has been successful in minimizing 80% to 90% of the behavior in cats so treated.[76,77] In addition, various long-acting progestogens have been successfully used to control this aggression, including medroxyprogesterone acetate and megestrol acetate. Several other drugs with similar actions can also be used. Specifics of male behaviors are discussed in Chapter 5.

Pain-induced aggression

Pain effectively elicits defensive aggression, and it can cause aggression at levels significantly greater than expected in certain situations.[90] Obvious causes of pain-induced aggression include attacks on humans when a cat's hair or tail is pulled or when its tail is stepped on. Continued application of pain eventually causes the cat to submit to the stimulus or try to escape it.[56] Early social play helps teach the kitten what pain is and how much pain it can inflict on others. If slight oral pressure elicits a pain reaction from a littermate, the kitten learns this by the victim's reaction. Singly raised orphans are deprived of this learning experience. Those who do not have the opportunity to play with littermates may also miss this important lesson.

Fear-induced aggression

Fear or stress can, if continued long enough, result in neurosis, and either can produce aggression. The aggression is usually preceded by attempts to avoid or escape, indicating that some degree of confinement is present in conjunction with a threatening situation.[33,137] Frightened animals can react aggressively if escape is not possible when their critical distance is reached by an approaching animal or object. The body posture is usually that of defensive threats, and the cat is growling or hissing.[36] Cats that have not been well socialized to humans or that must interact with small children are often unable to escape an approaching individual and become aggressive when the person gets too close. In either case the defensive attack lasts until escape is possible.

The most obvious methods of relieving or preventing this form of aggression are to eliminate the source of fear or allow escape from the situation. Extinction of the fear will occur over time if the stimulus does not reoccur. More often, it is necessary to use desensitization and counterconditioning to stop the problem.[33] The person could sit in the same room as the cat's food while it eats, getting gradually closer as the cat accepts the minimal presence over several days. Playful cats can be encouraged to interact with a chase toy at the end of a long string, which will be very gradually shortened as the fear dissipates.[39] Of course, that is not always possible, and drug therapy may be needed. Benzodiazepines can be used on a temporary basis, and tricyclic antidepressants (TCAs) or selected serotonin reuptake inhibitors (SSRIs) are preferred for long-term stress reduction, especially when desensitization and counterconditioning are being used.[151]

Carbamazepine, a TCA, has been shown to reduce fear aggression.[168] Some individuals never fully adapt and must be maintained on low doses of the drugs, and others need treatment only before exposure to the stimulus.

In a veterinary clinic, cats with fear-induced aggression can often be handled if surrounded by the familiar smells of the bottom half of their carrier. Reducing the visual and auditory stimulation, particularly that of other cats and dogs, will minimize aggression in most cats.[143] Benzodiazepines, particularly diazepam, can be helpful, because they reduce anxiety and increase the appetite, which in turn increases the significance of food treats.[123] Forced restraint, thick gloves, muzzles, cat bags, and a thrown blanket or towel tend to aggravate the situation instead of helping but are used on a one-time basis. As a last resort, one can use a bag on a collapsible frame, squeeze cage, fishnet, or oral spray of ketamine hydrochloride or acepromazine maleate.[143] These drugs can create a workable situation, even though the full dose may not have been delivered.

Maternal aggression

A female's defense of her young is another form of affective aggression. Queens with kittens are the least tolerant of approaches by other cats and intruders. This is one of the few times when the female cat is truly an aggressor, and the display tends to be one of threats over long distances rather than attacks.[147] Maternal aggression is regulated by hormonal influences on the appropriate hypothalamic centers of the brain and by environmental factors, particularly the presence of the kittens.[57,71,91]

Territorial aggression

Defense of territory is relatively common in the cat and can be directed toward humans and other cats.[149] It probably was developed to aid in social spacing.[76] A territory can be delineated by areas patrolled or marked via chin rubbing, urine, and perhaps feces. If the cat perceives an offender entering its space, it may threaten or attack. Both males and females can exhibit this aggression, but it is particularly noticeable in territorial males during the breeding season. It is also common when a new cat is introduced into a home with a resident cat.[88,128] Neighboring cats are often better tolerated than strange ones.[49] Encounters with the resident male usually involve threats but can easily escalate to fighting. The owner of the territory has a significant psychologic advantage, so strangers tend to flee or submit much sooner than residents.[49,76] The resident male first tries to threaten the floater male but will fight to maintain his territory if intimidation is unsuccessful. Losing to the stranger can significantly affect the resident, who may even lose primary breeding status or undergo psychologic castration.[45,76] Territorial aggression is observed in female cats who are very protective of the area near their kittens.[112]

An animal outside his own territory tends to be less aggressive in inverse proportion to the distance from its core area.[181]

Competitive aggression

Competitive aggression is normally controlled by dominance status and associated threat-submission postures, but the cat lacks clear dominant-subordinate relationships and dominance hierarchies. Generally animals that share a dominance position show frequent competition for a particular item such as food. This competition can be solved by fighting during the encounter or by reacting in a compatible, first-come, first-served basis. The latter is generally what happens in cats, because protection of food resources has not been seen.[4] Even in the groups with a dominant male, several nonspecifics, and pariahs, an early arriving low-ranking member usually finishes eating before the later-arriving dominant one begins if there is room for only one at a time.

Learned (instrumental) aggression

When an aggressive behavior is reinforced, a cat can learn to use the behavior to affect a desired result.[137] Cats are rarely trained to attack but have on occasion learned that aggression can produce results. When a child pulls a cat's tail, the cat shows pain-induced aggression by scratching or biting and the child responds by releasing the cat. Soon the cat acts aggressively toward the child even though the child applies no painful stimulus. Some cats will even generalize to all humans from an experience with one.

Play aggression

Kittens use social play to develop motor skills. The target of playful aggression is often a moving stimulus, such as a person walking by. In fact, the behavior is considered five times more of a problem when directed toward people than toward other cats[21] (Figure 4-8). The behavior may be directed only at certain people, and at times the cat may even seem to be stalking a particular individual.[36] Early weaned kittens do not learn to moderate their social play responses and so may not learn to sheathe claws and inhibit bites.[84,145,146] These lessons normally occur during social play and then are expressed as predation, activated in weeks 10 through 12, and as social fighting by week 14.[146,153] If they do not have littermates to interact with, kittens may direct the play aggression

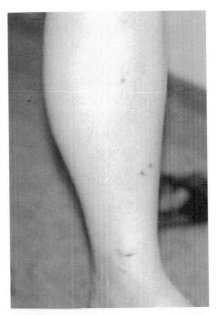

Figure 4-8 Aggression toward an owner, even in play, can cause severe injuries.

toward the owner. Without the thick fur, the owner is more likely to be injured and less likely to respond with deterrent types of responses.[33] Although most owners understand what to expect, a few kittens play fight harder than most, and a few owners do not recognize it as normal. Even older cats will occasionally cause unintentional injuries during play from sharp claws or teeth.

To prevent the unacceptable versions of play aggression, owners should avoid situations that tend to trigger it. If the attacks occur when the owner comes home from work, confine the cat to avoid access to the entrance or come in another way. The play should also be redirected to an inanimate object such as a "wing on a string" toy. That same type of mobile toy should be used to provide appropriate opportunities to use playful energy, especially before bedtime.[39,122,124,145] Punishment, such as a water sprayer or noise maker, can teach the cat to leave a specific person alone, provided that alternative play opportunities are provided. Getting another kitten of approximately the same age will provide a suitable outlet for the behavior too.

Sexual Aggression

Authorities disagree about the classification of sexual aggression. Some call it a type of affective aggression, and others believe it deserves separate classification.[47,48,161] The confusion is understandable when the areas of the brain associated with sexual aggression are compared with those associated with other types of affective behaviors.[179] Because additional tracts within the central nervous system are involved, sexual aggression is considered somewhat different and is covered in Chapters 5 and 6.

Predatory Aggression

Predatory aggression differs considerably from other forms for several reasons. These aggressive responses are not the result of either fear or threat, but prey capture. Emotions are not involved, so there is little autonomic arousal, making this a type of nonaffective aggression. One reason given for tomcats killing very young kittens is that the behavior is a form of predatory aggression,[147] because the kitten would be approximately the same size as mice. Kitten attacks on moving objects usually represent a play version of predatory aggression. This type of aggression is discussed with ingestive behavior in Chapter 7.

Redirected Aggression

Aggression evoked by any stimulus can be redirected to another target if the attack is prevented or if the primary target is no longer available. This is a common form of aggression representing about 50% of the cases of feline aggression toward people.[28] The initiating stress may be as subtle as the cat not receiving a bedtime snack, fear, noises, or unusual odors.[10,19,28] Outdoor cats roaming near a favorite window can also trigger an attack by the confined cat directed toward something it can reach—the owner or another pet. Once the cat has physically and psychologically been aroused to the point of attack, the accompanying emotion is not easily contained, even though the target is no longer available. The threshold for the behavior's release is very low, and substitute targets are easily found, especially when a third party interrupts the aggressive episode. This interruption could be intentional, as when trying to break up a cat fight, or unintentional, as when walking past an aroused cat.[21,61,124,153] A tomcat that is threatening another will quickly release its aggression on a cat or human who interferes. People should not interfere with an aroused cat, being particularly careful not to try to calm it.[28] Unfortunately cats tend to have long memories for victims, so they tend to remain aggressive toward the redirected target. Aggressive episodes can also result in fearful responses by the victim, which complicates the problem even more.[152] Changing that perspective can take a long time of behavioral and environmental modification.[148] The cat needs to calm down away from the person or animal primarily and secondarily targeted, perhaps while confined in a separate room. The initial stimulus must be removed so that the behavior is not triggered again. To help restore the relationships that were challenged, first exchange odors via a towel, with or without synthetic pheromones, while the cat is eating or being petted by an accepted person. Eventually the targeted person is made visible at a distance while the cat is fed, with the distance gradually reduced over time.

It is not always possible to predict or control those things that will trigger an episode of redirected aggression. To prevent the problem, however, the owner may have to confine the cat to a single room or even to a very large cage.[180]

Petting-Induced Aggression

Some cats, usually lying on a person's lap and being petted, suddenly claw and bite. The cat immediately jumps down, runs a short distance, and stops, perhaps to groom itself.[18] Generally these cats are male. The reason for the action is unknown; however, three theories are currently used to explain its occurrence. One theory is that the cat initially enjoys the handling and petting, which finally become excessive and reach a threshold level. The cat bites and claws when the handling is no longer acceptable because there is no other natural way for the cat to say, "Thanks, that is enough." Mutual grooming sessions between cats would normally be terminated by the one doing the licking. Humans may continue too long. The second theory holds that the petting and handling are so pleasurable that the cat falls into a light sleep, oblivious to its surroundings. The cat awakens suddenly and, still not completely oriented, is aware only of "confinement" and fights its way to freedom. By the time it has jumped clear of the person, it is totally aware, and to dissociate from the situation, the cat uses grooming as a displacement activity. The third theory is that the behavior is a desire or need to control the time when the attention begins or ends.[148] Treatment of this cat with progestins may be successful in some problem cases[76,79] but is generally not indicated. Because these cats are usually willing to sit on the owner's lap for long periods if not petted, this observation may also be part of the solution. Assume the cat will never be cuddly.[36,148] If it normally can be petted for 1 minute before showing aggression or the cat shows preaggression signs like a tail or skin twitch, the owner should limit all petting bouts to less than 1 minute or until the signs first appear. All other interaction will simply be the lap contact.

Feline Dispersion Aggression

As kittens reach the age of 6 to 12 months, their social play bouts begin to end with a fight. Over time the length of the play gets shorter and the fight segment becomes more intense. Eventually the frequent aggressive interactions result in the dispersion of the kittens from their home. It is the time of personality change from social kitten to a less social adult. If kittens have been separated from littermates previously, the aggressive interactions may still be expressed to owners or other animals. Many owners at least notice the personality change.

Feline Asocial Aggression

Feline asocial aggression is the type of aggression shown by older cats toward kittens. The usual situation where feline asocial aggression shows up is when one of two older cats that had been "friends" dies. Both the owners and the remaining cat miss the animal, so a new kitten is brought in to become a replacement. The older cat becomes very aggressive toward the kitten whenever it approaches. The kitten is social and readily approaches the older cat, which really just wants to be left alone. It responds aggressively to the approach. Management is difficult because it generally takes several months for the new kitten to become less interactive. Until then, the owner should keep the opportunities for interaction to a minimum. This has also been called *retaliatory aggression.*[27]

Medically Related Aggression

Certain medical changes may be manifested clinically only as aggression. Currently not all of these conditions are understood. Treatments for certain conditions have been successfully used, but the mechanisms of action are still uncertain.

Hypothyroid aggression

Although not common, hypothyroidism classically involves changes in a cat's appearance, but in one form of the disease, aggression is the clinical manifestation. The affected cat becomes "grumpy."[8] Although it may sleep on the bed with the owner at night, the cat might not allow the owner to sit on the sofa or walk past it. Thyroid hormone replacement is successful. Evaluations of T_4 values screen for the condition; however, other factors must also be considered, such as an excess of testosterone or estrogen in the circulating bloodstream, which can also decrease the normal levels.

Aggression of seizures

Another medical condition that may cause aggression is epilepsy. The history often gives other clues of this condition. During these episodes, the cat may seem oblivious to its surroundings, stare into space for short periods, or suddenly start chasing its tail. Electroencephalographic (EEG) recordings show changes from normal patterns in less than 40% of these cases. In humans, α-chloralose has been used to demonstrate EEG activation of a latent instability in the central nervous system.[133] Although treatment with anticonvulsants is approximately 80% successful, the drugs may have to be given at initially high doses, which are reduced according to clinical progress. Phenobarbital is usually used but occasionally may require combination with other anticonvulsants.

Feline ischemic encephalopathy has aggression as a common presenting sign. It and poorly controlled seizures are often residual problems.[175] Because of the proximity of the hypothalamus and the hormone system, the success of adrenocorticotropin and medroxyprogesterone acetate is not surprising. Frontal lobe epilepsy in humans does not always respond to anticonvulsants, but some cases have been successfully controlled by medroxyprogesterone acetate.[17]

Irritable aggression

Irritable aggression is the result of being less tolerant when the cat is not feeling well or is stressed.[8,137] The animal can become irritable if forced to interact when it is ill. Impacted anal sacs, oral ulcers, and feline lower urinary tract disease are among many initiating problems that need to be ruled out.

Other medically related aggressions

Other medical abnormalities are associated with aggression. Some are known to affect the central nervous system cells or neurotransmitters, and others are suspected of doing so.[44] In addition to being caused by irritative brain lesions such as encephalitis, aggression has been caused by tumors that bilaterally affect the hypothalamus.[56,76,81,191] For certain predictable hypothalamically mediated aggressions, pretreatment with chlordiazepoxide hydrochloride might be used for control.[99,174] Occasional individuals recover spontaneously.[106]

Blindness can affect the social relationship between cats. A change in dominance may be the only clinical sign that vision has been lost.[92]

Drugs have been implicated in personality changes involving aggression. Extremely vicious cats have had favorable personality changes after undergoing one or more episodes of prolonged deep barbiturate anesthesia.[135,136,157] In addition, personalities have been changed by withdrawing, during anesthesia, one third of the blood volume and then repeating the process 3 days later. Neural anoxia is the possible explanation for these occasional successes. The reduction of blood volume might also have been used occasionally on an individual with erythrocythemia, with resultant personality changes.[135] In some individuals diazepam causes a paradoxical reaction, and ketamine hydrochloride, known to cause postsedation hallucinations in humans, may cause the same in cats.

Food additives, including meat preservatives, have been incriminated as causes of aggression.[7,135] This condition is difficult to prove but should be considered whenever aggression begins or ceases after food brands or types are changed.

Genetics and Pigmentation

Epinephrine has the same metabolic pathway as the pigment melanin, and the same precursor is needed for the synthesis of both. Genetic manipulation of coat color could then be useful for breeding in or out certain behavioral characteristics, such as fear and aggression.[182]

Neural Regulation of Aggression

Numerous studies have been conducted to determine the central nervous system components of aggression. These studies often fail to differentiate the specific types of aggression under study, so results must be carefully evaluated. The hypothalamus is the primary area involved with the threat reactions of affective and irritable aggression.

With increasing electrical stimulation of the hypothalamus, characteristic components begin to appear sequentially: alerting, mydriasis, ear retraction, piloerection, hissing, and claw protrusion. These were blocked by lesions in several tegmental areas.[14] Periventricular fibers into the central gray area of the midbrain are probably also related.[51,176] The amygdala balances excitation and inhibition of external stimuli, is involved in fear reactions, and inhibits predatory and irritable aggression.[137] The defense reactions can be elicited from the hypothalamus as early as 12 days of age and from the amygdala by 21 days.[60,101] The neural substrate for escape in the hypothalamus and midbrain overlaps that for threat, and the amount of stimulation determines the resulting behavior.[1,24,30] Parts of the thalamus can also stimulate or inhibit a hypothalamic attack.[29,134] In addition, the septum, lateral aspect of the prefrontal cortex, and hippocampus probably have some inhibitory actions on agonistic behaviors.[30,134,142,176,177] A ragelike syndrome has been associated with several neural areas but is not fully understood.

Certain neurotransmitters have also been shown to influence affective aggression. Dopamine, norepinephrine, and acetylcholine are enhancers of this behavior, and serotonin, termed the *civilizing hormone,* has an inhibitory effect.[48,161] Serotonin levels may be less important than the ability to appropriately respond to serotonergic stimulation.[43] Predatory aggression is facilitated by *p*-chlorophenylalanine with a concurrent depletion in serotonin.[46] Irritable aggression is affected by changes in norepinephrine levels and metabolism, which in turn are affected by several drugs, including lithium, and by stress.[46] Acetylcholine is the primary neurotransmitter for predatory aggression, with serotonin and γ-aminobutyric acid being inhibitory.[43]

There are several explanations for the apparent inconsistency of threshold stimulus strength required to elicit aggression and other behaviors in various situations. Aggression may be evoked easily at times and only with great difficulty at other times. The primary explanation is motivation. This can be influenced by physiologic states, environment, eliciting stimuli, and previous experience.[20] Even before birth, behavior can be affected. Queens that are severely deprived nutritionally during gestation produce kittens that are less able to appropriately integrate, and thus are more reactive to, environmental and social stimuli.[149] Because we often do not know what the early nutritional history was or how it affected behavioral development, we cannot rule out its affect on inappropriate behaviors. Other influences on inconsistent aggressive reactions are explained by theories. One theory describes an innate energy that is associated with each behavior and is constantly being generated. After a certain amount of this energy has been produced but not used, the excess is used to produce an alternate behavior.[138] Unused sexual energy can give rise to excessive territorial aggression or its threat displays.[112] A second theory holds that certain neurotransmitters, such as serotonin, are produced, and the excess not used for a specific behavior results in a different behavior.[138] In the third theory, aggressive behavior is considered to be learned and thus does not originate internally.[138]

SOCIAL BEHAVIOR PROBLEMS

Social behavior, or relative lack thereof, has a profound effect on the behavior of the cat. Many changes in the environment as well as within the cat can result in abnormal behavior.

Restraint

Restraint of cats can be difficult because they may not recognize the person as an authority figure. In general, cats that are the least stressed are the most tolerant. Control of the dorsal neck initiates passive immobility, a remnant behavior from kittenhood. Thus an uncooperative animal can often be picked up by the back of the neck and held suspended. Subcutaneous injections can also take advantage of the passive immobility. While holding the cat by the loose skin just behind the head and sliding the cat slowly forward on the slippery examination table, the veterinarian can distract the cat's attention from the injection.

Intermuscular injections will often be tolerated if the cat can lean forward and away as the rear limb is held during the injection. The rear limb is held by the same hand holding the dorsal cervical skin, allowing the second hand to give the injection into the caudal thigh muscles of the restrained limb.

Collecting a blood sample from a jugular vein can often be accomplished with minimal restraint. One hand covers the top of the head and holds the mandible to maneuver it to tip the head back, while the second hand lightly covers or holds the forepaws. As the needle penetrates the skin, the holder can lightly blow air on the cat's face or gently tap the top of the head for distraction. As an alternative, most cats will lie peacefully on their side if the head and limbs are lightly restrained.

Temporary immobilization is often possible with another procedure that alters perception around the head, giving enough time for basic examination procedures. Hands can be cupped over the cat's face so that the darkness and human smells provide some stress relief. The cat muzzle has a somewhat similar effect. A rubber band can also be gently applied across the cat's ears.[109]

Social Stress

Social stress in any of its numerous forms can create problems or aggravate an existing situation. Forced situations can result in acute stress responses, and behavioral responses can be used to help identify affected cats.[189] These include events such as restraint and the invasion of territory by a new cat or human. This is particularly true for intact males if there is crowding of the living space or reduced food sources. Coping styles are based on different neurochemical brain states that may be affected by the cat's motivational state too.[103] Signs of social stress vary from aggression to catalepsy. They include failure to bury feces, housesoiling, insufficient grooming, excessive grooming, oral behaviors, scratching/shaking the head, overeating, anorexia, diarrhea, constipation, social withdrawal, vomiting, and chronic piloerection (Figure 4-9). Chronic stress of any kind, including excessive attention by well-meaning humans, can result in immunosuppression. A cat that is physically ill does not seek social relations with its peers, preferring instead the seclusion of a corner or isolated area. This behavioral tendency is useful in locating sick cats in a colony long before their illness would be obvious if they were housed individually.[55] Sick cats appear to have a lower pain threshold and a lower resistance to stress and other illnesses.[69,111] Increased susceptibility is not unique to this situation. Stress can be minimized by eliminating unnecessary handling and providing a box or sack for security in strange surroundings.

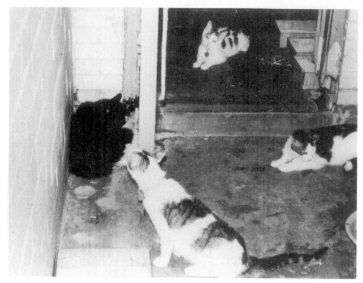

Figure 4-9 The resident male, forced into isolation by nonestrous females, shows both social withdrawal and insufficient grooming.

When old friends fight, it is usually preceded by an obvious disruption.[39] Initially the cats should be separated until both cats become calm. During this time of separation, which can be several days or weeks, it is helpful to transfer scents by rubbing each cat with the same towel.[39] After the initial few days, each cat gets to eat alone at a site that is neutral. Visual contact can be started with each cat in a carrier as they eat, with the carriers gradually being moved closer to each other with each meal. This should not happen in the core area, however.[34] Eventually one cat is fed outside the carrier, and then both. The initial goal is tolerance. In situations where the aggression is toward humans entering the territory, it may be easiest to confine the cat when guests come or to board it rather than trying to have a housesitter.[124]

The introduction of a new cat into a household or the reintroduction of a cat back into its home after it has been hospitalized or boarded can be problematic.[39,128,199] When introducing a new cat to a household that already has one or more cats, one should place the new cat in a separate room with food, water, litterbox, and a bed for a few days so the resident cat or cats become familiar with the new cat's odors and sounds. The older the resident cat is, the longer this adjustment period can take; in fact, some older cats never learn to accept newcomers. If there is a choice, it is easier to introduce a new cat of the opposite sex.[199] Acceptance will take time, so the introduction should be done gradually, beginning with physical separation lasting at least 5 to 15 days.[89] The purpose of this is to allow the newest addition to establish a miniterritory with hiding spots while both cats get used to the new odors and sounds. The new cat should get some time to roam throughout the larger space for orientation while the resident cat is confined. After the adjustment period, the owner should partially open the door to allow the cats to meet each other on their own initiative but still maintain an area where the new cat feels secure. The durations for interactions should be gradually increased over the next several days; time to destress in the miniterritories is helpful. Eventually the doors to the rooms are left open, and the cats are allowed to find each other on their own terms. With time the new cat will travel throughout the house. A cage or screen door between the cats has also been used for this introductory period.[26] A cat that has been away for a time, for example, while hospitalized, may have picked up additional odors and therefore may need to be reintroduced to the household. The previously mentioned methods can also be used under these circumstances.

A great deal of individual variation exists among cats in preference for group or individual living.[82] People who have not had problems introducing several cats into a home without special precautions often find that at some point the introduction of another cat results in behavioral changes in several of the resident cats. These changes occur when the point of overcrowding has been reached but can be altered by familiarizing the cats with each other. The new animal will probably be accepted after a period of confinement to a specific room, followed by introduction to the household as previously described. If the resident cats continue the undesirable behaviors, they too can be confined in small groups to various rooms and gradually reintroduced to the rest of the house by the controlled opening of doors. In colonies, an arrangement of shelves or boxes allows individuals the desired privacy.

The signs of stress associated with overcrowding are essentially the same as those associated with forced changes in routine and invasion of territory, whether by humans or cats. In fact, the combination of overcrowding and territorial invasion creates many problem situations. Because of their strong territorial attachments, cats are best left at home when the owner is gone. There is less change in the animal's environment, and the isolation usually is not as disturbing to the cat as it would be to dogs.

Moving can seriously affect the cat because of its strong attachment to its old home range. A cat taken to a new home all too often disappears and is never seen by its owners again. The homing instinct is so strong in most cats that new homeowners may find that an old cat is included with their new house. Cats have been reliably tracked over great distances in their efforts to reach their old home. After being taken to a new home, the cat should be placed in an enclosed area with food, water, litterbox, and bed and given several days to several weeks to adjust to the sounds and smells of the new location and to establish a feeling of security. Assurance and attention from the owner are helpful.[59] Eventually the door to that room or shed can then be left partially open so the animal can explore and still use the room for security. Even these precautions may not help older outdoor cats adjust, and they follow their strong tendency to search out their former home.

Physical changes, including immunosuppression, may accompany the translocation of the cat. In addition, a prolonged fear reaction may occur, which leads to a chronic increase in gastrointestinal motility or in constipation for a prolonged anger state.[56] It is obviously undesirable to maintain the cat in this state of psychologic and physical distress. The ideal solution is to remove the initiating factor and provide the quiet security desired by the cat. Unfortunately this option is not always possible, and the cat then must be desensitized to the environmental stimulus.

Antianxiety medications, such as the benzodiazepines, can be useful in any stress-related problem, but the dosage must be carefully monitored to avoid heavy sedation.[68,71] The TCAs and SSRIs are preferred for chronic problems because the learning of desensitization is more affective. While under the influence of the drug, the cat is repeatedly exposed to the stimulus for varying durations, from 2 to 10 weeks, depending on the problem's severity and on the cat's response. When a favorable response occurs and the cat is on a benzodiazepine, the dosage can be reduced by one third and exposure to the stimulus can be repeated. In 1 to 2 weeks more, the dosage can again be reduced by one third and the exposure repeated. In another week or so, the drug is stopped. If signs of stress reappear, the benzodiazepine can be used again and the procedure for desensitization repeated.[68] The progestins are also described for use with behavior problems caused by stress; however, their success is probably more a result of their calming effect than of specific hormonal actions.[66]

Converting an Outdoor Cat

Bringing a friendly outdoor cat into a home can be troublesome, so precautions taken early will help make the transition easier for both the cat and the human. Because the cat will be developing a new territory, it is best to confine it to a small area, like a small room, for a couple of weeks.[85] This allows the cat to establish its odors in the new territory by shedding hair and dander, making urine marking unnecessary. Encouraging activities like play will promote exercise and human interaction. When the cat seems relatively comfortable in this small new territory, allow it to have access to more of the house by letting it explore for gradually longer periods each day. It will be important not to reinforce attempts to go out by successful escapes.[126] Vocalizations also should not be rewarded by attention, food, or play. All interactions should occur when the cat is showing an acceptable behavior.

Many of these cats seem to retain an interest in going outside again, as evidenced by their spending long periods sitting in windows, retaining the tendency to escape through open doors or windows, and long periods of vocalization near doors or windows. Some owners ignore these behaviors, and others allow the cat outside for short periods as free roaming or under leash control. A few owners use cat-proof patios, porches, or small yard areas to restrain the cat but allow it some fresh air.

Improper Socialization

Young kittens that do not experience normal socialization will react in unusual ways later in life. Kittens obtained before 5 weeks of age may not socialize well to their own species and as a result will become overly attached to humans. As they mature, these cats often become aggressive toward other cats or show an abnormal behavior, such as self-mutilation, to gain attention. Such extreme behavior could become learned if reinforced by attention.[76] Mating and maternal behaviors will be affected because this animal does not recognize other cats or kittens as beings of the same species. Kittens raised without peers may not learn proper control of teeth or claws or may not learn to use them at all, because humans tend not to interact with the kitten as frequently as the mother would. Some of these youngsters develop timid or aggressive attitudes toward people and tend not to make suitable pets.[65,67,75] Orphans that do not mutilate each other by excessive sucking can partially compensate for the lack of maternal care.[75]

The cat that is minimally socialized to other species by 8 weeks may direct aggressive actions toward members of other species such as humans (both adults and children) or dogs. This cat is suffering from the "isolated syndrome," and social stress on such an animal causes problems. Adoption of an adult cat or older kitten is ill advised unless its background is known. Sedation with a great deal of handling to desensitize the cat may be useful in some extreme situations.[54] A cat poorly socialized to humans may learn to accept one or two as part of its environment but when confronted with strangers will crouch and growl in a pariah-like reaction. When extremely crowded, as when the owners give a party, the cat may even show aggression. Putting the cat in a quiet room away from the social activities can eliminate a great deal of tension on both sides. The isolated syndrome handicaps the individual in social situations and gives it a marked preference for an environment relatively barren of other beings.[58]

Runts in a litter should be carefully evaluated before being accepted as a pet. Possible intimidation by littermates during this critical early period may have affected that animal's capacity for socialization.

Overattachment and Separation Anxiety

Some cats are particularly demanding for attention, even from kittenhood. They may pace and vocalize if the owner is not immediately available, even to the point of interfering with the owner's sleep. The clingy behavior may increase as a cat gets older, and it has become one of the primary reasons for euthanasia of older, but otherwise healthy, cats.[86] Because most affected cats are older, a good medical checkup is important. It is also necessary to rule out a day/night activity shift, which can be treated with melatonin, and feline cognitive dysfunction. If separation anxiety is the diagnosis, behavior modification teaches the cat how to tolerate short but increasingly longer owner absences. Drug therapy with TCAs or SSRIs may be helpful too.

Separation anxiety has only recently been defined as a problem in cats, even though it has been recognized since first described in dogs. A study of 136 cats diagnosed with separation anxiety reports 32.4% are 3 to 5 years of age, 26.5% are 1 to 3 years, and 17.6% are 5 to 7 years.[169] The behaviors shown by these cats can vary widely, but inappropriate urination is most common, occurring in 70.6% of the cats, with 75% of those urinating on the owner's bed.[170] Just more than 35% of the cats show inappropriate defecation.[170] Destructive behaviors (8.8%), excessive vocalization (11.8%), and psychogenic grooming (5.9%) are also seen.[169,170] Factors that may contribute to the problem include long work hours, vacations, business travel, or changes that affect the cat's schedule.[169] About one fifth of the cats tend to follow the owners around the house (dogs with separation anxiety tend to follow owners, but cats generally do not).

Treating separation anxiety in cats may be more dependent on drug therapy than is typical for dogs. Several affected cats are described by owners as being very anxious, nervous individuals all the time, so drugs like the TCAs and SSRIs are appropriate. This is the same type of personality that tends to show excessive grooming when stressed by outdoor cats. Gradual desensitization to owner departures can be taught, and they can be coupled with food as a counterconditioner.

Extreme Timidity

The timid cat can also be an undesirable pet and a difficult patient. Timidity can be inherited, although the specific behavior may not express itself until a later age.[7,59]

Timid kittens dislike restraint, do not relax when picked up, tend to remain immobile instead of exploring a new area, do not follow people, are less playful, and fear noise.[7,59] Stimulus desensitization, with decreasing dosages of tranquilizers and continuous stimulus exposure, can be useful for some of these cats. Buspirone is the drug of choice because it tends to increase boldness while reducing anxieties. Occasionally cats that have undergone anesthesia become extremely timid or aggressive and require patient, careful handling to reverse the behavior. No correlation has yet been made between production of this behavior and handling techniques or use of a specific anesthetic agent. Care should be exercised, however, when using anesthetics that are known to cause psychic phenomena in human patients, such as ketamine hydrochloride.

REFERENCES

1. Adams DB: Cells related to fighting behavior recorded from midbrain central gray neuropil of cat, *Science* 159:894–896, Feb 23, 1968.
2. Baron A, Stewart CN, Warren JM: Patterns of social interaction in cats *(Felis domestica)*, *Behaviour* 11:56–67, 1956.
3. Barry K: Time-budgets and social behavior of the indoor domestic cat. Paper presented at American Veterinary Society Animal Behavior meeting, Pittsburgh, Penn, July 10, 1995.
4. Barry KJ: Gender differences in the social behavior of the indoor-only neutered domestic cat, PhD Dissertation, University of Georgia, May 1998.
5. Barry KJ, Crowell-Davis SL: Gender differences in the social behavior of the neutered indoor-only domestic cat, *Appl Anim Behav Sci* 64(3):193–211, 1999.
6. Beadle M: *The cat: history, biology, and behavior*, New York, 1977, Simon & Schuster.
7. Beaver BV: Feline behavioral problems, *Vet Clin North Am* 6:333–340, Aug 1976.
8. Beaver BV: Disorders of behavior. In Sherding RG, editor: *The cat: diseases and clinical management*, New York, 1989, Churchill Livingstone.
9. Beaver BV: Feline behavioral problems other than housesoiling, *J Am Anim Hosp Assoc* 25:465–469, July/Aug 1989.
10. Beaver BV: Psychogenic manifestations of environmental disturbances. In August JR, editor: *Consultations in feline medicine*, Philadelphia, 1991, WB Saunders.
11. Beaver BV: Differential approach to aggression by dogs and cats, *Vet Q* 16(suppl 1):48S, 1994.
12. Bernstein P, Strack M: Home ranges, favored spots, time-sharing patterns, and tail usage by 14 cats in the home, *Anim Behav Consult Newslett* 10(3):1–3, 1993.
13. Bernstein PL, Strack M: A game of cat and house: spatial patterns and behavior in 14 domestic cats *(Felis catus)* in the home, *Anthrozoös* 9(1):25–39, 1996.
14. Berntson GG: Blockade and release of hypothalamically and naturally elicited aggressive behaviors in cats following midbrain lesions, *J Comp Physiol Psychol* 81(3):541–554, 1972.
15. Blackshaw JK: Abnormal behaviour in cats, *Aust Vet J* 65:395–396, Dec 1988.
16. Blackshaw JK: Management of orally based problems and aggression in cats, *Aust Vet Practit* 21(3):122–125, 1991.
17. Blumer D, Migeon C: Hormone and hormonal agents in the treatment of aggression, *J Nerv Ment Dis* 160:127–137, Feb 1975.
18. Bond E, Mathews SL, Hart BL, Beaver B: Aggressive behavior, *Feline Pract* 15(5):29–30, 1985.
19. Borchelt PL, Voith VL: Diagnosis and treatment of aggression problems in cats, *Vet Clin North Am Small Anim Pract* 12:665–671, Nov 1982.
20. Borchelt PL, Voith VL: Aggressive behavior in dogs and cats, *Compend Contin Educ* 7(11):949–957, 1985.

21. Borchelt PL, Voith VL: Aggressive behavior in cats, *Compend Contin Educ* 9:49–57, Jan 1987.
22. Bradshaw JWS, Hall SL: Affiliative behaviour of related and unrelated pairs of cats in catteries: a preliminary report, *Appl Anim Behav Sci* 63(3):251–255, 1999.
23. Bradshaw JWS, Horsfield GF, Allen JA, Robinson IH: Feral cats: their role in the population dynamics of *Felis catus, Appl Anim Behav Sci* 65(3):273–283, 1999.
24. Brown JL, Hunsperger RW: Neurothology and motivation of agonistic behaviour, *Anim Behav* 11:439–448, Oct 1963.
25. Brunner F: The application of behavior studies in small animal practice. In Fox MW, editor: *Abnormal behavior in animals,* Philadelphia, 1968, WB Saunders.
26. Bryant D: *The care and handling of cats,* New York, 1944, Ives Washburn.
27. Chapman B, Voith VL: Geriatric behavior problems not always related to age, *DVM* 18(3):32, 33, 38, 39, 1987.
28. Chapman BL, Voith VL: Cat aggression redirected to people: 14 cases (1981–1987), *J Am Vet Med Assoc* 196:947–950, March 15, 1990.
29. Chi CC, Bandler RJ, Flynn JP: Neuroanatomic projections related to biting attack elicited from ventral midbrain in cats, *Brain Behav Evol* 13:91–110, 1976.
30. Clemente CD, Chase MH: Neurological substrates of aggressive behavior, *Annu Rev Physiol* 35:329–356, 1973.
31. Cole DD, Shafer JN: A study of social dominance in cats, *Behaviour* 27:39–53, 1966.
32. Collard RR: Fear of strangers and play behavior in kittens with varied social experience, *Child Dev* 38:877–891, 1967.
33. Crowell-Davis S: Aggressive behavior in cats, *Proc Am Anim Hosp Assoc* pp 29–33, March 10–14, 2001.
34. Crowell-Davis SL: Social behavior and aggression in the cat. Paper presented at American Veterinary Medical Association meeting, San Francisco, July 9, 1994.
35. Crowell-Davis SL: Social behavior and gender in domestic cats. Paper presented at American Veterinary Medical Association meeting, Reno, Nev, July 22, 1997.
36. Crowell-Davis SL: Social behavior in cats. Paper presented at Western Veterinary Conference, Las Vegas, February 22, 2000.
37. Crowell-Davis SL: Social organization and communication in cats, *Proc Am Anim Hosp Assoc* pp 24–28, March 10–14, 2001.
38. Crowell-Davis SL: Update on understanding cat social organization and communication. Available at www.avma.org/noah/members/convention/conv01/notes/04010102.asp.
39. Crowell-Davis SL, Barry K, Wolfe R: Social behavior and aggressive problems of cats, *Vet Clin North Am Small Anim Pract* 27(3):549–568, 1997.
40. Deag JM, Manning A, Lawrence CE: Factors influencing the mother-kitten relationship. In Turner DC, Bateson PPG, editors: *The domestic cat: the biology of its behaviour,* Cambridge, 1988, Cambridge University Press.
41. DeBoer JN: Dominance relations in pairs of domestic cats, *Behav Process* 2:227–242, 1977.
42. deMonte M, LePape G: Behavioural effects of cage enrichment in single-caged adult cats, *Anim Welfare* 6(1):53–66, 1997.
43. Dodman NH: Pharmacological treatment of behavioral problems in cats, *Vet Forum* pp 62–65, 71, April 1995.
44. Dow SW, Dreitz MJ, Hoover EA: Exploring the link between feline immunodeficiency virus infection and neurologic disease in cats, *Vet Med* 87(12):1181–1184, 1992.
45. Eaton RL: The evolution of sociality in the Felidae. In Eaton RL, editor: *The world's cats,* ed 3, Seattle, 1976, Carnivore Research Institute.
46. Eichelman BS Jr, Thoa NB: The aggressive monoamines, *Biol Psychiatry* 6(2):143–164, 1973.
47. Eleftheriou BE, Scott JP: *The physiology of aggression and defeat,* New York, 1971, Plenum Publishing.

48. Everett GM: The pharmacology of aggressive behavior in animals and man, *Psychopharmacol Bull* 13:15–17, Jan 1977.

49. Ewer RF: *Ethology of mammals,* London, 1968, Paul Elek Ltd.

50. Ewer RF: *The carnivores,* Ithaca, NY, 1973, Cornell University Press.

51. Ewert JP: *Neuroethology,* New York, 1980, Springer-Verlag.

52. Feldman HN: Domestic cats and passive submission, *Anim Behav* 47:457–459, 1994.

53. Feral cat colonies in Great Britain, *Bull Inst Study Anim Probl* 1:5, March/April 1979.

54. Fox MW: New information on feline behavior, *Mod Vet Pract* 56(4):50–52, 1965.

55. Fox MW: Natural environment: theoretical and practical aspects for breeding and rearing laboratory animals, *Lab Anim Care* 16(4):316–321, 1966.

56. Fox MW: Aggression: its adaptive and maladaptive significance in man and animals. In Fox MW, editor: *Abnormal behavior in animals,* Philadelphia, 1968, WB Saunders.

57. Fox MW: Ethology: an overview. In Fox MW, editor: *Abnormal behavior in animals,* Philadelphia, 1968, WB Saunders.

58. Fox MW: Neurobehavioral development and the genotype-environment interaction, *Q Rev Biol* 45:131–147, June 1970.

59. Fox MW: *Understanding your cat,* New York, 1974, Coward McCann & Geoghegan.

60. Fox MW: The behaviour of cats. In Hafez ESE, editor: *The behaviour of domestic animals,* ed 3, Baltimore, 1975, Williams & Wilkins.

61. Frank D: Diagnosis and treatment of intercat aggression. Available at www.avma.org/noah/members/convention/conv01/notes/04010103.asp.

62. Gittleman JL, Harvey PH: Carnivore home-range size, metabolic needs and ecology, *Behav Ecol Sociobiol* 10:57–63, 1982.

63. Griffiths AO, Silberberg A: Stray animals: their impact on a community, *Mod Vet Pract* 56(4):255–256, 1975.

64. Guyot GW, Bennett TL, Cross HA: The effects of social isolation on the behavior of juvenile domestic cats, *Dev Psychobiol* 13(3): 317–329, 1980.

65. Guyot GW, Cross HA, Bennett TL: The domestic cat. In Roy MA, editor: *Species identity and attachment: a phylogenetic evaluation,* New York, 1980, Garland STPM Press.

66. Hart BL: Gonadal hormones and behavior of the female cat, *Feline Pract* 2:6–8, July/Aug 1972.

67. Hart BL: Maternal behavior. II. The nursing-suckling relationship and the effects of maternal deprivation, *Feline Pract* 2(6):6–7, 10, 1972.

68. Hart BL: Psychopharmacology in feline practice, *Feline Pract* 3(3):6, 8, 1973.

69. Hart BL: Disease processes and behavior, *Feline Pract* 3(6):6–7, 1973.

70. Hart BL: Social interaction in cats, *Feline Pract* 4(3):12, 20, 1974.

71. Hart BL: Types of aggressive behavior, *Can Pract* 1(1):6, 8, 1974.

72. Hart BL: Behavioral patterns related to territoriality and social communication, *Feline Pract* 5(1):12, 14, 1975.

73. Hart BL: A quiz on feline behavior, *Feline Pract* 5(3):12, 14, 1975.

74. Hart BL: Social interactions between cats and their owners, *Feline Pract* 6(1):6, 8, 1976.

75. Hart BL: Behavioral aspects of selecting a new cat, *Feline Pract* 6(5):8, 10, 14, 1976.

76. Hart BL: Aggression in cats, *Feline Pract* 7(2):22, 24, 28, 1977.

77. Hart BL: Feline behavior problems, *Friskies Symp Behav* pp 28–39, 1994.

78. Hart BL, Hart LA: Selecting the best companion animal: breed and gender specific behavioral profiles. In Anderson RK, Hart BL, Hart LA, editors: *The pet connection: its influence on our health and quality of life,* Minneapolis, 1984, Center to Study Human-Animal Relationships and Environments, University of Minnesota.

79. Hart BL, Hart LA: *Canine and feline behavioral therapy,* Philadelphia, 1985, Lea & Febiger.

80. Heidenberger E: Housing conditions and behavioural problems of indoor cats as assessed by their owners, *Appl Anim Behav Sci* 52(3,4):345–364, 1997.

81. Henry JP: Mechanisms of psychosomatic disease in animals, *Adv Vet Sci Comp Med* 20:115–145, 1976.

82. Hetts S: Cats behaving badly, *Vet Pract News* 13(7):26–27, 2001.

83. Houpt KA: Animal behavior as a subject for veterinary students, *Cornell Vet* 66:73–81, Jan 1976.

84. Houpt KA: Companion animal behavior: a review of dog and cat behavior in the field, the laboratory and the clinic, *Cornell Vet* 75:248–261, 1985.

85. Houpt KA: Transforming an outdoor cat into an indoor cat, *Vet Med* 95(11):830, 2000.

86. Houpt KA: Cognitive dysfunction in geriatric cats. In August JR, editor: *Consultations in feline internal medicine,* vol 4, Philadelphia, 2001, WB Saunders.

87. Houpt KA, Beaver B: Behavioral problems of geriatric dogs and cats, *Vet Clin North Am Small Anim Pract* 11:643–652, Nov 1981.

88. Houpt KA, Honig SU, Reisner IR: Breaking the human-companion animal bond, *J Am Vet Med Assoc* 208(10):1653–1659, 1996.

89. Hunthausen WL: Rule out medical etiologies first in geriatric behavior problems, *DVM* 22(7):24, 38, 1991.

90. Hutchinson RR, Ulrich RE, Azrin NH: Effects of age and related factors on the pain-aggression reaction, *J Comp Physiol Psychol* 59(3):365–369, 1965.

91. Inselman-Temkin BR, Flynn JP: Sex-dependent effects of gonadal and gonadotropic hormones on centrally-elicited attack in cats, *Brain Res* 60:393–409, Oct 12, 1973.

92. James RB: Notes on blindness in cats, *Vet Med Small Anim Clin* 77(5):776, 778, 1982.

93. Jewell PA: The concept of home range in mammals, *Symp Zool Soc Lond* 18:85–109, 1966.

94. Jöchle W, Jöchle M: Reproductive and behavioral control in the male and female cat with progestins: long-term field observations in individual animals, *Theriogenology* 3(5):179–185, 1975.

95. Johnson PD, Pullen MM, Cox PD: The socio-economic implications of animal bites—St. Paul, Minnesota 1976, *University of Minnesota Veterinary Medical Reporter* 114:1, May/June 1978.

96. Jones E, Coman BJ: Ecology of the feral cat, *Felis catus* (l.), in Southern Australia. III. Home ranges and population ecology in semiarid North-West Victoria, *Aust Wildl Res* 9:409–420, 1982.

97. Karsh E: Factors influencing the socialisation of cats to people. In Anderson RK, Hart BL, Hart LA, editors: *The pet connection: its influence on our health and quality of life,* Minneapolis, 1984, Center to Study Human-Animal Relationships and Environments, University of Minnesota.

98. Karsh EB, Turner DC: The human-cat relationship. In Turner DC, Bateson P, editors: *The domestic cat: the biology of its behaviour,* Cambridge, 1988, Cambridge University Press.

99. Katz RJ, Thomas E: Effects of a novel anti-aggressive agent upon two types of brain stimulated emotional behavior, *Psychopharmacology* 48(1):79–82, 1976.

100. Kerby G, Macdonald DW: Cat society and consequences of colony size. In Turner DC, Bateson PPG, editors: *The domestic cat: the biology of its behaviour,* Cambridge, 1988, Cambridge University Press.

101. Kling A, Kovach JK, Tucker TJ: The behaviour of cats. In Hafez ESE, editor: *The behaviour of domestic animals,* ed 2, Baltimore, 1969, Williams & Wilkins.

102. Kolb B, Nonneman AJ: The development of social responsiveness in kittens, *Anim Behav* 23(2):368–374, 1975.

103. Koolhaas JM, de Boer SF, Bohus B: Motivational systems or motivational states: behavioural and physiological evidence, *Appl Anim Behav Sci* 53(1,2):131–144, 1997.

104. Kruuk H: Functional aspects of social hunting in carnivores. In Baerends G, Manning A, Beers C, editors: *Function and evolution in behaviour,* New York, 1975, Oxford University Press.

105. Kuo ZY: Studies on the basic factors in animal fighting. VII. Inter-species coexistence in mammals, *J Genet Psychol* 97:211–225, 1960.
106. Kydd AM, Boswood B, Watts AE: A new syndrome in cats? *Vet Rec* 87:518, Oct 24, 1973.
107. Landsberg G: Feline behavior and welfare, *J Am Vet Med Assoc* 208(4):502–505, 1996.
108. Laundré J: The daytime behaviour of domestic cats in a free-roaming population, *Anim Behav* 25:990–998, 1977.
109. Leedy MG, Fishelson BA, Cooper LL: A simple method of restraint for use with cats, *Feline Pract* 13(5):32–33, 1983.
110. Lehman HC: The child's attitude toward the dog versus the cat, *J Gen Psychol* 35:62–72, 1928.
111. Levinson BM: Man and his feline pet, *Mod Vet Pract* 53:35–39, Nov 1972.
112. Leyhausen P: Communal organization of solitary mammals, *Symp Zool Soc Lond* 14:249–263, 1965.
113. Leyhausen P: *Cat behavior: the predatory and social behavior of domestic and wild cats,* New York, 1978, Garland STPM Press.
114. Leyhausen P: The tame and the wild—another just-so story? In Turner DC, Bateson P, editors: *The domestic cat: the biology of its behaviour,* Cambridge, 1988, Cambridge University Press.
115. Liberg O: Spacing patterns in a population of rural free roaming domestic cats, *Oikos* 35(3):336–349, 1980.
116. Liberg O: Predation and social behaviour in a population of domestic cat. An evolutionary perspective, Dissertation, Sweden, 1981, Department of Animal Ecology, University of Lund.
117. Liberg O, Sandell M: Spatial organisation and reproductive tactics in the domestic cat and other felids. In Turner DC, Bateson P, editors: *The domestic cat: the biology of its behaviour,* Cambridge, 1988, Cambridge University Press.
118. Lorenz K, Leyhausen P: *Motivation of human and animal behavior,* New York, 1973, Van Nostrand Reinhold.
119. Lowe SE, Bradshaw JWS: Ontogeny of individuality in the domestic cat in the home environment, *Anim Behav* 61(1):231–237, 2001.
120. Macdonald DW: The ecology of carnivore social behaviour, *Nature Lond* 301:379–389, Feb 3, 1983.
121. Macdonald DW, Apps PJ, Carr GM, Kerby G: *Social dynamics, nursing coalitions and infanticide among farm cats,* Felis catus, Berlin, 1987, Paul Parey Scientific Publishers.
122. Marder A: Managing behavioural problems in puppies and kittens, *Small Anim Behav Friskies Pet Care,* 1997.
123. Marder AR: Psychotropic drugs and behavioral therapy, *Vet Clin North Am Small Anim Pract* 21(2):329–342, 1991.
124. Marder AR: Diagnosing and treating aggression problems in cats, *Vet Med* 88(8):736–742, 1993.
125. Martin P, Bateson P: Behavioural development in the cat. In Turner DC, Bateson P, editors: *The domestic cat: the biology of its behaviour,* Cambridge, 1988, Cambridge University Press.
126. Mathews S: An outdoor cat to an indoor cat, *Feline Pract* 12(6):6–10, 1982.
127. McCune S: The impact of paternity and early socialisation on the development of cats' behaviour to people and novel objects, *Appl Anim Behav Sci* 45(1–2):109–124, 1995.
128. McKeown DB, Luescher UA, Machum MA: Aggression in feline housemates: a case study, *Can Vet J* 29(9):742–744, 1988.
129. Mendl M, Harcourt R: Individuality in the domestic cat. In Turner DC, Bateson P, editors: *The domestic cat: the biology of its behaviour,* Cambridge, 1988, Cambridge University Press.
130. Mertens C: Human-cat interactions in the home setting, *Anthrozoös* 4(4):214–231, 1991.

131. Mertens C, Turner DC: Experimental analysis of human-cat interactions during first encounters, *Anthrozoös* 2(2):83–97, 1988.

132. Miller J: The domestic cat: perspective on the nature and diversity of cats, *J Am Vet Med Assoc* 208(4):498–502, 1996.

133. Monroe RR: Anticonvulsants in the treatment of aggression, *J Nerv Ment Dis* 160:119–126, Feb 1975.

134. Morgenson GJ, Huang YH: The neurobiology of motivated behavior, *Prog Neurobiol* 1:55–83, 1973.

135. Mosier JE: Personal communication, 1970.

136. Mosier JE: Common medical and behavioral problems in cats, *Mod Vet Pract* 56:699–703, Oct 1975.

137. Moyer KE: Kinds of aggression and their physiological basis, *Comm Behav Biol A* 2:65–87, 1968.

138. Moyer KE: A model of aggression with implications for research, *Psychopharmacol Bull* 13:14–15, Jan 1977.

139. Natoli E: Spacing pattern in a colony of urban stray cats (*Felis catus* L.) in the historic centre of Rome, *Appl Anim Behav Sci* 14(3).289–304, 1985.

140. Natoli E, De Vito E: Agonistic behaviour, dominance rank and copulatory success in a large multi-male feral cat, *Felis catus* L., colony in central Rome, *Anim Behav* 42:227–241, 1991.

141. Neville PF, Remfry J: Effect of neutering on two groups of feral cats, *Vet Rec* 114:447–450, May 5, 1984.

142. Nonneman AJ, Kolb BE: Lesions of hippocampus or prefrontal cortex alter species-typical behaviours in the cat, *Behav Biol* 12(1):41–54, 1974.

143. Norsworthy GD: Dealing with fractious feline patients, *Vet Med* 88(11):1053–1057, 1060, 1993.

144. Overall KL: Preventing behavior problems: early prevention and recognition in puppies and kittens, *Purina Specialty Review* pp 13–29, 1992.

145. Overall KL: Management related problems in feline behavior, *Feline Pract* 22(1):13–15, 1994.

146. Overall KL: Feline aggression, part 1, *Feline Pract* 22(4):25–26, 1994.

147. Overall KL: Feline aggression, part 2, *Feline Pract* 22(5):16–17, 1994.

148. Overall KL: Feline aggression, part 3, *Feline Pract* 22(6):16–17, 1994.

149. Overall KL: Cat aggression: client vigilance imperative in correcting serious behavior disorder, *DVM Newsmagazine* 26(10):3S, 18S, 1995.

150. Overall KL: Behavioral knowledge can help smooth introduction of new pet to household, *DVM Newsmagazine* 26(11):6S, 12S, 13S, 1995.

151. Overall KL: Rational behavior pharmacology. The Friskies Symposium on Behavior pp 18–28, 1996.

152. Overall KL: Managing an aggressive cat, *Vet Med* 93(12):1051–1052, 1998.

153. Overall KL: Master class case discussion: diagnosis and treatment of canine and feline aggression, *Proc Am Anim Hosp Assoc* pp 76–87, April 1–5, 2000.

154. Panaman R: Behaviour and ecology of free-ranging female farm cats (*Felis catus* L.), *Z Tierpsychol* 56:59–73, 1981.

155. Passanisi WC, Macdonald DW: Group discrimination on the basis of urine in a farm cat colony. In Macdonald DW, Müller-Schwarze D, Natynczwk SE, editors: *Chemical signals in vertebrates,* ed 5, New York, 1990, Oxford University Press.

156. Patience pays off for hero cat, *Friskies Research Digest* 14:14, Spring 1978.

157. Personality change in a Siamese cat, *Vet Med Small Anim Clin* 59:144, Feb 1964.

158. Podberscek AL, Blackshaw JK, Beattie AW: The behaviour of laboratory colony cats and their reactions to a familiar and unfamiliar person, *Appl Anim Behav Sci* 31(1–2):119–130, 1991.

159. Poe E, Hope K: Group housing products for cats, *Lab Anim* 29(4):40–43, 2000.

160. Poucet B, Thinus-Blanc C, Chapus N: Route planning in cats, in relation to the visibility of the goal, *Anim Behav* 31:594–599, May 1983.

161. Reis DJ: Central neurotransmitters in aggression, *Res Publ Assoc Res Nerv Ment Dis* 52:119–147, 1974.

162. Reisner IR, Houpt KA, Hollis NE, Quimby FW: Friendliness to humans and defensive aggression in cats: the influence of handling and paternity, *Physiol Behav* 55(6):1119–1124, 1994.

163. Rheingold HL, Eckerman CO: Familiar social and nonsocial stimuli and the kitten's response to a strange environment, *Dev Psychobiol* 4(1):71–89, 1971.

164. Romanes GJ: *Mental evolution in animals,* New York, 1969, AMS Press.

165. Rosenblatt JS: Sucking and home orientation in the kitten: a comparative developmental study. In Tobach E, Aronson LR, Shaw E, editors: *The biopsychology of development,* New York, 1971, Academic Press.

166. Rosenblatt JS: Learning in newborn kittens, *Sci Am* 227:18–25, 1972.

167. Rosenblatt JS, Turkewitz G, Schneirla TC: Development of suckling and related behavior in neonate kittens. In Bliss EL, editor: *Roots of behavior,* New York, 1962, Harper & Row.

168. Schwartz S: Carbamazepine in the control of aggressive behavior in cats, *J Am Anim Hosp Assoc* 30(5):515–519, 1994.

169. Schwartz S: Comparison of separation anxiety in the cat and dog. Available at www.avma.org/noah/members/convention/conv01/notes/040100104.asp.

170. Schwartz S: Separation anxiety syndrome in cats: 136 cases (1991–2000), *J Am Vet Med Assoc* 220(7):1028–1033, 2002.

171. Scott JP: The analysis of social organization in animals, *Ecology* 37:213–221, April 1956.

172. Scott JP: Critical periods in behavioral development, *Science* 138:949–958, Nov 30, 1962.

173. Seitz PFD: Infantile experience and adult behavior in animal subjects, *Psychosom Med* 21:353–378, 1959.

174. Sheard MH: Lithium in the treatment of aggression, *J Nerv Ment Dis* 160(2):108–118, 1975.

175. Shell L: Feline ischemic encephalopathy (cerebral infarct), *Virginia Vet Notes* 35:3, Sep/Oct 1988.

176. Siegel A, Edinger H: Neural control of aggression and rage behavior. In Morgane PJ, Panksepp J, editors: *Behavioral studies of the hypothalamus,* vol 3, pt B, New York, 1981, Marcel Dekker.

177. Siegel A, Edinger H, Dotto M: Effects of electrical stimulation of the lateral aspect of the prefrontal cortex upon attack behavior in cats, *Brain Res* 93(3):473–484, 1975.

178. Smith DFE, Bradshaw JWS: Social behaviour and stress in rescued cats, *Appl Anim Behav Sci* 31(3–4):291–292, 1991.

179. Sutin J, Rose J, Van Atta L, Thalmann R: Electrophysiological studies in an animal model of aggressive behavior, *Res Publ Assoc Nerv Ment Dis* 52:93–118, 1974.

180. Taliaferro L, Beaver BV: Animal behavior case of the month, *J Am Vet Med Assoc* 209(1):66–68, 1996.

181. Todd NB: Behavior and genetics of the domestic cat, *Cornell Vet* 53:99–107, Jan 1963.

182. Todd NB: Cats and commerce, *Sci Am* 237:100–107, Nov 1977.

183. Turner D, Appleby D, Magnus E: The Association of Pet Behaviour Counsellors: annual review of cases 2000. Available at www.apbc.org.uk/2000/report.htm.

184. Turner DC, Feaver J, Mendl M, Bateson P: Variation in domestic cat behaviour towards humans: a paternal effect, *Anim Behav* 34:1890–1892, Dec 1986.

185. Turner DC, Meister O: Hunting behaviour of the domestic cat. In Turner DC, Bateson P, editors: *The domestic cat: the biology of its behaviour,* Cambridge, 1988, Cambridge University Press.

186. Turner DC, Mertens C: Home range size, overlap, and exploitation in domestic arm cats *(Felis catus), Behaviour* 99:22–45, 1986.
187. Underman AE: Bite wounds inflicted by dogs and cats, *Vet Clin North Am Small Anim Pract* 17(1):195–207, 1987.
188. Ursin H: Flight and defense behavior in cats, *J Comp Physiol Psychol* 58:180–186, Oct 1964.
189. van den Bos R: Post-conflict stress-response in confined group-living cats *(Felis silvestris catus), Appl Anim Behav Sci* 59(4):323–330, 1998.
190. Voith VL, Borchelt PL: Social behavior of domestic cats, *Compend Contin Educ* 8:637–647, Sep 1986.
191. Voith VL, Marder AR: Feline behavioral disorders. In Morgan RV, editor: *Handbook of small animal practice,* New York, 1988, Churchill Livingstone.
192. Warner RE: Demography and movements of free-ranging domestic cats in rural Illinois, *J Wildl Manag* 49:340–346, 1985.
193. Weigel I: Small cats and clouded leopards. In Grzimek HCB, editor: *Grzimek's animal life encyclopedia,* vol 12, New York, 1975, Van Nostrand Reinhold.
194. Wemmer C, Scow K: Communication in the Felidae with emphasis on scent marking and contact patterns. In Sebeok TA, editor: *How animals communicate,* Bloomington, 1977, Indiana University Press.
195. Winslow CN: Observations of dominance-subordination in cats, *J Genet Psychol* 52:425–428, 1938.
196. Wolfe R, Crowell-Davis S: Developing a model of sociality for the free-ranging domestic cat, *Am Vet Soc Anim Behav* 22(3):7, 2000.
197. Wolfe RC: The social organization of the free-ranging domestic cat *(Felis catus),* PhD Dissertation, University of Georgia, 2001.
198. Wolfe RC, Sung W, Crowell-Davis S: Individual and gender preferences in association in a free-ranging population of domestic cats, *Am Vet Soc Anim Behav* 19(2):4, 1997.
199. Wolski TR: Feline behavioral problems: social causes and practical solutions, *Cornell Feline Health Center News* 3:1, 2, 4–6, May, 1981.
200. Wolski TR: Spatial distribution of free-ranging domestic cats. Paper presented at Animal Behavior Society meeting, Knoxville, Tenn, June 1981.
201. Worden AN: Abnormal behaviour in the dog and cat, *Vet Rec* 71:966–978, Dec 26, 1959.
202. Zaunbrecher KI, Smith RE: Neutering of feral cats as an alternative to eradication programs, *J Am Vet Med Assoc* 203(3):449–452, 1993.

Additional Readings

Adamec RE, Stark-Adamec C, Livingston KE: The expression of an early developmentally emergent defensive bias in the adult domestic cat *(Felis catus)* in non-predatory situations, *Appl Anim Ethol* 10:89–108, 1983.
Allen RP, Safer D, Covi L: Effects of psychostimulants on aggression, *J Nerv Ment Dis* 160:137–145, Feb 1975.
Allikmets LH: Cholinergic mechanisms in aggressive behaviour, *Med Biol* 52:19–30, Feb 1974.
Andy OJ, Giurintano L, Giurintano S, McDonald T: Thalamic modulation of aggression, *Pav J Biol Sci* 10:85–101, April/June 1975.
August JR: Dog and cat bites, *J Am Vet Med Assoc* 193:1394–1398, Dec 1, 1988.
Baron A, Stewart CM, Warren JM: Patterns of social interaction in cats *(Felis domestica), Behaviour* 11:56–66, 1957.
Berntson GG, Leibowitz SF: Biting attack in cats: evidence for central muscarinic mediation, *Brain Res* 51:366–370, 1973.

Blacklock GA: A cat's purr...on purpose? *Cat Fancy* 16:20–22, Aug 1973.

Blackshaw JK: Management of behavioral problems in cats, *Feline Pract* 22(3):25–29, 1994.

Candland DK, Milne DW: Species differences in approach-behavior as a function of developmental environment, *Anim Behav* 14:539–545, Oct 1966.

Collard RR: Fear of strangers and play behavior in kittens with varied social experience, *Child Dev* 38:877–891, Sep 1967.

Dallaire A: Stress and behavior in domestic animals: temperament as a predisposing factor to stereotypies, *Ann N Y Acad Sci* 697:269–274, Oct 29, 1993.

De Molina AF, Hunsperger RW: Organization of subcortical systems governing defense and flight reactions in the cat, *J Physiol* 160:200–213, Feb 1962.

Eichelman B: Neurochemical studies of aggression in animals, *Psychopharmacol Bull* 13:17–19, Jan 1977.

Feaver J, Mende M, Bateson P: A method for rating the individual distinctiveness of domestic cats, *Anim Behav* 34:1016–1025, 1986.

Fokin VF: Dynamics of active defensive reflex formation in cats, *Zh Vyssh Nerv Deiat* 25:752–759, July/Aug 1975.

Fox MW: Psychomotor disturbances. In Fox MW, editor: *Abnormal behavior in animals,* Philadelphia, 1968, WB Saunders.

Fox MW: Behavioral effects of rearing dogs with cats during the "critical period of socialization," *Behaviour* 35:273–280, 1969.

Fox MW: Psychopathology in man and lower animals, *J Am Vet Med Assoc* 159(1):66–77, 1971.

Glusman M: The hypothalamic "savage" syndrome, *Res Publ Assoc Res Nerv Ment Dis* 52:52–90, 1974.

Guyot GW, Cross HA, Bennett TL: Early social isolation of the domestic cat: responses during mechanical toy testing, *Appl Anim Ethol* 10:109–116, March 1983.

Hart BL: Gonadal hormones and behavior of the male cat, *Feline Pract* 2(3):7–8, 1972.

Hart BL: Genetics and behavior, *Feline Pract* 3(1):5, 8, 1973.

Hart BL: The brain and behavior, *Feline Pract* 3(5):4, 6, 1973.

Hart BL: Gonadal androgen and sociosexual behavior of male mammals: a comparative analysis, *Psychol Bull* 81:383–400, July 1974.

Hart BL: Behavioral aspects of raising kittens, *Feline Pract* 6(6):8, 10, 20, 1976.

Hart BL: Quiz on feline behavior, *Feline Pract* 7(3):20–21, 1977.

Hart BL: Feline life-styles: solitary versus communal living, *Feline Pract* 9(5):10, 14, 16, 1979.

Hart BL: *The behavior of domestic animals,* New York, 1985, WH Freeman and Company.

Heath S: Commonly encountered feline problems, *Vet Q* 16(S1):51S, April 1994.

Horwitz DF: Feline socialization: how environment and early learning influence behavior, *Vet Med* 88(8):743–747, 1993.

Houpt KA, Wolski TR: *Domestic animal behavior for veterinarians and animal scientists,* Ames, 1982, The Iowa State University Press.

Hubbert WT, McCulloch WF, Schnurrenberger PR, editors: *Diseases transmitted from animals to man,* ed 6, Springfield, Ill, 1975, Charles C Thomas Publisher.

Jewell PA, Loizos C, editors: *Play, exploration, and territory in mammals,* New York, 1966, Academic Press.

Joshua JO: Abnormal behavior in cats. In Fox MW, editor: *Abnormal behavior in animals,* Philadelphia, 1968, WB Saunders.

Kleiman DG, Eisenberg JF: Comparisons of canid and felid social systems from an evolutionary perspective, *Anim Behav* 21(4):637–659, 1973.

Kršiak M, Steinberg H: Psychopharmacological aspects of aggression: a review of the literature and some new experiments, *J Psychosom Res* 13(3):243–252, 1969.

Langworthy OR: Behavioral disturbances related to the decomposition of reflex activity caused by cerebral injury: an experimental study of the cat, *J Neuropathol Exp Neurol* 3:87–100, 1944.

Laundré J: The daytime behaviour of domestic cats in a free-roaming population, *Anim Behav* 25:990–998, Nov 1977.

Macy DW, Siwe ST: The use of ketamine as an oral anesthetic in cats, *Feline Pract* 7(1):44–46, 1977.

Maeda H, Kono E, Maki S: Lesions of the mediodorsal thalamic nucleus do not change thresholds for hypothalamic defensive attack in cats, *Exp Neurol* 82:64–72, 1983.

Mathews-Cameron S, Vogl JF: Diazepam treatment of fear-related aggression in a cat, *Comp Anim Pract* 1:4–6, 1987.

McDougall W, McDougall KD: Notes on instinct and intelligence in rats and cats, *J Comp Psychol* 7:145–175, 1927.

McKeown DB, Luescher UA, Halip J: Stereotypies in companion animals and obsessive-compulsive disorder. *Behavior Problems in Small Animals, Purina Specialty Review* pp 30–35, 1992.

Mintz NL: Demand qualities and social development: some experiments with puppies and kittens, *Lab Bull Harv Univ* 9:12–17, 1959.

Overall KL: Recognition, diagnosis, and management of obsessive-compulsive disorders. Part 1. A rational approach, *Canine Pract* 17(2):40–44, 1992.

Polsky RH: Diazepam-induced defensive aggression in a cat, *Feline Pract* 21(4):21–22, 1993.

Roldán E, Alvarez-Pelaez R, de Molina AF: Electrographic study of the amygdaloid defense response, *Physiol Behav* 13(6):779–787, 1974.

Romaniuk A, Brudzyński S, Grońska J: Comparison of defensive behavior evoked by chemical and electrical stimulation of the hypothalamus in cats, *Acta Physiol Pol* 26(1):23–31, 1975.

Rosenblatt JS, Turkewitz G, Schneirla TC: Early socialization in the domestic cat as based on feeding and other relationships between female and young. In Foss BM, editor: *Determinants of infant behavior,* New York, 1961, John Wiley and Sons.

Rothfield L, Harman PJ: On the relation of the hippocampal-fornix system to the control of rage responses in cats, *J Comp Neurol* 101:265–282, Oct 1954.

Schmidt JP: Psychosomatics in veterinary medicine. In Fox MW, editor: *Abnormal behavior in animals,* Philadelphia, 1968, WB Saunders.

Scott JP: *Aggression,* ed 2, Chicago, 1975, University of Chicago Press.

Spiegel EA, Miller HR, Oppenheimer MJ: Forebrain and rage reactions, *J Neurophysiol* 3:538–548, 1940.

Sprague JM, Chambers WW, Stellar E: Attentive, affective, and adaptive behavior in the cat, *Science* 133(3447):165–173, 1961.

Suehsdorf A: The cats in our lives, *National Geographic* 125:508–541, April 1964.

Svoboda L: Reduce the incidence of bitten fingers, *Vet Med* 80(5):6, 1986.

Thiessen DD, Rodgers DA: Population density and endocrine function, *Psychol Bull* 58(6):441–451, 1961.

Tsai LS: Peace and cooperation among "natural enemies": educating a rat-killing cat to cooperate with a hooded rat, *Acta Psychol Taiwan* 5:1–5, 1963.

Wilson M, Warren JM, Abbott L: Infantile stimulation, activity and learning by cats, *Child Dev* 36(4):843–853, 1965.

Winslow CN: Patterns of competitive, aggressive, and altruistic behavior in the cat, *Psychol Bull* 38:564, July 1941.

Wolski TR: Social behavior of the cat, *Vet Clin North Am Small Anim Pract* 12:693–706, Nov 1982.

5

Male Feline Sexual Behavior

Domestication has greatly altered the sexuality of animals, although probably less for dogs and cats than for other species. Sexual behavior is generally intensified and controlled so desired matings can be achieved, particularly in livestock species. Humans have selectively bred dogs for behavioral traits, like scent-tracking ability, or physical characteristics, like short noses or skin wrinkles. Highly successful reproduction has not been a priority for selection. Most feline reproduction has been dependent on the cats themselves with less human impact.

SEXUAL MATURATION

Puberty

Near the time of birth, a surge of testosterone brings about masculinization of neurons that will later direct male feline sexual behavior; however, the Leydig cells remain inactive after this surge until the kitten is approximately 3 months of age.[91] By $3\frac{1}{2}$ months of age, the male kitten has sufficient testosterone to initiate the growth of penile spines, which reach full size between 6 and 7 months of age. Growth or recession of the spines has been positively correlated with androgen-dependent mating activity.[6] By 5 months the kitten's testes are mature enough for early spermatogenesis, but usually another 1 or 2 months must pass before spermatozoa can be found in the seminal tubules.[91]

Behavioral sexual maturity, as demonstrated by complete copulations, occurs sometime after sperm enter the seminal tubules, generally between 9 and 12 months (see Appendix D). In the wild, however, cats may not reach this degree of maturity until 18 months of age.[11,63] Certain patterns associated with sexual behavior appear before true sexual maturity and are often associated with play. Although young kittens do not commonly mount or perform the neck grip in social play, some males begin mounting, pelvic thrusts, and neck biting as early as 4 months of age (Figure 5-1). They cannot yet achieve intromission, however. Owners are often aware of increased roaming, intermale aggression, and scent marking with urine, all of which accompany the increase in testosterone at puberty.

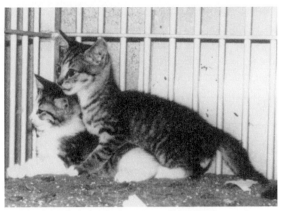

Figure 5-1 A 4-month-old male kitten mounting an uncooperative littermate in prepubertal play.

Reproductive Cycle

Intact males typically leave the homes where they were raised between $1\frac{1}{2}$ and 3 years of age.[59,71] They have been called "outcasts" if they settle away from other male cats and "challengers" if they are peripheral to other tomcats.[71]

Male cats are generally regarded as polygamous, fertile, and sexually active throughout the year; however, studies indicate that males do have subtle cyclic patterns. The sexual activity cycle reaches a peak in the spring and a low point during the late fall in the northern hemisphere, when the female is also naturally nonreceptive.[5,26,78] This low point may be noticed behaviorally as only a decreased eagerness to mate, so in a breeding operation it is the most difficult time to keep males sufficiently vigorous.[78] Changes in sensory feedback from the penis have also been reported in association with reproductive cycles.[5]

Longevity

Mature male cats not only are likely to show sexual interests beyond their mating capabilities but also are likely to maintain this desire even though reproductive functions may decrease with age.[89] Male behavior will usually be evident throughout the animal's adult life and has been observed in cats 27 years old.[23,99]

PREMATING BEHAVIOR

Territorial Effect

Territory is very important in male sexual behavior. Upon arriving at a breeding area, the tomcat spends a variable amount of time investigating it, and most will not breed in a strange place. Occasionally the tomcat may require more than a month to become familiar with his new surroundings, but the insecurity generally lasts only a few days. For the best results, the female should be brought to the area with which the male is familiar. If the territory is too small or the tomcat is confined to a small cage, reproductive capacity may be decreased.

Once an area is selected, the tomcat often sprays urine on prominent sites. He backs up to objects of about nose level, extends his pelvic limbs, raises his tail, and sprays (see Figure 3-17). He occasionally assumes a front-end–down, rear-end–up posture, possibly to spray higher, and as urine forcefully leaves the caudally directed penis, the tomcat usually wiggles his tail characteristically.[98] Other locations may be marked by cheek rubbing.[12,66,70] The increased frequency of marking during the mating season may help reassure the male of his surroundings, attract estrous females, and reinforce the resident's odor for the benefit of wandering males that seem oblivious to territories. Thus marking is associated with response to psychologic disturbances, such as the invasion of territory.

Intermale Aggression

Territorial males become increasingly irritable and protective of their areas during mating season. This is partly because other males wander great distances, with less recognition of territories, interacting with several groups of females.[26,71,96] The increased contact between males can result in increased intermale aggression, particularly during encounters between individuals sharing an area. In a home or laboratory setting, irritability is minimized if tomcats can neither see nor hear estrous females and if there are hiding spaces for individuals. Intermale aggression, which is controlled by testosterone, can be violent and even take precedence over sexual behavior. The environment does not seem to be particularly important, and the attack is not provoked except by the physical presence of another intact male.[80]

After the initial intermale encounter, subsequent meetings usually do not involve fights, and courting males do not fight around estrous females.[82] This system generally allows all healthy males a chance to mate an estrous female, with territorial males having the best opportunity, especially for the first mating. Certain territorial males do not permit other males to mate within their area or in their presence, which causes the intruder to flee or become a psychologic castrate. An occasional male does not leave home at sexual maturity but is usually restless in the presence of the resident tomcat.[63] Under controlled conditions, one tomcat is usually sufficient for 20 females.[32]

Courtship

For an individual tomcat, the amount of breeding experience and the familiarity with the breeding area are the primary influences on the duration and displays of courtship behavior. This period of mating is variable, lasting between 10 seconds and 5 minutes, and it occurs primarily at night. Initially the tomcat calls with a loud, harsh vocalization, commonly termed *caterwauling*. This mating or courtship call serves to advertise the tomcat's availability to estrous females and to warn wandering males of his territoriality. Increased roaming and urine spraying are also part of the very early stages of mating.

Up to six male cats will follow an estrous female, but only one third of the time is there more than one male present.[65] They are attracted by olfactory cues from her urine and vaginal secretions or by her vocalizations. When several males are around, there may be a "central male" that tends to stay much closer and will perform most of the copulations with this female.[71,72] At some point, the male then takes the initiative for mating,

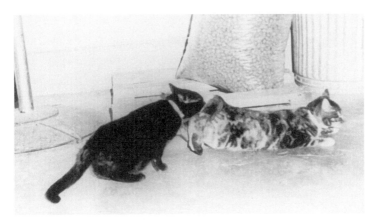

Figure 5-2 The anogenital approach of an estrous female by the territorial male.

using either the facial or anogenital approach (Figure 5-2). Thus chin and face rubbing may be more like greeting and courtship behavior than territorial marking.[29] Sniffing urine from or the genital area of proestrous and estrous females often results in flehmen, an extension of the head, neck, and upper lip (see Figure 2-8). Because flehmen is more easily elicited by urine from estrous queens than from anestrous ones,[95] it probably makes the female estrous odor more accessible to the openings of the vomeronasal organ and associated brain areas. Lack of olfactory ability decreases the time spent smelling the environment and prolongs time used for mating.[7,27] A softer mating call, which has been described as an imitation of the female's "heat cry," indicates readiness to mate.[94] The male usually circles the female before directly approaching her. However, more experienced tomcats may follow the moderate mating call with running directly to the female and initiating mating behavior.[29,33,34] An experienced tomcat may run directly to any cat presented in the breeding area and mount, whereas untrained ones may be partial to certain females and ignore others.[11] Only one in three healthy males become vigorous reliable breeders, and even testosterone injections are not effective in increasing low sex drive.[77]

Mating Behavior

Neck Grip

Although each tomcat has an individual style, a general pattern is often seen, with the neck grip the most consistent behavior (Figure 5-3). An experienced tomcat achieves the grip within 16 seconds.[97] Biting the skin of the dorsum of the neck is a remnant behavior used to immobilize the female and provide proper orientation for mounting.[29,99] The neck grip is not a form of male aggression. In fact, the male is extremely inhibited from showing aggression to an estrous female, and the mating neck bite may represent the inhibited form of the predatory neck bite.[31] Even being aggressively struck by a proestrous queen does not elicit retaliation. Rarely does the male's bite penetrate the skin, and his balance is shifted too far forward to indicate aggression.[31] The strong inhibition is probably due to the female's low posture with more weight carried on the forelimbs, representing a signal to mount, not fight.[30,78] The neck grip has been compared with the way a queen carries her kittens and with the lick-grooming behavior.[55,68]

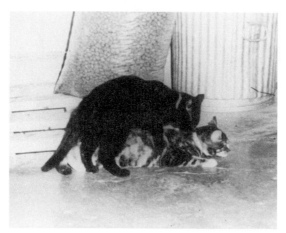

Figure 5-3 A tomcat achieving a neck grip on an estrous female before mounting her.

Copulation

Mounting is the beginning of the mating copulatory sequence. False mounts, those without intromission, do occur, with some males having a higher rate than others.[82] False mounts occur normally in many species and may be a way to test receptiveness of the female, to prepare the female for true mounts, or to show dominance, or they may simply represent a failed attempt at copulation.

The tomcat eventually mounts the female, straddling her first with his forelimbs and then with his hindlimbs (Figure 5-4). The treading or stepping movements of the pelvic limbs help the male arch his back and move caudally to position his perineal area for successful intromission. Pelvic thrusts, dorsoventral movements of the pelvic region, begin as he nears the proper posture, and the penis becomes erect. Intromission occurs after a final, slightly more forceful thrust, the pelvic lunge. This is followed by ejaculation. The neck grip is released, the penis withdrawn, and the female rapidly dismounted.

The preliminary positioning-straddling-treading sequence takes 0.3 to 8 minutes.[69] The entire mating behavior sequence generally lasts between 1 and 9 minutes, with experienced males achieving intromission in an average of 1.8 minutes.[69,85,97] The neck grip–mounting sequence lasts 5 to 50 seconds, and intromission-ejaculation-withdrawal takes only 5 to 18 seconds of this period (mean 8.2 seconds).[69,77]

Repeated Matings

The pattern of repeated matings between a pair of cats varies considerably with the individuals. After each mating the male goes though a postejaculatory refractory period before mounting again. The duration of this latent period varies from 5 to 15 minutes, increasing after each mating. The female must play a more active role in courtship. If the repeated matings continue long enough, the male may mount without using the neck grip.[30] The physiologic component of the postejaculatory refractory period

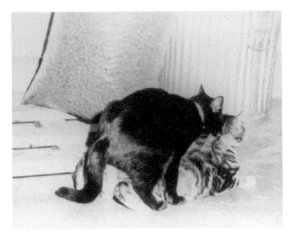

Figure 5-4 The breeding postures of the male cat.

is relatively constant because of its relation with the neural regulation of mating. The psychologic portion is primarily responsible for the changes in refractory time.[42,48] Mating enthusiasm can be renewed by introducing a new estrous female during the psychologic phase. Otherwise the fatigue will dissipate within 24 hours. During the first 2 hours, tomcats may copulate three to six times.[69] The average number of intromissions per hour is 5.3, with 8.9 mounts during that time.[10] In subsequent 2-hour periods the rate drops to 0 to 4 copulations, with the frequency generally not exceeding 15 per 24 hours or 20 to 36 per 36 hours.[69,71,72]

Miscellaneous Influences

Although experienced tomcats are very eager to mate and may mount anything presented, rape is rare.[70] The female's presentation of an elevated perineum is almost physically essential for intromission to occur.

A male to be used as a stud can be trained through habituation to mount and mate an artificial vagina.[78] To condition a tomcat to mate quickly in a colony, one should bring receptive females to him in a special area, allow several matings, and then remove the female first.[55]

POSTMATING BEHAVIOR

Postmating behavior varies because of the latent period, but the tomcat begins by leaping away from the female's striking "afterreaction," which may be accompanied by her growling.[29] The male then licks his penis and forepaws before he goes to sit near the female, but out of her clawing distance.

Pair bonds of long duration are seldom formed. The tomcat often remains with the female only during a few matings, although some males will extend that time for one estrous period. Rarely does a bond last between estrous cycles.

PATERNAL BEHAVIOR

Although most males do not show interest in newborn kittens, there are a few that do. This paternal behavior is probably seen more in the Siamese breed, where the tomcats will lay with and groom the young.[11] At the other extreme are tomcats that indiscriminately kill the kittens. This behavior may be an inherited predisposition for bringing the female back into estrus so that the next litter would be sired by that male.[45,58] In species that have a high turnover of breeding males, a male has a greater chance of his genes being passed on if he can get females pregnant with his offspring instead of having them use energy resources on the offspring of another male. Infanticide is not as common in domestic cats compared with the large felids, possibly because the female does not actually return to estrus faster.[81] Another explanation for infanticide is that the size and shape of the newborn approximate those of natural prey. This appearance then initiates the normal prey-killing instincts of the male, which does not have the hormonal inhibiting influence. He also may mistake the kitten for a crouching female and thus inflict a fatal nape bite.[58]

NEURAL REGULATION

Brain

The relationship of the brain to male sexual behavior has undergone a great deal of study. As expected, the limbic system, specifically the medial preoptic-rostral hypothalamic region, is primarily responsible. Bilateral ablation of these hypothalamic areas eliminates mounting and pelvic thrusts, a result that is not affected by testosterone.[37,41,53] Bilateral removal of the neocortex produces variable results, which probably reflect disturbances in motor coordination rather than deficits in mating behavior. Because these motor capabilities are more important for male mating behavior than for female mating or maternal behavior, differences associated with neocortical control probably reflect the differences in motor needs rather than true sexual neurologic differences.[17]

Neural and Hormonal Interrelationships

The complex interrelationship between the brain and body hormones complicated many early reports. It has been shown in a number of species that gonadal steroids can have a profound affect on behavior, both with morphogenesis and with specific neuron survival.[3] The late prenatal or neonatal male kitten receives a surge of testosterone, which masculinizes the brain. This may be a result of a direct testosterone effect or testosterone converted to estradiol. At the same time, an estrogen-binding plasma protein works to prevent estrogen from entering the brain.[3] Without this surge, the infant develops female behavior patterns and responds primarily to female hormones. The differences between males and females are relative, even though they are under a specific hormone's control.

At maturity, three levels of hormonal control exist.[42] Certain hypothalamic nuclei produce gonadotropic-releasing factors that go to the pituitary gland. At the rostral lobe of the pituitary gland, these releasing factors cause production of the gonadotropins: follicle-stimulating hormone (FSH) and luteinizing hormone (LH). FSH and LH work at the testes, where FSH stimulates the production of sperm cells and LH stimulates testosterone production by interstitial cells. Negative feedback mechanisms regulate hypothalamic production so low FSH or LH levels are stimulatory. In castrates, these levels are therefore quite high.[42]

At puberty, maturing interstitial cells begin producing adult levels of testosterone, which initiates male behaviors from the premasculinized brain. Regions of the hypothalamus actually contain and respond to concentrations of testosterone. Specific androgen-related behaviors include male sexual behavior, intermale aggression, roaming, and scent-marking patterns.

Spinal Cord and Peripheral Nerves

Part of the male's sexual behavior is mediated by specific segments of the spinal cord. Spinal transection in the thoracic region may partially affect posturing but not the capacity for erection and ejaculation or associated caudosacral responses.[9,22] Erection can be induced by stimulation of the second sacral nerve, and ejaculation is mediated by the lumbosacral spinal cord at the internal pudendal nerves and is triggered by tactile stimulation of the penile body via the dorsal nerve of the penis.[8,42,43,87] Androgens appear to intensify low spinal reflexes.[8]

Sympathetic fibers via the hypogastric nerves cause erection to subside and stop emission of prostatic fluids into the urethra, but the exact roles of the autonomic nervous system are not clearly defined.[8]

CASTRATION EFFECTS ON BEHAVIOR

Approximately 34% to 38% of male cats are castrated.[74] The rate tends to be lower in rural areas when compared with urban areas and in shelter cats compared with licensed cats.[74,84]

Neutering at an early age has become popular, particularly for kittens surrendered at animal shelters. Although most cats coming into animal shelters are euthanized, compliance for neutering those intact male cats adopted out with prepaid neutering contracts is only 45%.[2] Despite this concern for compliance, some people remain skeptical of problems that might arise later. Risk factors for relinquishment of a cat to a shelter include being sexually intact, the frequency of inappropriate elimination, and aggression.[83]

Studies comparing cats castrated around 6 weeks or 6 months with intact males showed differences only between intact and neutered animals. No difference was found in the incidence of infectious diseases, behavior problems, or problems associated with any body system over a 3-year period in the group of cats castrated early or at 6 months.[60] Intact males weighed significantly less than the other two groups at 7 months and had earlier closure of the distal radial physis.[19,92] They usually catch up in weight later. Intact cats also show significantly more intraspecies aggression and were less affectionate to humans.[19,92] Physically, castrates had no penile spine development (7-week-old castrates) or atrophied spines (7-month-old castrates).[19,92] Behaviorally, owners of early neutered cats are generally pleased with their pet's behavior, reporting that only 2.5% spray.[73]

This is compared with the general population, in which 26% to 29% of castrated male cats develop some type of behavior problem, mainly destructive behavior, shyness, elimination problems, and aggression to people.[60]

Because male sexually dimorphic behaviors include mating behavior, roaming, urine marking, and intermale aggression, one expects that if these behaviors are primarily controlled by testosterone, castration at any age would significantly reduce their incidence; it does. This means learning, age, and environmental factors have minimal influence on the expression of these behaviors. The male behaviors are reduced by 80% to 90% with castration, half rapidly and half gradually.[51] Prepubertal castration is no more effective in preventing these behaviors than postpuberal castration is in eliminating them.[67]

MALE SEXUAL BEHAVIOR PROBLEMS

Behavior Problems in Intact Males

Much of the normal behavior of the intact male cat may be objectionable to the owner. The male sprays urine mainly to mark his territory, particularly during mating season, and its strong odor is often offensive to humans. The increased activity associated with the mating season can result in a house cat that is difficult to live with or that is subject to injuries. Mating behavior can also be undesirable under a bedroom window at night.

Each of the intact male behaviors is enhanced by postpubertal androgens, and castration is therefore the treatment of choice. Male cats castrated as adults may show a rapid decrease, a gradual decrease over about 3 months, or no decrease in sexually related fighting, roaming, and/or spraying, despite essentially undetectable blood testosterone levels by 6 hours after surgery.[39,46,49,94]

Changes in mating behavior after castration can be divided into three types: rapid, gradual, and minimal decline. All three are characterized first by the disappearance of intromission; followed by increasingly longer mounts; then by only short mounts without the neck bite, stepping, or pelvic thrusts. The first of the three types of changes, rapid decline, involves disappearance of all sexual behavior shortly after castration.[86] The second type, gradual decline, is characterized by the cessation of intromissions within 2 or 3 months after surgery, although mounting persists for several more months.[42] In the third type of change, an initial decrease in frequency of intromissions occurs, but sexual behavior persists for 8 months to $3\frac{1}{2}$ years and mounting continues indefinitely. Penile sensory thresholds are unaltered by castration.[24] Sexual experience preceding castration has a small influence on how long mating behavior is retained after surgery. This is not, however, a predictor of the success of surgery in stopping the behavior.[46,50]

Other male behaviors respond independently of age and sexual experience. Prepubertal castration usually prevents androgen-dependent behavior, and the cat does not ordinarily develop other secondary sexual characteristics, such as the thicker skin of the cheeks and neck. In addition, body weight may increase by the addition of a subcutaneous fat layer, especially in the inguinal region.[64]

Progestins can usually control such undesirable behaviors as roaming, fighting, and spraying in cats that do not change behaviors with castration or that cannot be castrated for some reason. As long as the initiating stimulus is present, however, the objectionable behavior resumes as soon as hormone therapy is discontinued. Progestins counter male behaviors because they are both antiandrogenic and tranquilizing, possibly because of their suppression of neural components normally responsive to testosterone.[20,40,44] The antiandrogenic effect includes decreased spermatogenesis and a lowered social status, so the use of progestins in a breeding tomcat should be discouraged.[20,40,62] Medroxyprogesterone acetate, megestrol acetate, delmadinone acetate, methyloestrenolone, and chlormadinone acetate have also been useful.[*] Observed side effects of short-term use of progestins in the males are increased appetite and food intake. Long-term use has several potentially serious side effects (discussed in Chapter 1) and is rarely indicated.[14,56]

Other factors may also affect a tomcat's sexual behavior. For example, experienced queens may show aggressive tendencies and inhibit a tomcat, and catnip may increase the male's sexual aggression.[21,91] Population density is also known to affect reproduction. In addition to increased suprarenal (adrenal) activity, crowding negatively affects gonadal function.[93]

Tomcat urine is noted for its distinctive odor, which is apparently testosterone dependent.[98] This odor, useful to mark territories and facilitate estrus in females, may be a pheromone or sulfur compound.[1,18] It is present in bladder urine and so may be the sulfur-containing amino acid felinine, which enters urine through the kidneys.[1] Castration minimizes the odor, and other products help reduce it when surgery is not feasible. Cleaning compounds that contain ammonia should not be used to clean up areas with cat urine, because the ammonia of the cleanser is the same as that of the urine. Newer commercial products specifically made to break up the source of urine odors work the best.[13] Specifics are discussed in Chapter 8.

Another problem behavior of intact tomcats is the killing of kittens not sired by the male. The result is that in many species the female may return to estrus sooner if she is not lactating to increase the chances of producing offspring of his own. Kittens also may be killed because they are mistaken for a crouching female and die from the nape bite, or kittens may fail to inhibit the male's predatory drive because they are the size of typical prey animals. Prevention can be ensured only by keeping males away from kittens.

Disinterest in mating can occur for several reasons. Young males can be psychologically castrated in the presence of older males or in their odors.[58] Environmental factors like slippery floors, pain, or memory of pain can also reduce libido.[58] Experienced queens, a new breeding area, and observed learning can be tried. In the medical evaluation, the veterinarian looks for physical reasons. Rings of hair around the penis and congenital abnormalities can be present. Laboratory tests should show serum testosterone levels of at least 1 ng/ml.[58]

Behavior Problems of Castrated Males

Castrated male cats have been known to suddenly show male sexual behaviors, including spraying, fighting, mounting, neck grips, pelvic thrusting, and erection, after a period without them. Mounting behavior is diagnosed as a problem in 19% to 20% of

---

*References 35, 36, 47, 61, 62, 90.

cat behavior cases.[57,58] There are several causal factors for each behavior, but all are based on neonatal masculinizing of the brain, which makes the cat neurologically male. Sexually dimorphic behaviors are primarily dependent on serum testosterone levels but can be learned or activated by certain intense environmental stimuli such as invasion of territory. Notably, about 10% of all cats castrated retain behaviors associated with intact tomcats.

Testosterone administration to castrated cats results in resumption of typical male behaviors, but there are individual differences, based primarily on the cat's precastration experience. Although testosterone is not likely to be administered clinically, anabolic steroids might be. These steroids can be metabolized into progesterone and testosterone, which can produce male behaviors.[12] Because of the progesterone pathway, anabolic agents have also been successfully used to limit typical male behaviors,[79] but the results of this usage are not predictable.

Resumption of male behaviors by castrated individuals can be generally controlled by the short-term use of progestins, provided the psychologic stressor causing the male behavior is removed. The cat should continue normal castrated-male behavior once the drug has worn off. Tension-relieving drugs such as the benzodiazepines, tricyclic antidepressants, and selected serotonin reuptake inhibitors may work as well or better, because they reduce situational anxieties with fewer potential side effects.

Hypersexuality

Hypersexuality includes five feline behaviors: (1) male cats indiscriminately mounting other male cats or humans, (2) multiple mounting, (3) mounting of small kittens, (4) tenaciously clinging to females during copulation, and (5) masturbation.[77]

The mounting of male cats by male cats, although often observed, rarely represents true homosexual behavior, because tomcats prefer female sexual partners if females are available. A dominant, territorial male may mount any cat that enters his territory as a social rather than a sexual behavior. The visiting cat, whether male or female, crouches with partial lordosis while the resident male mounts, treads, and neck grips. If the resident male is placed in the visiting male's territory, the reverse happens: The visitor will show lordosis while the previously mounted cat now does the mounting.[78,94] Mounting is common between male kittens at about 3 months of age, as is common in pubertal males of many species. The presence of an estrous female usually stops it. Experimental depletion of serotonin from the feline brain has caused males to mount other males; however, pretreatment with chlordiazepoxide at doses that do not interfere with muscle activity prevents this behavior.[88] Tomcats housed under a great deal of sexual stress might be managed by pretreatment with this drug.

Occasionally a cat will direct sexual behavior toward an owner's arms or legs.[25] This can require punishment, diversion, or even drug therapy to control. Simply the threat of carrying a squirt bottle of water around may be enough to keep this behavior in check.

The remaining four categories of hypersexual behavior are usually seen in confined tomcats that have no access to an estrous female. These behaviors have been linked to specific brain lesions, but all can be observed in situations of environmental deprivation. Cats that are not used as breeding animals can be spared much of this trauma by castration. The threshold stimulus to mate decreases under experimentally deprived conditions to the point that a minimal stimulus can elicit mating behaviors. Eventually, inappropriate mating can occur spontaneously if the tomcat does not mate for a prolonged time. As a result, a normal behavior is expressed in atypical situations. Multiple mountings of males by males, the mounting of young kittens that do not normally initiate the mating response, the mounting of other species, the clinging to females during copulation to the point that attempts to pull them apart result in both being suspended in midair, masturbation, and the mounting of inanimate objects are expressions of this depressed threshold stimulus. Aberrant mounting can be self-perpetuating, and erection, occasionally with ejaculation, can result.

Masturbation and the mounting of inanimate objects usually develop in young, isolated males or when young males are housed in pairs.[77,78] As a complaint, it is most common in castrated males.[15] A house cat usually chooses to mount a furry toy. Masturbation is more common in laboratory animals than in homed cats and is often accomplished by rubbing the perineal area on the cage floor in a pendulum fashion or rubbing the area against the front paws.[66]

Although spontaneous emissions are apparently not common, a case has been reported.[4,11]

Genetic Problems

Three genetically determined conditions are known to affect the tomcat's ability to mate. Male tortoiseshell and calico cats are almost always sterile and show no interest in estrous females. These XXY individuals may be treated like kittens by their peers.[28] Occasionally, however, males of these colors are fertile and express normal libido.

The autosomal-dominant W gene associated with the blue-eyed, white cat produces semisterility. These deaf, semisterile, poorly sighted cats also have a lower disease resistance.[16] Natural selection is against this gene.

Cryptorchidism is rare in the cat and thus has not been well studied. Strong evidence exists, however, especially in other species, that the condition may be heritable.[76] Retained testicles produce testosterone but not sperm cells, so a bilaterally affected male acts like an intact tomcat but cannot produce offspring. A unilaterally affected tomcat can produce male offspring, which may or may not have the trait, and female offspring, which may be carriers of the trait.

Other Problems

Few males show persistent mounting with intense, prolonged pelvic thrusting but no intromission. In some cases this condition is caused by the formation of a hair ring around the base of the glans penis.[38,42,52,54] The caudally directed penile spines sometimes collect hair from the female's perineum, which may not have been removed by normal grooming. In other tomcats, the problem might be due to improper pelvic orientation, which usually results from lack of experience.

Feminizing syndromes are rare in male cats but have been reported.[75] In male cats so affected, several possibilities should be considered: a genetic XXY male; a true hermaphrodite; a female pseudohermaphrodite; a cat with a Sertoli cell tumor, particularly if it has a retained testicle; and cats that have had massive female hormone therapy.

Unusually low testosterone levels might play a role in lack of libido, but once the brain has been masculinized in the kitten, very low concentrations are necessary to activate libido and other male behaviors in the adult.[55]

REFERENCES

1. Albone ES: *Mammalian semiochemistry: the investigation of chemical signals between mammals,* New York, 1984, John Wiley and Sons.
2. Alexander SA, Shane SM: Characteristics of animals adopted from an animal control center whose owners complied with a spaying/neutering program, *J Am Vet Med Assoc* 205(3):472–476, 1994.
3. Arnold AP, Gorski RA: Gonadal steroid induction of structural sex differences in the central nervous system, *Annu Rev Neurosci* 7:413–442, 1984.
4. Aronson LR: Behavior resembling spontaneous emission in the domestic cat, *J Comp Physiol Psychol* 42:226–227, June 1949.
5. Aronson LR, Cooper ML: Seasonal changes in mating behavior in cats after desensitization of glans penis, *Science* 152:226–230, April 8, 1966.
6. Aronson LR, Cooper ML: Penile spines of the domestic cat: their endocrine-behavior relations, *Anat Rec* 157:71–78, Jan 1967.
7. Aronson LR, Cooper ML: Olfactory deprivation and mating behavior in sexually experienced male cats, *Behav Biol* 11:459–480, 1974.
8. Beach FA: *Hormones and behavior,* New York, 1961, Cooper Square Publishers.
9. Beach FA: Cerebral and hormonal control of reflexive mechanisms involved in copulatory behavior, *Physiol Rev* 47:289–316, April 1967.
10. Beach FA, Zitrin A, Jaynes J: Neural mediation of mating in male cats. I. Effects of unilateral and bilateral removal of the neocortex, *J Comp Physiol Psychol* 49:321–327, 1956.
11. Beadle M: *The cat: history, biology, and behavior,* New York, 1977, Simon & Schuster.
12. Beaver BV: Mating behavior in the cat, *Vet Clin North Am* 7:729–733, Nov 1977.
13. Beaver BV: The marking behavior of cats, *Vet Med Small Anim Clin* 76:792–793, June 1981.
14. Beaver BV: Disorders of behavior. In Sherding RG, editor: *The cat: diseases and clinical management,* New York, 1989, Churchill Livingstone.
15. Beaver BV: Feline behavioral problems other than housesoiling, *J Am Anim Hosp Assoc* 25:465–469, July/Aug 1989.
16. Bigbee HG: Personal communication, 1977.
17. Bjursten LM, Norrsell K, Norrsell U: Behavioural repertory of cats without cerebral cortex from infancy, *Exp Brain Res* 25:115–130, May 28, 1976.
18. Bland KP: Tom-cat odor and other pheromones in feline reproduction, *Vet Sci Commun* 3:125–136, 1979.
19. Bloomberg MS: Surgical neutering and nonsurgical alternatives, *Am Vet Med Assoc* 208(4):517–519, 1996.
20. Blumer D, Migeon C: Hormone and hormonal agents in the treatment of aggression, *J Nerv Ment Dis* 160(2):127–137, 1975.
21. Bryant D: *The care and handling of cats,* New York, 1944, Ives Washburn.
22. Campbell B, Good CA, Kitchell RL: Neural mechanisms in sexual behavior. I. Reflexology of sacral segments of cat, *Proc Soc Exp Biol Med* 86(3):423–426, 1954.
23. Comfort A: Maximum ages reached by domestic cats, *J Mammal* 37(1):118–119, 1956.
24. Cooper KK, Arnson LR: Effects of castration on neural afferent responses from the penis of the domestic cat, *Physiol Behav* 12(1):93–107, 1974.

25. Crowell-Davis SL, Barry K, Wolfe R: Social behavior and aggressive problems of cats, *Vet Clin North Am Small Anim Pract* 27(3):549–568, 1997.

26. Dards JL: The behaviour of dockyard cats: interactions of adult males, *Appl Anim Ethol* 10:133–153, March 1983.

27. Doty RL: *Mammalian olfaction, reproductive processes, and behavior,* New York, 1976, Academic Press.

28. Ehrman L, Parons PA: *The genetics of behavior,* Sunderland, Mass, 1976, Sinauer Associates.

29. Ewer RF: *Ethology of mammals,* London, 1968, Paul Elek Ltd.

30. Ewer RF: *The carnivores,* Ithaca, NY, 1973, Cornell University Press.

31. Ewer RF: Viverrid behavior and the evolution of reproductive behavior in the Felidae. In Eaton RL, editor: *The world's cats,* Seattle, 1974, Feline Research Group.

32. Fox MW: Natural environment: theoretical and practical aspects for breeding and rearing laboratory animals, *Lab Anim Care* 16:316–321, Aug 1966.

33. Fox MW: *Understanding your cat,* New York, 1974, Coward, McCann & Geoghegan.

34. Fox MW: The behaviour of cats. In Hafez ESE, editor: *The behaviour of domestic animals,* ed 3, Baltimore, 1975, Williams & Wilkins.

35. Gerber HA, Jochle W, Sulman FG: Control of reproduction and of undesirable social and sexual behaviour in dogs and cats, *J Small Anim Pract* 14:151–158, March 1973.

36. Gerber HA, Sulman FG: The effect of methyloestrenolone on oestrus, pseudopregnancy, vagrancy, satyriasis, and squirting in dogs and cats, *Vet Rec* 76:1089–1093, 1964.

37. Hart BL: Abolition of mating behavior in male cats with lesions in the medial preoptic-anterior hypothalamic region, *Am Zool* 10(3):296, 1970.

38. Hart BL: Gonadal hormones and behavior of the male cat, *Feline Pract* 2(3):7–8, 1972.

39. Hart BL: Behavioral effects of castration, *Feline Pract* 3(2):10–12, 1973.

40. Hart BL: Behavioral effects of long-acting progestins, *Feline Pract* 4(4):8, 11, 1974.

41. Hart BL: Gonadal androgen and sociosexual behavior of male mammals: a comparative analysis, *Psychol Bull* 81(7):383–400, 1974.

42. Hart BL: Normal behavior and behavioral problems associated with sexual function, urination, and defecation, *Vet Clin North Am* 4(3):589–606, 1974.

43. Hart BL: Physiology of sexual function, *Vet Clin North Am* 4(3):557–571, 1974.

44. Hart BL: Medication for control of spraying, *Feline Pract* 7(3):16, 1977.

45. Hart BL: The client asks you: a quiz on feline behavior, *Feline Pract* 8(2):10–13, 1978.

46. Hart BL: Problems with objectionable sociosexual behavior of dogs and cats: therapeutic use of castration and progestins, *Compend Contin Educ Small Anim Pract* 1:461–465, 1979.

47. Hart BL: Objectionable urine spraying and urine marking in cats: evaluation of progestin treatment in gonadectomized males and females, *J Am Vet Med Assoc* 177:529–533, Sep 15, 1980.

48. Hart BL: *The behavior of domestic animals,* New York, 1985, WH Freeman and Company.

49. Hart BL, Barrett RE: Effects of castration on fighting, roaming, and urine spraying in adult male cats, *J Am Vet Med Assoc* 163:290–292, Aug 1, 1973.

50. Hart BL, Cooper L: Factors relating to urine spraying and fighting in prepubertally gonadectomized cats, *J Am Vet Med Assoc* 184(10):1255–1258, 1984.

51. Hart BL, Eckstein RA: The role of gonadal hormones in the occurrence of objectionable behaviours in dogs and cats, *Appl Anim Behav Sci* 52(3,4):331–344, 1997.

52. Hart BL, Hart LA: *Canine and feline behavioral therapy,* Philadelphia, 1985, Lea & Febiger.

53. Hart BL, Haugen CM, Peterson DM: Effects of medial preoptic-anterior hypothalamic lesions on mating behavior of male cats, *Brain Res* 54:177–191, 1973.

54. Hart BL, Peterson DM: Penile hair rings in male cats may prevent mating, *Lab Anim Sci* 21:422, June 1971.

55. Hart BL, Voith VL: Sexual behavior and breeding problems in cats, *Feline Pract* 7(1):9–10, 12, 1977.

56. Henik RA, Olson PN, Rosychuk RA: Progestogen therapy in cats, *Compend Contin Educ* 7(2):132–142, 1985.

57. Houpt KA: Problems in maternal and sexual behaviors. Paper presented at American Veterinary Medical Association meeting, Minneapolis, July 18, 1993.

58. Houpt KA: Sexual behavior problems in dogs and cats, *Vet Clin North Am Small Anim Pract* 27(3):601–615, 1997.

59. Houpt KA, Wolski TR: *Domestic animal behavior for veterinarians and animal scientists,* Ames, 1982, The Iowa State University Press.

60. Howe LM, Slater MR, Boothe HW, et al: Long-term outcome of gonadectomy performed at an early age or traditional age in cats, *J Am Vet Med Assoc* 217(11):1661–1665, 2000.

61. Jöchle W: Progress in small animal reproductive physiology, therapy of reproductive disorders, and pet population control, *Folia Vet Lat* 4:706–731, Oct/Dec 1974.

62. Jöchle W, Jöchle M: Reproductive and behavioral control in the male and female cats with progestins: long-term field observations in individual animals, *Theriogenology* 3(5):179–185, 1975.

63. Joshua JO: Abnormal behavior in cats. In Fox MW, editor: *Abnormal behavior in animals,* Philadelphia, 1968, WB Saunders.

64. Joshua JO: Some conditions seen in feline practice attributable to hormonal causes, *Vet Rec* 88:511–514, May 15, 1971.

65. Kerby G, Macdonald DW: Cat society and the consequences of colony size. In Turner DC, Bateson PPG, editors: *The domestic cat: the biology of its behavior,* Cambridge, 1988, Cambridge University Press.

66. Kling A, Kovach JK, Tucker TJ: The behavior of cats. In Hafez ESE, editor: *The behavior of domestic animals,* ed 2, Baltimore, 1969, Williams & Wilkins.

67. Knol BW, Egberink-Alink ST: Treatment of problem behavior in dogs and cats by castration and progestogen administration: a review, *Vet Q* 11(2):102–107, 1989.

68. Langworthy OR: Behavioral disturbances related to the decomposition of reflex activity caused by cerebral injury: an experimental study of the cat, *J Neuropathol Exp Neurol* 3:87–100, 1944.

69. Lein D, Concannon PW, Hodgson BG: Reproductive behavior in the queen, *J Am Vet Med Assoc* 181(3):275, 1982.

70. Leyhausen P: *Cat behavior: the predatory and social behavior of domestic and wild cats,* New York, 1978, Garland STPM Press.

71. Liberg O: Predation and social behaviour in a population of domestic cat. An evolutionary perspective, Dissertation, Sweden, 1981, Department of Animal Ecology, University of Lund.

72. Liberg O: Courtship behavior and sexual selection in the domestic cat, *Appl Anim Ethol* 10:117–132, March 1983.

73. Lieberman LL: A case for neutering pups and kittens at two months of age, *J Am Vet Med Assoc* 191(5):518–521, 1987.

74. Mahlow JC: Estimation of the proportions of dogs and cats that are surgically sterilized, *J Am Vet Med Assoc* 215(5):640–643, 1999.

75. Mason KV: Oestral behaviour in a bilaterally cryptorchid cat, *Vet Rec* 99:296–297, Oct 9, 1976.

76. McFarland C, Herron M, Burke RJ, Richkind M: Cryptorchidism and fertility, *Feline Pract* 8(4):14, 1978.

77. Michael RP: "Hypersexuality" in male cats without brain damage, *Science* 134:553–554, Aug 25, 1961.

78. Michael RP: Observations upon the sexual behavior in the domestic cat (*Felis catus* L.) under laboratory conditions, *Behaviour* 18:1–24, 1961.

79. Mosier JE: Common medical and behavioral problems in cats, *Mod Vet Pract* 56(10):699–703, 1975.

80. Moyer KE: Kinds of aggression and their physiological basis, *Commun Behav Biol* 2(pt A):65–87, 1968.

81. Natoli E: Mating strategies in cats: a comparison of the role and importance of infanticide in domestic cats, *Felis catus* L., and lions, *Panthera leo* L., *Anim Behav* 40(1):183–186, 1990.

82. Natoli E, DeVito E: Agonistic behaviour, dominance rank and copulatory success in a large multi-male feral cat, *Felis catus* L., colony in central Rome, *Anim Behav* 42:227–241, 1991.

83. Patronek GJ, Glickman LT, Beck AM, et al: Risk factors for relinquishment of cats to an animal shelter, *J Am Vet Med Assoc* 209(3):582–588, 1996.

84. Pet sterilization, *Bull Inst Study Anim Probl* 1(3):4, 1979.

85. Root MV, Johnston SD, Olson PN: Estrous length, pregnancy rate, gestation and parturition lengths, litter size, and juvenile mortality in the domestic cat, *J Am Anim Hosp Assoc* 31(5):429–433, 1995.

86. Rosenblatt JS, Aronson LR: The decline of sexual behavior in male cats after castration with special reference to the role of prior sexual experience, *Behaviour* 12:285–338, 1958.

87. Semans JH, Langworthy OR: Observations on the neurophysiology of sexual function in the male cat, *J Urol* 40:836–846, Dec 1938.

88. Sheard MH: Lithium in the treatment of aggression, *J Nerv Ment Dis* 160(2):108–118, 1975.

89. Smithcors JF: Sexual capacity of males, *Mod Vet Pract* 58(7):579–580, 1977.

90. Stansbury RL: Altered behavior in castrated male cats, *Mod Vet Pract* 46:68, July 1965.

91. Stein BS: The genital system. In Catcott EJ, editor: *Feline medicine and surgery*, ed 2, Santa Barbara, Calif, 1975, American Veterinary Publications.

92. Stubbs WP, Bloomberg MS, Scruggs SL, et al: Effects of prepubertal gonadectomy on physical and behavioral development in cats, *J Am Vet Med Assoc* 209(11):1864–1871, 1996.

93. Thiessen DD, Rodgers DA: Population density and endocrine function, *Psychol Bull* 58(6):441–451, 1961.

94. Todd NB: Behavior and genetics of the domestic cat, *Cornell Vet* 53:99–107, Jan 1963.

95. Verbene G, Ruardy L: Sniffing and flehmen reactions on pheromonal scent sources in domestic male cats. In Breipohl W, editor: *Olfaction and endocrine regulation*, London, 1982, IRL Press.

96. Weigel I: Small cats and clouded leopards. In Grzimek HCB, editor: *Grzimek's animal life encyclopedia*, vol 12, New York, 1975, Van Nostrand Reinhold.

97. Whalen RE: Sexual behavior of cats, *Behaviour* 20(3–4):321–342, 1963.

98. Whitehead JE: Tomcat spraying, *Mod Vet Pract* 46(2):68, 1965.

99. Worden AN: Abnormal behaviour in the dog and cat, *Vet Rec* 71:966–978, Dec 26, 1959.

ADDITIONAL READINGS

Andy OJ: Catecholamine effects on limbic induced hypersexuality, *Anat Rec* 187(4):525, 1977.

Aronsohn MG, Faggella AM: Surgical techniques for neutering 6- to 14-week-old kittens, *J Am Vet Med Assoc* 202(1):53–55, 1993.

Bard P, Macht MB: The behaviour of chronically decerebrate cats. In Wolstenholme GEW, O'Connor CM, editors: *Neurological basis of behaviour*, Boston, 1952, Little, Brown and Company.

Barton A: Sexual inversion and homosexuality in dogs and cats, *Vet Med (Praha)* 54:155–156, March 1959.

Beach FA, Zitrin A, Jaynes J: Neural mediation of mating in male cats. II. Contributions of the frontal cortex, *J Exp Zool* 130:381–402, 1956.

Beaver BV: Feline behavioral problems, *Vet Clin North Am* 6(3):333–340, 1976.

Beaver BV, Terry ML, LaSagna CL: Effectiveness of products in eliminating cat urine odors from carpet, *J Am Vet Med Assoc* 194:1589–1591, June 1, 1989.

Bergsma DR, Brown KS: White fur, blue eyes, and deafness in the domestic cat, *J Hered* 62(3):171–185, 1971.

Boudreau JC, Tsuchitani C: *Sensory neurophysiology,* New York, 1973, Van Nostrand Reinhold.

Brunner F: The application of behavior studies in small animal practice. In Fox MW, editor: *Abnormal behavior in animals,* Philadelphia, 1968, WB Saunders.

Burke TJ: Feline reproduction, *Vet Clin North Am* 6(3):317–331, 1976.

Chalifoux A, Gosselin Y: The use of megestrol acetate to stop urine spraying in castrated male cats, *Can Vet J* 22(7):211–212, 1981.

Cooper KK: Cutaneous mechanoreceptors of the glans penis of the cat, *Physiol Behav* 8:793–796, 1972.

Doering GG: "Stud tail" in cats, *Feline Pract* 6(5):28, 1976.

Dunbar IF: Behaviour of castrated animals, *Vet Rec* 96(4):92–93, 1975.

Eleftheriou BE, Scott JP: *The physiology of aggression and defeat,* New York, 1971, Plenum Publishing.

Fox MW: Ethology: an overview. In Fox MW, editor: *Abnormal behavior in animals,* Philadelphia, 1968, WB Saunders.

Fox MW: The veterinarian: mercenary, Saint Frances—or humanist, *J Am Vet Med Assoc* 166(3):276–279, 1975.

Gessa GL, Tagliamonte A: Role of brain monoamines in male sexual behavior, *Life Sci* 14(3):425–436, 1974.

Goodrowe K, Chakraborty PK, Wildt DE: Pituitary and gonadal response to exogenous LH-releasing hormone in the male domestic cat, *J Endocrinol* 105:175–181, 1985.

Green JD, Clemente CD, DeGroot J: Rhinencephalic lesions and behavior in cats, *J Comp Neurol* 108:505–545, Dec 1957.

Hagamen WD, Zitzmann EK, Reeves AG: Sexual mounting of diverse objects in a group of randomly selected, unoperated male cats, *J Comp Physiol Psychol* 56(2):298–302, 1963.

Hart BL: The brain and behavior, *Feline Pract* 3(5):4, 6, 1973.

Hart BL: Types of aggressive behavior, *Canine Pract* 1:6, 8, May/June 1974.

Hart BL: Gonadal androgen and sociosexual behavior of male mammals: a comparative analysis, *Psychol Bull* 81:383–400, July 1974.

Hart BL: Behavioral patterns related to territoriality and social communication, *Feline Pract* 5(1):12, 14, 1975.

Hart BL: Spraying behavior, *Feline Pract* 5(4):11–13, 1975.

Hart BL: Quiz on feline behavior, *Feline Pract* 6(3):10, 13, 1976.

Hart BL: Behavioral aspects of raising kittens, *Feline Pract* 6(6):8, 10, 20, 1976.

Hart BL: Aggression in cats, *Feline Pract* 7(2):22, 24, 28, 1977.

Hart BL: Olfaction and feline behavior, *Feline Pract* 7(5):8–10, 1977.

Johnstone I: Electroejaculation in the domestic cat, *Aust Vet J* 61(5):155–158, 1984.

Kleiman DG, Eisenberg JF: Comparisons of canid and felid social systems from an evolutionary perspective, *Anim Behav* 21(4):637–659, 1973.

Kuo ZY: Studies on the basic factors in animal fighting. VII. Inter-species coexistence in mammals, *J Genet Psychol* 97:211–225, 1960.

Kustritz MVR: Elective gonadectomy in the cat, *Feline Pract* 24(6):36–39, 1996.

Levinson BM: Man and his feline pet, *Mod Vet Pract* 53:35–39, Nov 1972.

Leyhausen P: The communal organization of solitary mammals, *Symp Zool Soc Lond* 14:249–263, 1965.

Marvin C: Hormonal influences on the development and expression of sexual behavior in animals, In Fox MW, editor: *Abnormal behavior in animals,* Philadelphia, 1968, WB Saunders.

Memon MA, Ganjam VK, Pavletic MM, Schelling SH: Use of human chorionic gonadotropin stimulation test to detect a retained testis in a cat, *J Am Vet Med Assoc* 201(10):1602, 1992.

Michael RP: Sexual behaviour and the vaginal cycle in the cat, *Nature* 181:567–568, Feb 22, 1958.

Mitchell RA, Hart BL, Voith VL, et al: Roaming behavior, *Feline Pract* 15(4):31–32, 1985.

Mykytowycz R: Reproduction of mammals in relation to environmental odours, *J Reprod Fertil* 19(suppl):433–446, 1973.

Neville PF, Remfry J: Effect of neutering on two groups of feral cats, *Vet Rec* 114(18):447–450, 1984.

Pfaff DW: Interactions of steroid sex hormones with brain tissue: studies of uptake and physiological effects. In Segal SJ, editor: *The regulation of mammalian reproduction,* Springfield, Ill, 1973, Charles C Thomas Publisher.

Platz CC Jr, Seager SWJ: Semen collection by electroejaculation in the domestic cat, *J Am Vet Med Assoc* 173(10):1353–1355, 1978.

Romatowski J: Use of megestrol acetate in cats, *J Am Vet Med Assoc* 194(5).700–702, 1989.

Rosenblatt JS: Effects of experience on sexual behavior in male cats. In Beach FA, editor: *Sex and behavior,* New York, 1965, John Wiley and Sons.

Rosenblatt JS, Aronson LR: The influence of experience on the behavioural effects of androgen in prepuberally castrated male cats, *Anim Behav* 6(3–4):171–182, 1958.

Schwartz AS, Whalen RE: Amygdala activity during sexual behavior in the male cat, *Life Sci* 4:1359–1366, July 1965.

Scott PP: The domestic cat as a laboratory animal for the study of reproduction, *J Physiol* 130:47P–48P, 1955.

Smith RC: *The complete cat book,* New York, 1963, Walker and Company.

Spraying by castrated tomcats, *Mod Vet Pract* 56(10):729–731, 1975.

West M: Social play in the domestic cat, *Am Zool* 14:427–436, Winter 1974.

Zitrin A, Jaynes J, Beach FA: Neural mediation of mating in male cats. III. Contributions of occipital, parietal and temporal cortex, *J Comp Neurol* 105:111–125, Aug 1956.

6

Female Feline Sexual Behavior

Throughout the years when cats have been closely associated with humans, selective breeding has accentuated certain color patterns and physical features. At the same time, codependent genes related to other features such as reproductive behavior and physiology can also be changed. This means variability is a common and normal feature in all phases of female sexual behavior of *Felis catus,* even among purebreds. Selective breeding for both domestication and breed development has tended to intensify feline sexuality and enhance the diversity of female sexual behaviors.

SEXUAL MATURATION

The developing prenatal or early neonatal kitten that is not exposed to a testosterone surge develops the female nervous system, and at puberty the female behavior characteristics become apparent. The onset of puberty in the cat varies considerably, depending on several factors: The presence of a tomcat or estrous female, the time of year, and climate are more influential than age alone.[62,83] For the tame domestic cat, the first signs of estrus appear between $3\frac{1}{2}$ and 12 months of age, usually at 5 to 9 months. (See Appendix D.) Burmese cats tend to be the youngest cycling breed, and Persian and free-ranging cats are apt to reach puberty at an older age, even as late as 15 to 18 months.[30,58] Behavioral signs of the first estrus are usually associated with the physiologic ability to conceive.[6]

Environmental factors can also affect the onset of puberty. Young females that are born early in the season or that are exposed to tomcats, cycling females, or increasing amounts of light generally show signs of first estrus before similar individuals born later or not exposed to these factors. Kittens born in early spring may show estrus in the fall instead of waiting through a winter season.

REPRODUCTIVE CYCLES

Seasonal Variations

The female cat is seasonally polyestrous and has several estrous cycles during each of its two or three seasons per year. In the latitudes of the United States and Europe, cats are generally anestrous from late September through late December or January and may show reduced sexual activity for a few months on either side of this period. Seasonal cycle peaks tend to occur between February and early April and between June and August, although they tend to be delayed in the northern latitudes and hastened in the south. A great deal of individual variation exists, and some cats, particularly short-haired varieties, cycle all year.[13,53,58] At the other extreme, a wildcat may have only one seasonal cycle each year so that more time can be spent teaching skills to the young.[5,13]

The use of artificial light from September to March to lengthen "daylight" hours has been successful in many colonies to get females to cycle year round. Increasing the length of daily light from 12 to 14 hours will induce estrus in 44 to 45 days.[83] If an additional 1 hour of exposure to light during the dark period is provided, estrus will occur in 15 to 16 days instead.[83]

Estrous Cycle

Anestrus

The anestrous female may rebuff an approaching tomcat by hissing and striking out. If she accepts the tomcat with relative indifference, she flexes her spine when he mounts and covers the perineum tightly with her tail, almost achieving a sitting position instead of the lordosis seen during estrus. The same behavior is exhibited by prepubertal kittens weighing more than 1500 g when mounted by a male. Kittens weighing less than 1000 g remain passive to the neck grip because it resembles the carrying grip used by the queen.[81] The anestrous female also exhibits aggressive behaviors in attempting to free herself from an undesired mounting. Olfactory signals from her vulvar area apparently are repulsive to some tomcats, which will quickly turn away after smelling her perineum.[81]

Proestrus

The onset of estrous behavior may seem rather sudden to the owner because of a relatively short proestrous phase. Proestrus lasts between 1 and 3 days, and the associated behavior is highly variable among individuals. Only 16.1% of cats show proestrus.[105] For these, it typically begins as a subtle increase in general activity and progresses to increased rubbing against objects, especially with the head and neck. This behavior may prompt owners to report that their cat has become friendlier. A tomcat's approach no longer results in immediate sexual aggression by the female. The male cat's neck grip and mount may initially cause the female to crouch partially and tread temporarily. His advances during proestrus eventually initiate her aggression. During this time owners may witness more aggressive interactions between the male and female than between tomcats.[20] Amicable behaviors are also more often initiated by the female, and she is more likely to interact with a male that she knows.[20] Her rubbing the chin and cheek on objects, including the tomcat, becomes very marked within 36 hours of the onset of proestrus, and when done to a person, it may be related to courtship rather than marking.[24] Rubbing progresses to rolling, either gentle or violent, which is usually associated with purring, rhythmic opening and closing of the claws, squirming, and stretching[81,111] (Figure 6-1). Catnip may evoke a somewhat similar behavior.

The female begins calling to a male using the "heat cry," a vocalization unique to proestrus and estrus. This sound is a monotone howling that lasts up to 3 minutes at one time. Approximately 12% of the females eventually call continuously, although this

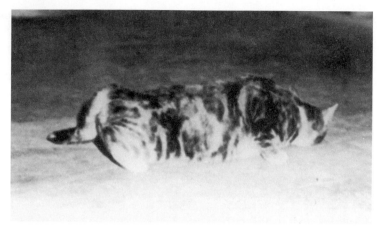

Figure 6-1 The characteristic rolling behavior of proestrus and estrus.

behavior is more prevalent in Siamese females. Another 14% vary considerably in the frequency of the call.[58] Some estrous females apparently do not call at all.[20] This cry is mimicked by the tomcat, answered by the female, and again mimicked by the male. The female may spray urine,[8] so that both the urine and the sebaceous secretions left by rubbing serve to attract males, particularly in areas where cats live relatively close together.[24,116]

Estrus

As the female enters estrus, a dramatic change occurs in her behavior toward the male. She still rolls and rubs, but no longer does she aggressively refuse the male's attempts to mount, exhibiting a crouching lordosis instead. In this position the ventral thorax and abdomen touch the floor, and the perineum is elevated because the hindlimbs are positioned caudal to the body and extended perpendicular to the ground (Figure 6-2). This copulatory stance can be induced by stroking the queen's back, thighs, or neck. Her tail is laterally displaced, and there may be a small amount of sanguineous discharge on the vulva.[111]

The behavioral events of mating begin with appetitive sexual behavior, or courtship. The elaborate courtship behaviors are important to bring males and females together. To ensure that males will be available and can succeed in intermale competition (although the winner may not be the one she eventually chooses) the female starts advertising before she is fully receptive. This courtship period also helps give the greatest number of healthy males an equal chance at reproduction.[70] The female usually sits some distance away from the competition. She may show preference or dislike for an interested male. This choice probably has an olfactory basis, because changes in the nasal mucosa occur in association with the estrous cycle.[84] Evidence indicates that odors affect reproduction in several mammals by means of the nervous and endocrine systems, and theories to the contrary fail to take the learning process into account.[84,114]

Lordosis is necessary if intromission is to occur and can be stimulated by the treading of the mounted male. While the male performs copulatory thrusts, the female adjusts her position slightly by alternate treading with her hindlimbs. During estrus,

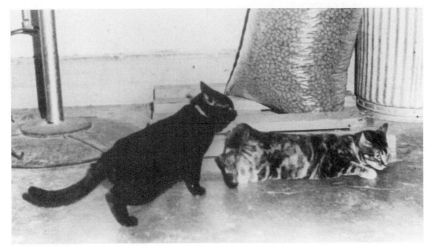

Figure 6-2 The natural lordosis posture of an estrous cat.

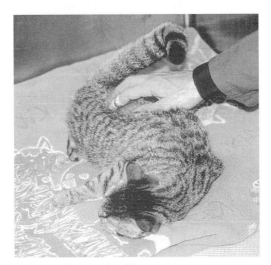

Figure 6-3 Estrous behavior can be stimulated by petting.

this rhythmic step, tail deviation, and rolling can be initiated by gently petting or tapping the female's perineum, flank, or back (Figure 6-3). The facial expression associated with mating is often intense, similar to that seen in aggressive cats and some that are fearful. In addition, the ears are positioned rostrolaterally. The crouching, rubbing, rolling, and treading portions of courtship last between 10 seconds and 5 minutes, tending to be shorter with repeated breedings.[5,31]

Postmating behavior of the female is characteristically dramatic. As the male starts to withdraw his penis after ejaculation, the female's pupils suddenly dilate. Immediately after, 53.8% of queens will utter the copulatory cry, a shrill piercing vocalization.[96] Then 76.9% of queens will turn aggressively on the male.[96] To a familiar male, the

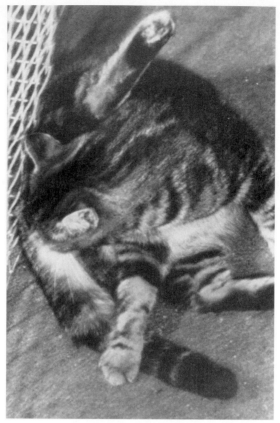

Figure 6-4 The female licks her external genitalia following mating.

female may be less aggressive and might instead proceed directly into the "afterreaction." During the afterreaction, the consummatory portion of the female's sexual behavior, she again rolls on the floor, stretches, and licks her vulva (Figure 6-4). This period lasts from 1 to 7 minutes.[68]

Typical estrous mating behavior resumes in 11 to 95 minutes (mean 19 minutes). Experienced pairs may mate as frequently as 8 times in 20 minutes, or 10 times per hour.[5,30,31] Female cats have been known to mate more than 50 times during an estrous period.[51] As mating continues over the next few days, the refractory period (the time between these behaviors) becomes longer. The female mating interval, however, actually decreases, and she becomes more active in encouraging the male to mount. This is particularly true of naive females.[122] Thus the male is primarily responsible for the increased time lapse between breedings. An estrous female can be conditioned to assume the estrous posture whenever she is placed in the mating area, even in the absence of a male.[81,122]

A mutual attraction between tomcat and queen can last for extended periods. A female will generally accept a number of males during her estrous period, and many litters have multiple sires.[24,26,30] If there is a central tomcat, he is the primary breeder of that female group, even with other peripheral males courting the females.[72] This is because of his proximity to the queens. He is not likely to fight off other males though, because it would be too dangerous for any one male to attempt to keep them all away.[85] When females are in the proximity of related males, they are more likely to leave their home areas during estrus than are those without related males nearby.[73]

The cat is an induced ovulator, so an estrous female generally does not ovulate unless mating occurs. Ovulation occurs approximately 24 hours after copulation—the same amount of time needed for sperm to capacitate.[85] The ovulation is probably induced by vaginal stimulation from the male's penile spines or by artificial means, such as with a glass rod. More than one natural mating may be necessary for conception.[104] Artificial stimulation requires several insertions of approximately 10 seconds in duration, 5 to 10 minutes apart, over a 48-hour period. Successful stimulation by either method causes the typical postcopulation aggression. The number of ovulation sites on the ovary varies directly with the number of matings and can include as many as 86.6% of the follicles with repeated matings.[124] All eggs leave the ovary at the same time.[26]

Ovulation has been prevented by a systemic shock factor such as abdominal surgeries but only if the shock occurs within 55 minutes after mating.[2]

The female remains in estrus for 2.5 to 11.1 days (range 2 to 19 days), a period that may include proestrus and metestrus.[96,105] She is most receptive on the third and fourth days if mated during that time. Estrus ends rather abruptly, within 24 hours after coitus. If pregnant, the cat usually will not return to estrus again until the next seasonal peak or the next year. However, about 10% of the pregnant queens display estrous behavior and produce a vaginal smear typical of estrus during the third to sixth week of gestation, possibly because of estrogen secretion by the placenta.[3,102,109] Mating at this time can result in superfetation.[57,109] Nursing queens have also been known to exhibit estrus 7 to 10 days after parturition, but estrus generally does not occur during lactation, so most do not return to estrus until 6 to 8 weeks after giving birth. It can be delayed as long as 21 weeks.[58,102] Postpartum estrus has a shorter duration than the initial estrus, averaging 3.8 days.[99]

When no tomcat is present, the female remains in estrus for 10 to 14 days, although the first estrus might last only 5 to 10 days.[51] She returns to estrus in 9.0±7.6 days (range 5 to 22 days).[105] Some studies suggest a minimal difference between bred and open estrus duration.[96,105] The average estrous cycle is 21 to 29 days long, but it can vary from 5 to 73 days. Young females tend to exhibit minimal estrous signs; become hyperexcitable, anorectic, or withdrawn; and have a shorter estrous period. In contrast, older females continue to cycle, even though the interval between estrous periods might increase and duration and intensity of estrous behavior decrease. Approximately 35% of the time, ovulation will occur without coitus.[66] In such a cat or in one that mated but did not conceive, the luteal phase will last 30 to 36 days and the interestrous interval is 35 to 76 days.[96,105,124]

Because some of the environmental factors that affect the onset of puberty in the female can also affect the onset of estrus, the nonpregnant female has been described as being in "potential" estrus during the mating season.[30,31] The result of exposure to certain factors, such as a tomcat or other cycling females, is the appearance of proestrus and estrus within a few hours to 3 or 4 days and a synchronization with female groups.[22,72,73] Valeric acid is plentiful in vaginal secretions during estrus and may be associated with the synchronization.[11] Other factors, such as a colony relocation, can result in coordinating estrous cycles for 42% to 77% of the females.[123]

Estrous behavior has been controlled with vasectomized male cats. In females mated to such tomcats, estrus lasts approximately 7 days and is followed by a 36- to 44-day interestrous period of pseudopregnancy.[31,69,86,93]

The behavior of a female cat, her vaginal smear, and her phase in the reproductive cycle are very closely correlated. Of the cats exhibiting estrous behavior in one study, 78% had a fully cornified estrous vaginal smear and another 18% were in proestrus.[81]

Metestrus

The behavior of metestrus begins with the appearance of leukocytes in the vaginal smear.[80] This phase rarely lasts more than 24 hours and is generally included in time ranges given for estrus because all of the postural responses continue and mounting is allowed. The female aggressively rejects the male during this phase only when he attempts intromission.

INTERSPECIES MATINGS

Periodically, newspapers carry articles about the offspring of cats that have mated with other animals, but they are generally not substantiated. A reported cat-rabbit cross that hopped around one town was really a tailless Manx cat with spinal cord problems. *F. catus* has 38 diploid chromosomes, as do most of the large cats of the Felidae family.[25,121] Ocelots are the noted exception, with 36 chromosome pairs. Crosses of domestic cats with larger cats having 38 chromosome pairs have been reported, but the fertility of the offspring is variable.[36]

PREGNANCY

In a laboratory setting, the pregnancy rate is 73.9% of bred queens, but because of reabsorptions, the queening rate is somewhat lower (65.2%).[96] In general then, the uncontrolled female cat is always pregnant, nursing, or both, except possibly in the late fall, and her entire body is geared for these conditions. In a home environment where the female is not allowed to breed, she is probably healthier physiologically and psychologically if ovariohysterectomized.

Gestation

The duration of gestation in the cat ranges from 60 to 68 days, with an average of 65 to 66 days. Gestation periods of 52 to 71 days have been reported; however, births before 60 days should be regarded as premature because they are often accompanied by a higher than normal rate of stillbirths and early postnatal deaths.[90,104]

During the last third of pregnancy, obvious behavioral changes occur, although some queens have already been showing increased docility. Along with a rapid weight gain, primarily a result of fetal growth, come an increase in appetite, a decrease in activity, and a decrease in agility. A slight distention of the mammae may also occur.

In the week immediately preceding parturition, the queen will seek a dark, dry area where she can remain relatively undisturbed. Ideally, this place will also contain shelter from the elements and a soft bedding material. A queen can choose a single, hidden nest site, or if she is associated with a group, she may share a communal nest.[76] Site selection may relate to the degree of cover available or the proximity to food sources for the queen or her older kittens. Perhaps it may even be chosen for the possible social interactions.[27] This early selection of the nesting area allows for the time required for the site to take on the female's odor so that she can relax in a familiar environment. This is somewhat similar to the function of sprayed urine in the tomcat's environment. The amount of seclusion preferred by a female during parturition is highly individual. Some actually seek out human companionship at this time and may finally choose the owner's bed as the queening area. Most prefer seclusion and would find the hayloft of a barn more acceptable. Queens living with several other related and unrelated females may use a communal nest.[19,22,27,52] During the last week the queen drives off kittens from the previous litter that are still with her. After queening, however, she may accept them back to nurse with her new offspring. During this period before delivery, the queen usually spends an increasing amount of time in self-grooming, particularly of her mammary and perineal areas, perhaps because of the increased cutaneous sensitivity in those regions.[5,24,100] Her personality may also become more irritable or defensive.

As parturition becomes imminent, the female becomes increasingly restless, digs at the floor or nesting material, and assumes a defecation posture without defecating. There may be calling vocalizations, particularly by Siamese cats, and a few queens become excessively anxious, almost frantic.[30]

Parturition

Most births occur at night, often in isolated locations, so parturition is not always observed. Because the cat is multiparous, the four phases normally associated with parturition are repeated several times. The termination of a kitten's birth occurs at the onset of contractions for the next. With multiparous animals, the delivery of a placenta does not necessarily mark the termination of parturition. The total time for normal parturition ranges from 4 to 42 hours (16.1 ± 14.3 hours is average).[96]

Each of the four phases of parturition is highly variable, but their order holds true for the majority of births. The initiation of each new phase is usually marked by an abrupt behavioral change, from contractions causing genitoabdominal licking to placental delivery resulting in the consumption of the placenta.

Contraction phase

During the first phase, contraction, the queen spends a great deal of time licking herself or the newborns already delivered. The abdominal musculature shows obvious contractions, which are considered to accompany uterine contractions. Pelvic limb movements by the queen should help distinguish these abdominal contractions from fetal movements.[100] Other signs of restlessness are obvious. In addition to squatting and scratching, the queen may circle, rearrange bedding, roll, or rub. She generally appears uncomfortable and seems to be constantly trying to adjust for some disturbance at the caudal portion of her body, even bracing her body against various objects. The duration of the contraction phase is variable, ranging from 12 seconds to $1\frac{1}{2}$ hours.[18,100]

Emergence phase

During the emergence phase, uterine contractions cause the kitten to pass through the birth canal and pause in the vulva (Figure 6-5). Usually the amniotic sac has been broken by uterine contractions, but if not, the queen's licking soon breaks it. The release of fluids from the amniotic sac causes the queen to spend additional time licking the fluids and coincidentally herself and the newborn.[43,53,100] Experienced queens may direct more attention to the newborn, but other behaviors are quite similar to those of the contraction phase.

Delivery phase

The third phase, delivery, represents passage of the fetus from the vulva[100] (Figure 6-6). Licking directed specifically at the newborn increases, although the queen may not begin immediately after the delivery. This licking supplies the stimulus for initiation of the newborn's respiration if passage through the birth canal did not. A first-litter queen tends to be the most restless and is less likely to lick herself and each kitten correctly.[22] Experience apparently is needed to refine these behaviors. From lateral recumbency the queen may try to reposition herself after the delivery and may coincidentally drag the kitten around by the still-attached umbilical cord, perhaps even stepping or sitting on it. Distress cries from this newborn or others are often ignored by the queen at this time, perhaps because of the excitement associated with parturition, or incomprehension of the vocal cue, or both.[22,100] Kittens can be injured during this period. Shortly after parturition, generally 1 to 4 minutes later, the female becomes responsive to the kittens.[18,100] She will sever the umbilical cord shortly after the delivery in about one third of the births (Figure 6-7).

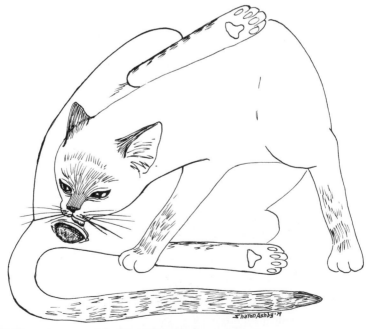

Figure 6-5 The emergence of the kitten through the queen's vulva.

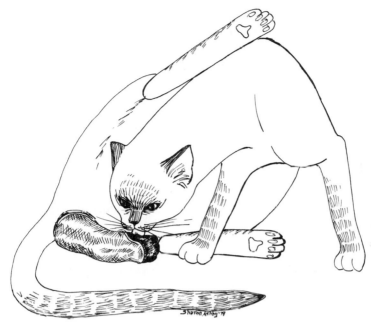

Figure 6-6 The delivery of the neonate, still partially covered by the amniotic sac.

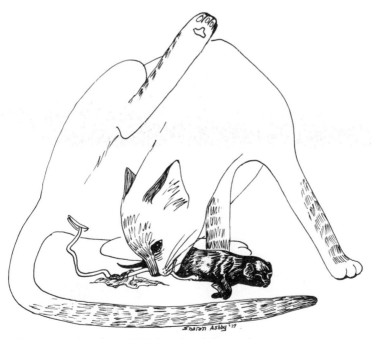

Figure 6-7 The queen severs the umbilical cord with her teeth.

There is tremendous variation in the intervals between kitten births, ranging normally from 32 seconds to more than 50 minutes.[53,100] Most kittens are born within 15 to 30 minutes of each other, with a total delivery time of 1 to 2 hours.[13,14] Some normal queens will take as much as 33 hours to complete the deliveries, but usually external disturbances, such as the absence of an owner or the moving of a nesting area, cause this extreme delay. Uterine inertia is relatively rare in cats.[61] There is no relationship between the sequence of a kitten's birth and the interval between its birth and that of its littermates.

Placental phase

The last of the four phases of parturition, as they usually occur, is the placental phase. During this time the placenta is expelled from the genital tract. Immediately before this expulsion, the female becomes restless, again appearing to focus her attention toward the caudal part of her body. She responds promptly to the emergence of this tissue, sometimes eating it before it has completely emerged[100] (Figure 6-8). No relationship has been shown between the sequence of the births and either the interval of response to the placentas or the rate and completeness of its consumption.[100] At times, a second or even third kitten is born before the umbilical cord of the first is severed or the placenta passed, but each will be attended to as time permits. Nutritive value from the afterbirth is considerable and allows the queen to spend more time with her offspring for the first few days than if she had to seek food as usual. In addition, this behavior minimizes the soiling of the nest area. The queen continues genital and neonatal licking during the placental phase but takes time to sever the umbilical cord with her carnassial teeth. Their crushing action, the stretching of the vessels, or both prevent fatal

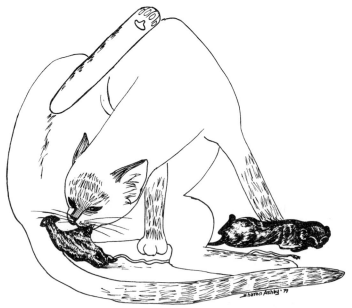

Figure 6-8 The queen responds to placental emergence by consuming the tissue.

umbilical hemorrhage.[40,100] The queen's care during this phase makes cannibalism as a consequence of overzealous eating of the placenta and cord very rare.

For those queens sharing a communal nest, one may be assisted immediately post-partum by another female.[19] The help usually is to clean and dry the young, but it can include severing the umbilical cord.[22]

Litter Size

The number of kittens born to a queen varies considerably, usually ranging between one and nine. Record litters of 13 kittens and one unusual incidence of a queen carrying 18 fetuses have been reported.[9,125] Of the kittens born alive, between 72% and 87% will be successfully raised to weaning.[58,89,96,101] Three to five then is an average litter, even for artificially induced pregnancies, and the male/female ratio of these kittens varies from 1:1 to 4:3. Although 7% of the older queens will litter three times a year, the mean is $2\frac{1}{2}$ litters.[73,95] Most litters result from several matings on consecutive days. Even though this increases the number of ovulation sites, litter size is not affected by the number of days the queen mates.[90] A queen then will normally bear between 50 and 150 kittens in a breeding life of about 10 years if allowed to mate naturally.[127] Some may produce for 13 or more years, but peak productivity is generally between the ages of 2 and 8 years.[5,60] One cat is known to have produced 420 kittens in 17 years, and another is said to have been pregnant at 26 years of age.[17,125] At 8 kittens per year per generation, a queen could ultimately be responsible for 174,760 cats in 7 years.[12]

Normal birth weight varies between 80 to 120 g, averaging about 113 g.[35,47,59] Also, the total birth weight relative to the queen's weight is significantly greater for kittens born to smaller queens compared with that of kittens born to larger females. This is despite the fact that larger queens tend to produce a larger number of kittens in each litter.[35]

In cats, abortion and stillbirths are common; one or two often occur per litter.[58,101] The incidence is 4.7% stillbirths.[96] These events may be difficult to observe, because the queen normally eats these fetuses. The stillborn rate is higher in older queens; in overweight cats; and in the Persian, Maine coon, Himalayan, and Manx breeds.[59,75,89,90,101] Other losses are associated with queens having nest sites away from the center of a farm.[63] This may be due to the queen not having others to help guard the nest site, increased vulnerability of the nest, and/or greater likelihood of disease. Some peripheral queens may not have any descendants, even over a 7-year span.[63]

MATERNAL BEHAVIOR

Mother-Young Interactions

The primary social pattern exhibited by the female cat is maternal behavior. In general, this behavior involves exaggerated licking of self and young, as well as the care of the young.[100] For the first few days after the completion of parturition, the queen remains almost continuously with the kittens, seldom leaving for more than 2 hours at a time, and then mainly to eat and exercise. During these early days, the kittens are particularly dependent on their mother for her warmth. A little while later they are able to maintain body temperatures in the warmth of the kitten huddles.[32] Much of the queen's time during the first few days is spent nursing the offspring, although the kittens may not nurse for as long as 2 hours postpartum. For nursing, the queen "presents," assuming lateral recumbency with her limbs and body completely enclosing the kittens (Figure 6-9). She may even twist her body to expose more of the mammary region. To stimulate the young to begin nursing, the female licks and often awakens them. Initially the direction of licking helps orient the blind kittens to her mammary region, but later, licking is concentrated on the kitten's anogenital region to stimulate eliminations. The queen's ingestion of this waste also helps keep the home area unsoiled. Once the queen presents the mammae, the entire litter usually nurses, but occasionally it may be only one or two individuals. During the first week, about 90% of the female's time is spent with her kittens, and as much as 70% is spent nursing them. By the fifth week, her time with the kittens decreases to 16%.[92,100] Initially each kitten spends about 25% of its time nursing, which decreases to about 20% by the fifth week.[64] Kittens spend almost all their time in contact with each other or the queen for the first 3 weeks, and contact time only decreases to 85% over the next few weeks.[92]

Cooperative nursing, grooming, and carrying between queens has been reported without preference to which kittens belong to which mother.[19,76] The advantages of communal nesting to the kittens include being guarded better, having multiple caregivers, and faster development.[19] These kittens will leave the nest approximately a week earlier than kittens raised in a solitary litter. Potential disadvantages of communal nesting include potential attraction of predators, increased aggression resulting from cat density, missing offspring because of combined litters, rapid disease and parasite transmission, premature displacement of a queen from the nest site, and increased competition for food or mates.[27]

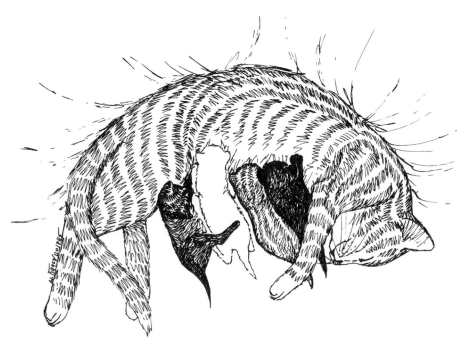

Figure 6-9 The "presenting" posture of a queen to her kittens.

The queen's nursing relationship to her young changes with time.[52,67] During the first 4 weeks she initiates and stimulates their interest in nursing, but eventually she actually runs away from their advances. The mother-young feeding relationships are covered in more detail in the discussion of ingestive behavior in Chapter 7.

Kitten vocalizations increase the likelihood that a queen will approach her kittens and present for nursing.[45,46] She will even carry them back to the nest first if she finds them elsewhere.

The mother-kitten interaction continues to change as the young gain mobility and independence. They may include her in their play, even though she increasingly avoids interaction with the kittens as they get older, paralleling her changes in nursing behavior. To control their biting and chewing of her, she may bat the kittens on the nose, drag them away, or turn and move away from them if a growl warning does not work. This same discipline technique, a bat on the nose and a "no," can be used by a human; however, experimental data indicate that this training must be initiated before 6 weeks of age if it is to be retained in adulthood.[30]

Kitten Relocation

Kittens that wander from the home area are usually retrieved by the queen, who carries them back to the nest by the dorsum of the neck (Figure 6-10). Retrieval is probably initiated by the kitten's distress vocalizations of a certain minimal intensity. The response is probably generalized to any distress vocalization because the queen probably cannot differentiate individuals by their distress calls. All queens in a colony show anxiety upon hearing the wails of kittens from other litters. The cries are a necessary signal to alert the queen of trouble, so deaf queens may totally ignore their misplaced young. This anxiety production in the queen is of significant survival value for the kittens and explains why the female becomes so concerned when one of the kittens is removed from the nest,

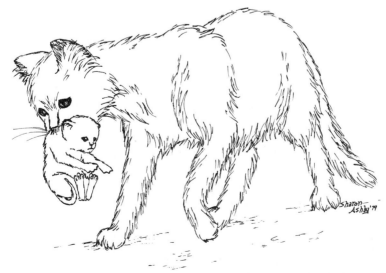

Figure 6-10 A queen carries her young, which assumes reflexive immobility, by the dorsum of its neck.

vocalizing as it is moved. The queen will usually approach whoever or whatever is holding the youngster, retrieve it from the intruder, and carry it back to the nest. This latency between kitten retrievals increases dramatically after the behavior has been used several times in succession.[71] Retrieval behavior peaks at about 1 week postpartum, possibly reflecting decreasing vocalization by kittens as they get older.[100] Reaction to the kitten cries lasts at least 30 days and influences the rate of various maternal behaviors.[45,46]

Over the weeks that follow parturition, the nest site will be moved several times. Queens sharing communal nests occupy approximately eight nests in 6 weeks for every four occupied by a solitary litter.[27] These moves are probably made to prevent predators and tomcats from finding the kittens, rather than to avoid the accumulation of ectoparasites, waste food, and kitten elimination products.[27] A female commonly moves her litter sometime around the third or fourth week postpartum, which is when this behavior seems to peak.[5,52] Multiple queens are more efficient at moving kittens to a new nest site, and with one at each site, there is an extra margin of safety too.[27]

Distressing situations, created by such things as loud noises or overcrowding, can cause the queen to move her young, which she carries by the dorsum of the neck. A few inexperienced females may hold other portions of a kitten, such as its leg. Some cats can be so nervous in an environment that they will move their litter four or five times a night. Whenever all the kittens have been transferred to the new location, the mother returns at least one more time to the old nest, indicating that she is not aware the move has been completed.[5,71]

Maternal Aggression

Maternal aggression in defense of young can be one of the fiercest forms of aggression shown by a cat. The female may attack humans, other species, or other cats without a threat display, almost eagerly.[24] Aggression toward male cats is normal and probably evolved as a way to protect kittens from being killed.[22] Even a very placid, human-loving cat can become highly aggressive toward people she knows if they try to remove her very young kittens from the home area. Because this is probably a function of her hormonal state, caution should always be exercised in any attempt to handle young kittens. Another factor that may contribute to the ferocity of maternal behavior is that in the effort to keep her group together, the queen must block her own flight response to danger. Thus she is more excitable and reactive to situations within her reach.[5] Because the domestic cat is normally not allowed to release her aggressions, when maternity lowers the aggression threshold, all the repressed energy of hostility is released at once.[24] Maternal aggression may be expressed as intolerance of other queens and their kittens unless raised in a communal nest. Selective breeding has helped reduce this undesirable behavior and other forms of maternal aggression.[29]

Infant Adoption

When two or more females give birth at approximately the same time and are housed in the same area, they may take turns nursing each other's kittens. It is also common, if one of the two females is the daughter of the other, for the daughter to nurse her own kittens while she and her half-siblings nurse the older female.[30] A more forward-acting female, whether she has queened or will do so soon, may take kittens from the more timid queen.

The early contact between mother and young results in a bond that continues their successful relationship until the time of the kittens' final dispersal. Much of this bond is probably formed because of licking. During the first week, particularly immediately after birth, most queens will readily accept any kitten. A queen's fostering of kittens is most successful before the maternal bond is established with her own kittens and when the foster kittens are about the same age as her own. Care must be taken if the kittens to be fostered are older than 1 week because females are known to react to young according to their size and not according to the age of the female's own young. The foster kittens may be ignored or attacked rather than accepted. Another factor influencing a queen's acceptance of foster kittens is the appearance the kitten presents to the approaching queen. If the female approaches the caudal area of a kitten, she may respond with anogenital licking. But if a cranial view of the same kitten is presented, she may display aggression.[5,24]

During the first week after littering, the queen may accept the young of other species, so pictures of cats nursing bunnies, rats, and puppies are often seen. Despite raising young of another species, a queen can still be a hunter of that species, even bringing the prey home to feed her "offspring."

Another time when the female may accept kittens other than her own is when hers start leaving the home area. At this time, the maternal bond decreases sharply and the queen ceases to differentiate between her young and other kittens.[25] That is also a common time for young housed together to begin sharing mothers. Ingestive patterns of the kittens are changing, in that the female starts bringing solid food to the kittens. In certain situations other cats will also bring food to kittens, indicating that this behavior may be initiated by kitten size or activity patterns.[25]

Miscellaneous Influences

The queen serves several functions during kitten development, but during the latter portions of her contact with the young, she teaches them that in dangerous situations a specific growl signals a "run for cover" message.[5] She also demonstrates hunting skills and other fundamentals necessary for an independent existence so that her offspring may learn by observation.

Early care, as well as the health of both neonate and mother, can have a profound effect on clinical entities in the older kitten. For example, Himalayan queens are generally poor milk producers, and supplements may be necessary to prevent neonatal starvation and poor nervous system development.[75] Other studies have shown that kittens of queens on a protein-restricted diet vocalize more.[33] Increased emotionality in adult cats is also associated with decreased queen-kitten interactions and retarded early attachments.[33]

Although domestication often prolongs mother-young interactions, evidence suggests that feral queens and kittens normally separate about 4 months postpartum.

NEUROLOGIC AND HORMONAL CONTROLS

Female sexual behavior in the cat is governed primarily by the central nervous system. This occurs either directly or through hormonal influence.

Spinal Cord

The lumbar spinal cord contains short reflex arcs associated with certain portions of estrous behavior, even in anestrous females and in males.[64,126] Stimulation of the perineum causes reflex elevation of the pelvis, treading, and lateral deviation of the tail, although facilitation of these reflexes in normal cats is strictly associated with the hormonal state of that animal.[39,77]

Peripheral Nerves

Connection by sensory portions of peripheral nerves to the lumbar spinal area is also regulated by hormones because estrogens facilitate posturing by the female.[41] Although the role of the clitoris is uncertain in the cat, deep pressure and tactile sensations to the vaginal walls result in the copulatory cry.[41] Removal of the pelvic nerve plexus, which supplies both the uterus and the vagina, results in fewer copulatory cries, less postcoital rolling, and fewer ovulations.[23] The afferent fibers carrying this information centrally are believed to be associated with the hypogastric nerves, which are more active during estrus.[115]

The sympathetic portion of the nervous system controls the smooth muscle around the ovary and uterine tube in particular. With emotional stress these muscles can be forced into a prolonged contraction, which can block ovulation. Another result could be a tubal pregnancy, although this has not been documented in the cat. Clitoral engorgement is under parasympathetic control, and sensation is via the pudendal nerve.

If the genitalia of the estrous cat are denervated, mating behavior remains the same, but postmating activity is eliminated.[1] This suggests that the peripheral nervous system initiates the postmating response in the central nervous system.

Brain

Several areas of the brain regulate sexual behavior in the cat. Within the hypothalamus, the supraoptic region controls sexual responses, particularly those mediated by estrogen, and lesions of this rostral hypothalamus result in permanent anestrus. The caudal hypothalamic region and the caudal brainstem are responsible for reflexes essential to copulation.[64] Ovarian function is also maintained by a normal caudal hypothalamus, probably because of its interrelationship with the gonadotropic activities of the pituitary, and ovulation can be induced in hormonally primed cats by stimulation of the hypothalamus.[64,97] By contrast, lesions of the rostral tuberal or caudal portions of the hypothalamus block ovulation.[97]

The ventromedial hypothalamus demonstrates a generalized response to vaginal stimulation, and portions of the lateral reticular nucleus and medullary reticular formation show a more specific response and are influenced by hormonal variations.[112] Stilbestrol placed directly in the caudal hypothalamus results in estrous behavior but without the normal vaginal cellular changes.[38] The highest amount of peripheral hormone uptake by selected brain sites occurs in the preoptic and ventromedial hypothalamus. The greatest effects from vaginal electrical stimulation are seen in the rostral hypothalamus, and the caudal cell response is influenced by estrogen. This suggests that the caudal hypothalamus plays a role in the regulation of postcopulatory behavior and ovulation.[91]

After coitus, electrical activity in the arcuate nucleus of the caudal hypothalamus increases norepinephrine levels, which then release luteinizing hormone–releasing factor (LHRF) to stimulate the pituitary to produce luteinizing hormone (LH). Ovulation then occurs 1 to 3 days after coitus, following the LH peak.[93] These data, however, are from a study that indicates no relation exists between either the cortical or the hypothalamic electroencephalographic activity and the behavioral or hormonal status of the animals.[111]

The hypothalamus is also the reception area from the retina and/or pineal gland for environmental light. When the amounts of orange and red intensities in daylight fall below a certain level, the anestrous portion of the reproductive cycle begins.[108] Input from this light to the hypothalamus releases gonadotropin-releasing hormone (GnRH), a neurohumoral factor that regulates the pituitary gland.[41,108] The pituitary responds by producing follicle-stimulating hormone (FSH), which with ovarian estrogens affects the genital system. It in turn feeds back to the hypothalamus. Special timed lighting can eliminate this anestrous season, and the lighting conditions of a home may be sufficient to keep the cat cycling year round.

Control of the estrous behaviors of rolling and vocalization is exerted by the amygdaloid nuclei and the pyriform cortex.[64] In addition, the amygdala shows electroencephalographic changes during the postcoital reaction, suggesting that it may be involved in ovulation.[41] Lesions of the lateral medulla or lateral midbrain stop the copulatory cry and afterreaction of an estrous female, although she will tolerate being mounted and exhibit lordosis, pelvic elevation, and lateral tail deviation even when anestrous.[4,112]

The hypophysis regulates the ingestion of placentas for a short period postpartum.[24]

Brain and hormone interactions are so closely related that it is almost impossible to separate one from the other. Without estrogen the behaviors of a normal, intact female do not occur. It can be concluded then that estrogen has its primary effect on specific, complex brain areas and results in specific behaviors.

Hormones

Even before puberty, female fetuses are probably affected by hormones. The neonatal testosterone surge in males can have an affect on adjacent female fetuses in several species. Freemartin cows that were born twins to a bull calf are well known to veterinarians. Similar results have been shown in species with multiple young, including mice, ferrets, gerbils, rats, and hamsters.[*] Female fetuses that grew next to males showed more male characteristics than females carried next to other females. The resulting slight androgen influence can partially affect neighboring females. Although this type of study has not been reported in cats, indirect evidence has been found. In one study, only 2 of 5 female cats that sprayed and 4 of 14 that fought frequently were from all-female litters.[42] Also, of 22 female cats that did not spray or fight, only 8 came from litters with at least 3 male littermates.[42]

The interaction of hormones is complicated in the queen, just as it is in the females of other species. Gonadotropin is released from the hypothalamus. LH release begins

[*]References 16, 34, 54, 55, 65, 79, 94, 118–120.

within minutes of breeding, and ovulation will begin about 24 hours later and continue for 8 to 52 hours.[106,124] The LH release continues for approximately 16 hours before returning to baseline.[106] Gestation lasts 64 days after the LH peak.[51]

Because the cat is usually an induced ovulator, the only time progesterone is important is during pregnancy or after a nonfertile mating. In nonfertile matings, the corpus luteum (CL) is active for several weeks, resulting in a pseudopregnancy during that time. By day 21 of pregnancy or pseudopregnancy, the progesterone levels peak between 24 and 35 ng/ml.[117] In the pseudopregnant queen, the levels then fall rapidly and the CL becomes inactive by day 35.[107] In the pregnant queen, progesterone levels fall slowly to approximately 5 ng/ml just before parturition.[117] Progesterone is even lower (<1 ng/ml) in the nonpregnant cat and just after parturition if pregnancy had occurred.[117]

Without the influence of estrogens, as after ovariectomy, the cat will not display the behaviors associated with estrus, pregnancy, parturition, or motherhood but will increase the size of her territory. No differences are seen in activity levels, playfulness, excitement, or vocalization between those cats that have undergone an ovariohysterectomy (OHE) and those that have not, and no difference is seen in cats that had the an OHE surgery at 7 weeks or those that had an OHE at 7 months.[110] Even the aggressive component of anestrous behavior gradually decreases after surgery, so after 5 or 6 months the cat will passively tolerate mounting. If the ovaries are removed during estrus, blood levels of estrogen and behaviors typical of anestrus return within 24 hours.[81] Later external supplementation of estrogens to this female results in the return of estrous behavior, with both onset of action and duration of action being closely dependent. Vaginal epithelial changes also occur, even at dosage levels lower than those necessary for behavioral changes.[82] Estrous behavior continues in these treated, ovariectomized animals as long as supplementation is continuous; however, once the animal no longer receives the exogenous gonadal hormone and is allowed to return to the anestrous state, she proves highly refractive to additional estrogen.[2]

During pregnancy, hormone production will be taken over by the placenta. The ovarian luteal function peaks by day 21 and then decreases, so by day 45 the ovaries can be removed and the pregnancy still maintained.[93,103] Progesterone is produced by the placenta after 21 days, indicating an interaction between the fetus and the placenta, which governs hormone production.[93,103]

Another hormone that affects estrus is oxytocin released by vaginal cells. Oxytocin functions to increase mobility of uterine and uterine tube smooth muscle, thus facilitating sperm transport.[41]

Certain drugs have been used to control estrus in the cat over the years but have generally not been too successful. Regulation of endogenous hormones with exogenous hormones must be very carefully controlled, and real success will probably require more sophisticated knowledge of the neural-hormonal interactions. Anabolic steroids and hormones may suppress the release of FSH to affect the queen or act directly on the fetal kittens.[21]

Approximately one third of the female cats in the United States have undergone an OHE.[78,88] This in part reflects owner concerns about how the cat may ultimately change. Over the years, the removal of the genital tract of the female cat in general, and ovariectomy in particular, has been associated with certain physical and behavioral changes. Research into whether these changes do occur was not done until the 1990s.

The rate of surgical sterilization is lower for rural female cats than for urban ones.[78] One life-saving discovery is that neutering reduces the risk of the cat being relinquished to an animal shelter by approximately one third.[78,87] Weight gain is often cited as a problem of neutering.[12] In addition to generalized subcutaneous layering, a characteristic fat deposit in the inguinal skinfolds has been associated with neutering.[61] It is, however, highly controversial whether the lack of the activity normally associated with estrogen can have such a great effect on fat deposition because estrogens are influential only two or three times a year. In some cases this added weight can be attributed to decreased roaming and increased accessibility of food, but newer studies suggest that the surgery does affect metabolism.[28] Where the 6-month-old recommendation for age of neutering came from is unknown. Research also shows that weight gain and other behavior changes do not occur any more often in early neutered cats than in those who had an OHE at the more traditional age.[56] A survey of owners of 120 cats neutered before 12 weeks indicated all have been pleased, and only three cats showed any problems.[74]

FEMALE SEXUAL BEHAVIOR PROBLEMS

Stress-Related Problems

Stress on the female cat can create a number of different behavior problems, depending on the individual and her hormonal state. Inhibition of innate releasing mechanisms, as for prey killing, can result in some very unusual reactions, particularly in queens. Such stresses as noise, malnutrition, or moving can result in varied reactions, including anestrus, lack of milk production, failure to deliver, extreme fearfulness, frantic running, increased restlessness, abandonment of young, chronic diarrhea, epileptic-like seizures, excessive moving of kittens, excessive neonatal grooming, urine spraying, redirected aggression, or cannibalism. Work in several species has shown that high population density has a negative effect on gonadal and mammary activity, with concurrent adrenal hypertrophy.[113] To some individual cats, small numbers may constitute overcrowding.

For stressful situations, removal of the inducing factors is necessary to eliminate the problem. Antianxiety medications, tranquilizers, or progesterone also may help the queen return to normal. In addition to supplying the hormone whose level has suddenly fallen at parturition, progesterone has a calming effect by suppressing the dorsomedial hypothalamic center that is related to rage.[48]

Maternal neglect

Maternal neglect has several causes, but the results are similar: Without proper care, the kittens die. Typically, these queens are excessively human oriented and neglect their kittens in favor of human attention. A kitten also may be singled out because it is too cold, is slow to move, or is nonvocal.[52] In cases in which dead kittens remain in the box, the queen may totally ignore the body, sometimes even lying on top of it.[46] Necropsies of the neglected young usually reveal empty stomachs and full urinary bladders, implying failure of the queen to nurse the kittens and to stimulate elimination by anogenital licking. Of the neonatal deaths, 8% to 19% result from maternal neglect.[43,128]

Relocation of the kittens by the queen can also be affected by stress. The desire to move kittens is strongest within the first few hours after parturition and again at 25 to 35 days after queening, but stress factors can increase the incidence of this moving behavior. On rare occasions, a queen forgets where she moved her kittens and becomes highly vocal and restless.

Cannibalism

Eating of the young occurs often in cat colonies, and certain forms of it are normal. Queens routinely consume aborted fetuses and stillborn kittens, probably to keep the nest unsoiled and to prevent attracting predators to the area. When one queen in an open colony gives birth, others that are not pregnant or near term may consume the neonates. It is theorized that the infant's size and shape closely resemble those of natural prey and may initiate a normal prey-killing instinct. An increased incidence of cannibalism has been associated with a very large litter, the second pregnancy, and illness in the kittens.[43] It is also more likely to occur to an injured kitten than to a newborn.[52] Other situations can provoke cannibalism, such as stress produced by the queen's inability to find an appropriate queening area.[30] Also, if extremely malnourished, a queen may cannibalize her young. This situation represents one in which self-preservation finally overrules maternalism. Still another type of cannibalism is hormonal cannibalism, which results from incomplete hormonal inhibition of the prey-killing instinct in a female cat. The same hormones that are responsible for maternal behavior are probably responsible for inhibition of the prey-killing instinct. Cannibalism can account for 12.5% of preweaning kitten losses.[128] Eviscerating and ingesting part of a kitten while chewing the umbilical cord too closely are not true cannibalism, and although this does occur, especially with the nervous cat, it is rare.

Correction of problem cannibalism depends on the initiating factors. At least 2 weeks before the expected littering date, the minimization of stress is highly desirable, as is the provision of an isolated queening area or even a separate cage in a colony situation. Progestins are successful in preventing hormonal cannibalism.

Delayed parturition

The interruption or prolongation of parturition is a common sequela to stress. Human-dependent cats very commonly have a prolonged labor, and when a kitten is first presented with its head protruding from the vulva, this type of queen may make no attempt to complete the delivery or to clean the kitten after the delivery is completed. This behavior may be repeated with each kitten. Disturbances to a delivering queen can delay further births, but normal parturition usually resumes within 12 to 24 hours. Mild sedation is helpful in initiating resumption of normal parturition. However, it is best that the owner give the medication at home rather than cause a disturbance to the queen by bringing her to a veterinary clinic. Delays in parturition caused by uterine inertia are rare in the cat.[61]

Stealing kittens

It is not uncommon for queens that share a communal nest to nurse and care for kittens from another litter. Occasionally though, a cat without a litter of her own will steal one or more kittens to raise as her own. This would be expected to occur near the end of pregnancy or pseudocyesis, as hormone levels begin to change. Lactation can follow an OHE performed near the regression or termination of the corpora lutea. Sometimes a spayed female will show interest in the kittens, and if they try to nurse her long enough, she will begin to lactate.[52]

Pseudocyesis

Pseudocyesis is another condition that is common but rarely observed in felids.[7] A functional CL remains after ovulation with or without pregnancy. That makes pseudocyesis a normal sequela to estrus. Because corpora lutea start regressing around 21 days after ovulation in the nonpregnant animal, after peak luteal production at 16 to 17 days, false pregnancy seldom lasts more then 45 days. Signs of the condition, although typically mild in the cat, may range from physical signs of pregnancy to "kitten tending," the adoption of other animals or soft toys. Milk production and labor can also occur. Nonfertilized ovulation is necessary to induce pseudopregnancy, and merely petting an estrous female has on rare occasions induced ovulation.[49] When this physiologic situation occurs, it produces psychologic manifestations and illustrates the extent to which the cat's body is adapted for a pregnant state. Pseudocyesis is self-limiting, so drug therapy is generally unnecessary. Tranquilizers, reposital testosterone, or reposital stilbestrol have been used in extreme cases.[109] The cat is typically in estrus again within 44 days.[93]

Hypersexuality

Nymphomania is a relatively common variation of female sexual behavior, especially in Siamese and Persian cats.[31,98] This prolonged, exaggerated, easily aroused estrous behavior often accompanies cystic ovaries.[30] The caudate nucleus of the brain has also been implicated with this form of feline hypersexuality, which along with other personality extremes induced by excitement has been classified as a hysterical disorder.[15,93]

True homosexual behavior in female cats is unusual. Females will occasionally mount other females, and this represents about 16% of cat sexual behavior problems.[50] This behavior can be a consequence of sexual energy not released during estrus rather than preference for the same sex. As a result of tension and frustration, an estrous female may suddenly mount another female or even a passive male. Prepubertal kittens may also engage in play behavior partially resembling sexual patterns, with indiscriminate mounting between sexes (see Figure 5-1).

Masturbation is unusual except in cats with high estrogen levels or prolonged estrogen exposure and is accomplished mainly by rubbing the anogenital region against the floor while suspending the body with the forelimbs. In addition, the cat usually vocalizes and licks her genital area.[64]

Other Problems

Pseudohermaphroditism does occur in felids. The male pseudohermaphrodite has testicles, but the external genitalia appear feminine, perhaps slightly modified. The female pseudohermaphrodite has male external genitalia with female internal organs and gonads, but this condition is extremely uncommon. Because testosterone influence is needed for the male physique, the condition is rare without gonads.[37]

An estrous female may not mate with a particular tomcat for several reasons, including environmental stress, invasion of her territory, and undesirability of the tomcat. Time together for such individuals may eventually result in successful copulations, although owners may not be aware of them. Physical restraint of an objecting female can permit an experienced tomcat to mate her.[44] In addition, tranquilizers and catnip have been successfully used to calm nervous female cats.[14] The cat subjected to controlled but infrequent matings may undergo endometrial and psychosomatic changes. If prolonged, this situation can lead to chronic diarrhea, aggression, or seizures.[60]

Blue-eyed, deaf white cats are perpetuated primarily by selective breeding. In addition to their other problems, females with this genetic makeup are semisterile.[10]

Progestational hormone therapy for any of a variety of clinical entities, from treatment of skin conditions to estrus prevention, has been accompanied by a myriad of complications. Some female cats fail to start cycling once drug therapy has been terminated, and others develop endometrial hyperplasia and pyometra. These conditions can occur in ovariohysterectomized females if any uterine tissue remains, as when the uterus is severed proximal to the cervix. In addition, neutered cats have exhibited mild estrous signs after cessation of the hormone therapy. Other adverse reactions from progestin use are described in Chapter 1.

REFERENCES

1. Bard P: Effects of denervation of the genitalia on the oestrous behavior of cats, *Am J Physiol* 113:5–6, Sep 1935.
2. Beach FA: *Hormones and behavior,* New York, 1961, Cooper Square Publishers.
3. Beach FA, editor: *Sex and behavior,* New York, 1965, John Wiley and Sons.
4. Beach FA: Cerebral and hormonal control of reflexive mechanisms involved in copulatory behavior, *Physiol Rev* 47:289–316, April 1967.
5. Beadle M: *The cat: history, biology, and behavior,* New York, 1977, Simon & Schuster.
6. Beaver BV: Mating behavior in the cat, *Vet Clin North Am* 7(4):729–733, 1977.
7. Beaver BV: Feline behavioral problems other than housesoiling, *J Am Anim Hosp Assoc* 25(4):465–469, 1989.
8. Beaver BV: Psychogenic manifestations of environmental disturbances. In August JR, editor: *Consultations in feline medicine,* Philadelphia, 1991, WB Saunders.
9. Beaver BVG: Supernumerary fetation in the cat, *Feline Pract* 3(3):24–25, 1973.
10. Bergsma DR, Brown KS: White fur, blue eyes, and deafness in the domestic cat, *J Hered* 62(3):171–185, 1971.
11. Bland KP: Tom-cat odour and other pheromones in feline reproduction, *Vet Sci Commun* 3:125–136, 1979.
12. Bloomberg MS: Surgical neutering and nonsurgical alternatives, *J Am Vet Med Assoc* 208(4):517–519, 1996.
13. Boudreau JC, Tsuchitani C: *Sensory neurophysiology,* New York, 1973, Van Nostrand Reinhold.
14. Bryant D: *The care and handling of cats,* New York, 1944, Ives Washburn.
15. Chertok L, Fontaine M: Psychosomatics in veterinary medicine, *J Psychosom Res* 7:229–235, 1963.
16. Clark MM, Malenfant SA, Winter DA, Galef BG Jr: Fetal uterine position affects copulation and scent marking by adult male gerbils, *Physiol Behav* 47(2):301–305, 1990.
17. Comfort A: Maximum ages reached by domestic cats, *J Mammal* 37(1):118–119, 1956.
18. Cooper JB: A description of parturition in the domestic cat, *J Comp Psychol* 37:71–79, 1944.
19. Crowell-Davis SL, Barry K, Wolfe R: Social behavior and aggressive problems of cats, *Vet Clin North Am Small Anim Pract* 27(3):549–568, 1997.

20. Dards JL: The behavior of dockyard cats: interactions of adult males, *Appl Anim Ethol* 10:133–153, 1983.
21. Davis LE: Adverse effects of drugs on reproduction in dogs and cats, *Mod Vet Pract* 64(12):969–974, 1983.
22. Deag JM, Manning A, Lawrence CE: Factors influencing the mother-kitten relationship. In Turner DC, Bateson PPG, editors: *The domestic cat: the biology of its behaviour,* Cambridge, 1988, Cambridge University Press.
23. Diakow C: Effects of genital desensitization on mating behavior and ovulation in the female cat, *Physiol Behav* 7:47–54, July 1971.
24. Ewer RF: *Ethology of mammals,* London, 1968, Paul Elek Ltd.
25. Ewer RF: *The carnivores,* Ithaca, NY, 1973, Cornell University Press.
26. Ewer RF: The evolution of mating systems in the Felidae. In Eaton RL, editor: *The world's cats,* Seattle, 1974, Feline Research Group.
27. Feldman HN: Maternal care and differences in the use of nests in the domestic cat, *Anim Behav* 45(1):13–23, 1993.
28. Flynn MF, Hardie EM, Armstrong PJ: Effect of ovariohysterectomy on maintenance energy requirement in cats, *J Am Vet Med Assoc* 209(9):1572–1581, 1996.
29. Fox MW: Aggression: its adaptive and maladaptive significance in man and animals. In Fox MW, editor: *Abnormal behavior in animals,* Philadelphia, 1968, WB Saunders.
30. Fox MW: *Understanding your cat,* New York, 1974, Coward, McCann & Geoghegan.
31. Fox MW: The behaviour of cats. In Hafez ESE, editor: *The behavior of domestic animals,* ed 3, Baltimore, 1975, Williams & Wilkins.
32. Freeman NCG, Rosenblatt JS: The interrelationship between thermal and olfactory stimulation in the development of home orientation in newborn kittens, *Dev Psychobiol* 11(5):437–457, 1978.
33. Gallo PV, Werboff J, Knox K: Protein restriction during gestation and lactation: development of attachment behavior in cats, *Behav Neural Biol* 29:216–223, 1980.
34. Gandelman R, vom Saal FS, Reinisch JM: Contiguity to male fetuses affects morphology and behaviour of female mice, *Nature* 266:722–724, April 21, 1977.
35. Hall VE, Pierce GN: Litter size, birth weight, and growth to weaning in the cat, *Anat Rec* 60:111–112, 1934.
36. Halsema LJ: Living room leopard cat, *Friskies Res Dig* 11:6–7, Summer 1975.
37. Hare WCD: Female pseudohermaphroditism, *Feline Pract* 9(1):4, 6, 1979.
38. Harris GW, Michael RP, Scott PP: Neurological site of action of stilboestrol in eliciting sexual behavior. In Wolstenholme GEW, O'Connor CM, editors: *Neurological basis of behaviour,* Boston, 1952, Little, Brown and Company.
39. Hart BL: Facilitation by estrogen of sexual reflexes in female cats, *Physiol Behav* 7(5):675–678, 1971.
40. Hart BL: Maternal behavior. I. Parturient and postparturient behavior, *Feline Pract* 2(5):6–7, 1972.
41. Hart BL: Physiology of sexual function, *Vet Clin North Am* 4(3):557–571, 1974.
42. Hart BL, Eckstein RA: The role of gonadal hormones in the occurrence of objectionable behaviours in dogs and cats, *Appl Anim Behav Sci* 52(3,4):331–344, 1997.
43. Hart BL, Hart LA: *Canine and feline behavioral therapy,* Philadelphia, 1985, Lea & Febiger.
44. Hart BL, Voith VL: Sexual behavior and breeding problems in cats, *Feline Pract* 7(1):9, 10, 12, 1977.
45. Haskins R: Effect of kitten vocalizations on maternal behavior, *J Comp Physiol Psychol* 91(4):830–838, 1977.
46. Haskins R: A causal analysis of kitten vocalizations: an observational and experimental study, *Anim Behav* 27(3):726–736, 1979.

47. Hemmer H: Gestation period and postnatal development in felids. In Eaton RL, editor: *The world's cats,* ed 3, Seattle, 1976, Carnivore Research Institute.

48. Henik RA, Olson PN, Rosychuk RA: Progestogen therapy in cats, *Compend Contin Educ* 7(2):132–142, 1985.

49. *Histochemistry* 43(3):191–202, 1975.

50. Houpt KA: Problems in maternal and sexual behaviors. Paper presented at meeting of the American Veterinary Medical Association, Minneapolis, July 18, 1993.

51. Houpt KA: Sexual behavior problems in dogs and cats, *Vet Clin North Am Small Anim Pract* 27(3):601–615, 1997.

52. Houpt KA: Maternal behavior and its aberrations. In Houpt KA, editor: *Recent advances in companion animal behavior problems,* International Veterinary Information Service. Available at www.ivis.org.

53. Houpt KA, Wolski RR: *Domestic animal behavior for veterinarians and animal scientists,* Ames, 1982, Iowa State University Press.

54. Houtsmuller EJ, Juranek J, Gebauer CE, et al: Males located caudally in the uterus affect sexual behavior of male rats in adulthood, *Behav Brain Res* 62:119–125, 1994.

55. Houstmuller EJ, Slob AK: Masculinization and defeminization of female rats by males located caudally in the uterus, *Physiol Behav* 48(4):555–560, 1990.

56. Howe LM, Slater MR, Boothe HW, et al: Long-term outcome of gonadectomy performed at an early age or traditional age in cats, *J Am Vet Med Assoc* 217(11):1661–1665, 2000.

57. Hunt HR: Birth of two unequally developed cat fetuses *(Felis domestica), Anat Rec* 16:371–377, 1919.

58. Jemmett JE, Evans JM: A survey of sexual behaviour and reproduction of female cats, *J Small Anim Pract* 18:31–37, Jan 1977.

59. Johnson CA, Grace JA: Care of newborn puppies and kittens, *Forum* 6(1):9–16, 1987.

60. Joshua JO: Abnormal behavior in cats. In Fox MW, editor: *Abnormal behavior in animals,* Philadelphia, 1968, WB Saunders.

61. Joshua JO: Some conditions seen in feline practice attributable to hormonal causes, *Vet Rec* 88:511–514, May 15, 1971.

62. Joshua JO: Feline reproduction: the problem of infertility in purebred queens, *Feline Pract* 5(5):52–54, 1975.

63. Kerby G, Macdonald DW: Cat society and the consequences of colony size. In Turner DC, Bateson PPG, editors: *The domestic cat: the biology of its behaviour,* Cambridge, 1988, Cambridge University Press.

64. Kling A, Kovach JK, Tucker TJ: The behaviour of cats. In Hafez ESE, editor: *The behaviour of domestic animals,* ed 2, Baltimore, 1969, Williams & Wilkins.

65. Krohmer RW, Baum MJ: Effect of sex, intrauterine position and androgen manipulation on the development of brain aromatase activity in fetal ferrets, *J Neuroendocrinol* 1(4):265–271.

66. Lawler DF, Johnston SD, Hegstad RL, et al: Ovulation without cervical stimulation in domestic cats, *J Reprod Fertil Suppl* 47:57–61, 1993.

67. Lawrence C: Individual differences in maternal behaviour in the domestic cat, *Appl Anim Ethol* 6:387–388, 1980.

68. Lein D, Concannon PW, Hodgson BG: Reproductive behavior in the queen, *J Am Vet Med Assoc* 181(3):275, 1982.

69. LeRoux PH: The use of a teaser tom to terminate oestrum in female cats, *J S Afr Vet Med Assoc* 42(2):195, 1971.

70. Leyhausen P: Communal organization of solitary mammals, *Symp Zool Soc Lond* 14:249–263, 1965.

71. Leyhausen P: *Cat behavior: the predatory and social behavior of domestic and wild cats,* New York, 1978, Garland STPM Press.

72. Liberg O: Predation and social behaviour in a population of domestic cat. An evolutionary perspective, Dissertation, Sweden, 1981, Department of Animal Ecology, University of Lund.
73. Liberg O: Courtship behaviour and sexual selection in the domestic cat, *Appl Anim Ethol* 10:117–132, March 1983.
74. Lieberman LL: A case for neutering pups and kittens at two months of age, *J Am Vet Med Assoc* 191(5):518–521, 1987.
75. Lott JN, Herron M: Sudden death syndrome in kittens, *Feline Pract* 7(3):16, 19, 1977.
76. Macdonald DW, Apps PJ, Curr GM, Kerby G: *Social dynamics, nursing coalitions, and infanticide among farm cats,* Felis catus, Berlin, 1987, Paul Parey Scientific Publishers.
77. Maes JP: Neural mechanism of sexual behaviour in the female cat, *Nature* 144:598–599, Sep 30, 1939.
78. Mahlow JC: Estimation of the proportions of dogs and cats that are surgically sterilized, *J Am Vet Med Assoc* 215(5):640–643, 1999.
79. Meisel RL, Ward IL: Fetal female rats are masculinized by male littermates located caudally in the uterus, *Science* 213:239–242, July 10, 1981.
80. Michael RP: Sexual behaviour and the vaginal cycle in the cat, *Nature* 181:567–568, Feb 22, 1958.
81. Michael RP: Observations upon the sexual behavior of the domestic cat (*Felis catus* L.) under laboratory conditions, *Behaviour* 18(1–2):1–24, 1961.
82. Michael RP, Scott PP: The activation of sexual behaviour in cats by the subcutaneous administration of oestrogen, *J Physiol* 171(2).254–274, 1964.
83. Michel C: Induction of oestrus in cats by photoperiodic manipulations and social stimuli, *Lab Anim* 27(3):278–280, 1993.
84. Mykytowycz R: Reproduction of mammals in relation to environmental odours, *J Reprod Fertil* 19(suppl):433–446, Dec 1973.
85. Natoli E, DeVito E: Agonistic behaviour, dominance rank and copulatory success in a large multi-male feral cat, *Felis catus* L., colony in central Rome, *Anim Behav* 42:227–241, 1991.
86. Paape SR, Shille VM, Seto H, Stabenfeldt GH: Luteal activity in the pseudopregnant cat, *Biol Reprod* 13:470–474, Nov 1975.
87. Patronek GJ, Glickman LT, Beck AM, et al: Risk factors for relinquishment of cats to an animal shelter, *J Am Vet Med Assoc* 209(3):582–588, 1996.
88. Pet sterilization, *Bull Inst Study Anim Probl* 1(3):4, 1979.
89. Povey RC: Reproduction in the pedigree female cat. A survey of breeders, *Can Vet J* 19(8):207–213, 1978.
90. Prescott CW: Reproduction patterns in the domestic cat, *Aust Vet J* 49(3):126–129, 1973.
91. Ratner A, Koenig JQ, Frazier DT: Hypothalamic unit activity in the cat: effects of estrogen and vaginal stimulation, *Proc Soc Exp Biol Med* 137:321–326, May 1971.
92. Rheingold HL, Eckerman CO: Familiar social and nonsocial stimuli and the kitten's response to a strange environment, *Dev Psychobiol* 4:71–89, 1971.
93. Richkind M: The reproductive endocrinology of the domestic cat, *Feline Pract* 8(5):28–31, 1978.
94. Richmond G, Sachs BD: further evidence for masculinization of female rats by males located caudally *in utero, Horm Behav* 18:484–490, 1984.
95. Robison R, Cox HW: Reproductive performance in a cat colony over a 10-year period, *Lab Anim* 4(1):99–112, 1970.
96. Root MV, Johnston SD, Olson PN: Estrous length, pregnancy rate, gestation and parturition lengths, litter size, and juvenile mortality in the domestic cat, *J Am Anim Hosp Assoc* 31(5):429–433, 1995.
97. Sawyer CJ, Robison B: Separate hypothalamic areas controlling pituitary gonadotropic function and mating behavior in female cats and rabbits, *J Clin Endocrinol Metab* 16(7):914–915, 1956.

98. Schmidt JP: Psychosomatics in veterinary medicine. In Fox MW, editor: *Abnormal behavior in animals,* Philadelphia, 1968, WB Saunders.

99. Schmidt PM, Chakraborty PK, Wildt DE: Ovarian activity, circulating hormones and sexual behavior in the cat. II. Relationships during pregnancy, parturition, lactation and the postpartum estrus, *Biol Reprod* 28:657–671, April 1983.

100. Schneirla TC, Rosenblatt JS, Tobach E: Maternal behavior in the cat. In Rheingold HL, editor: *Maternal behavior in mammals,* New York, 1963, John Wiley and Sons.

101. Scott FW, Geissinger C, Peltz R: Kitten mortality survey, *Feline Pract* 8(6):31–34, 1978.

102. Scott PP: The domestic cat as a laboratory animal for the study of reproduction, *J Physiol* 130:47P–48P, 1955.

103. Scott PP: Diet and other factors affecting the development of young felids. In Eaton RL, editor: *The world's cats,* ed 3, Seattle, 1976, Carnivore Research Institute.

104. Scott PP, Lloyd-Jacob MA: Some interesting features in the reproductive cycle of the cat, *Stud Fertil* 7:123–129, 1955.

105. Shille VM, Lundstrom KE, Stabenfeldt GL: Follicular function in the domestic cat as determined by estradiol-17β concentrations in plasma: relation to estrous behavior and cornification of exfoliated vaginal epithelium, *Biol Reprod* 21:953–963, 1979.

106. Shille VM, Munro C, Farmer SW, et al: Ovarian and endocrine responses in the cat after coitus, *J Reprod Fertil* 69(1):29–39, 1983.

107. Stabenfeldt GH: Physiologic, pathologic and therapeutic roles of progestins in domestic animals, *J Am Vet Med Assoc* 164(3):311–317, 1974.

108. Stapley R: Factors affecting the reproductive behavior of the feline. I. Photoperiodicity and controlled exposure to light, *Friskies Res Dig* 14:8, Spring 1978.

109. Stein BS: The genital system. In Catcott EJ, editor: *Feline medicine and surgery,* ed 2, Santa Barbara, Calif, 1975, American Veterinary Publications.

110. Stubbs WP, Bloomberg MS, Scruggs SL, et al: Effects of prepubertal gonadectomy on physical or behavioral development in cats, *J Am Vet Med Assoc* 209(11):1864–1871, 1996.

111. Sutin J, Michael RP: Changes in brain electrical activity following vaginal stimulation in estrous and anestrous cats, *Physiol Behav* 5(9):1043–1051, 1970.

112. Sutin J, Rose J, Van Atta L, Thalmann R: Electrophysiological studies in an animal model of aggressive behavior, *Res Publ Assoc Rec Nerv Ment Dis* 52:93–118, 1974.

113. Thiessen DD, Rodgers DA: Population density and endocrine function, *Psychol Bull* 58:441–451, Nov 1961.

114. Todd NB: Behavior and genetics of the domestic cat, *Cornell Vet* 53:99–107, Jan 1963.

115. Varbanova A, Doneshka P, Vassileva-Popova JG: Changes in EEG and in the activity of the whole cervical vagus upon application of sex hormones. In Vassileva-Popova JG, editor: *Physical and chemical bases of biological information transfer,* New York, 1975, Plenum Publishing.

116. Verberne G, DeBoer J: Chemocommunication among domestic cats, mediated by the olfactory and vomeronasal senses. I. Chemocommunication, *Z Tierpsychol* 42:86–109, Sep 1976.

117. Verhage HG, Beamer NB, Brenner RM: Plasma levels of estradiol and progesterone in the cat during polyestrus, pregnancy and pseudopregnancy, *Biol Reprod* 14:570–585, 1976.

118. Vomachka AJ, Lisk RD: Androgen and estradiol levels in plasma and amniotic fluid of late gestational male and female hamsters: uterine position effects, *Horm Behav* 20:181–193, 1986.

119. vom Saal FS: Variation in phenotype due to random intrauterine positioning of male and female fetuses in rodents, *J Reprod Fertil* 62:633–650, 1981.

120. vom Saal FS, Bronson FH: In utero proximity of female house mouse fetuses to males: effect on reproductive performance during later life, *Biol Reprod* 19:842–853, 1978.

121. Weigel I: Small cats and clouded leopards. In Grzimek HCB, editor: *Grzimek's animal life encyclopedia,* vol 12, New York, 1975, Van Nostrand Reinhold.

122. Whalen RE: The initiation of mating in naive female cats, *Anim Behav* 11:461–463, Oct 1963.

123. Wildt DE: Effect of transportation on sexual behavior of cats, *Lab Anim Sci* 30:910–912, Oct 1980.

124. Wildt DE, Chan SY, Seager SWJ, Chakraborty PK: Ovarian activity, circulation hormones, and sexual behavior in the cat. 1. Relationships during the coitus-induced luteal phase and the estrous period without mating, *Biol Reprod* 25:15–28, 1981.

125. Wood GL: *Animal facts and feats,* New York, 1972, Doubleday.

126. Worden AN: Abnormal behaviour in the dog and cat, *Vet Rec* 71:966–978, Dec 26, 1959.

127. Wynne-Edwards VC: *Animal dispersion in relation to social behaviour,* Edinburgh, 1962, Oliver & Boyd.

128. Young C: Preweaning mortality in specific pathogen-free kittens, *J Small Anim Pract* 14(7):391–397, 1973.

ADDITIONAL READINGS

Alexander SA, Shane SM: Characteristics of animals adopted from an animal control center whose owners complied with a spaying/neutering program, *J Am Vet Med Assoc* 205(3):472–476, 1994.

Aronsohn MG, Faggella AM: Surgical techniques for neutering 6- to 14-week-old kittens, *J Am Vet Med Assoc* 202(1):53–55, 1993.

Bard P, Macht MB: The behaviour of chronically decerebrate cats. In Wolstendholme GEW, O'Connor CM, editors: *Neurological basis of behaviour,* Boston, 1952, Little, Brown and Company.

Barton A: Sexual inversion and homosexuality in dogs and cats, *Vet Med* 54:155–156, March 1959.

Beaver BV: Feline behavioral problems, *Vet Clin North Am* 6:33–40, Aug 1976.

Beaver BV: Disorders of behavior. In Sherding RG, editor: *The cat: diseases and clinical management,* New York, 1989, Churchill Livingstone.

Beyer C: Effect of estrogen on brain stem neuronal responsivity in the cat. In Sawyer CH, Gorski RA, editors: *Steroid hormones and brain function,* Berkeley, 1971, University of California Press.

Brunner F: The application of behavior studies in small animal practice. In Fox MW, editor: *Abnormal behavior in animals,* Philadelphia, 1968, WB Saunders.

Burke TJ: Feline reproduction, *Vet Clin North Am* 6:317–331, Aug 1976.

Burke TJ: Pharmacologic control of estrus in the bitch and queen, *Vet Clin North Am Small Anim Pract* 12(1):79–84, 1982.

Centonze LA, Levy JK: Characteristics of free-roaming cats and their caretakers, *J Am Vet Med Assoc* 220(11):1627–1633, 2002.

Cerny VA: Failure of dihydrotestosterone to elicit sexual behavior in the female cat, *J Endocrinol* 75:173–174, Oct 1977.

Chakraborty PK, Wildt DE, Seager SW: Serum luteinizing hormone and ovulatory response to luteinizing hormone-releasing hormone in the estrous and anestrous domestic cat, *Lab Anim Sci* 29(3):338–344, 1979.

Chesler P: Maternal influence in learning by observation in kittens, *Science* 166:901–903, Nov 14, 1969.

Cline EM, Jennings LL, Sojka NJ: Breeding laboratory cats during artificially induced estrus, *Lab Anim Sci* 30(6):1003–1005, 1980.

Colby ED: Induced estrus and timed pregnancies in cats, *Lab Anim Care* 20:1075–1080, Dec 1970.

Dawson AB: Early estrus in the cat following increased illumination, *Endocrinology* 28:907–910, June 1941.

Diegmann FG, Loo BJ, Grom PA: Female pseudohermaphroditism in the cat, *Feline Pract* 8(5):45, 1978.

Eleftheriou BE, Scott JP: *The physiology of aggression and defeat,* New York, 1971, Plenum Publishing.

Evans I: Suppression of estrus in cats, *Feline Pract* 2(6):10, 1972.

Ewer RF: Viverrid behavior and the evolution of reproductive behavior in the Felidae. In Eaton RL, editor: *The world's cats,* Seattle, 1974, Feline Research Group.

Failla ML, Tobach E, Frank A: A study of parturition in the domestic cat, *Anat Rec* 111:482, Nov 1951.

Fox MW: New information on feline behavior, *Mod Vet Pract* 56(4):50–52, 1965.

Fox MW: Natural environment: theoretical and practical aspects for breeding and rearing laboratory animals, *Lab Anim Care* 16:316–321, Aug 1966.

Fox MW: The veterinarian: mercenary, Saint Francis or humanist? *J Am Vet Med Assoc* 166(3):276–279, 1975.

Fraser AF: Behavior disorders in domestic animals. In Fox MW, editor: *Abnormal behavior in animals,* Philadelphia, 1968, WB Saunders.

Friedgood HB: Induction of estrous behavior in anestrous cats with the FSH & LH of the anterior pituitary gland, *Am J Physiol* 126:229–233, 1939.

Gerber HA, Jochle W, Sulman FG: Control of reproduction and of undesirable social and sexual behaviour in dogs and cats, *J Small Anim Pract* 14(3):151–158, 1973.

Gottlieb G: Ontogenesis of sensory function in birds and mammals. In Tobach E, Aronson LR, Shaw E, editors: *The biopsychology of development,* New York, 1971, Academic Press.

Green JD, Clemente CD, DeGroot J: Rhinencephalic lesions and behavior in cats, *J Comp Neurol* 108:505–545, 1957.

Hart BL: Facilitation by estrogen of sexual reflexes in female cats, *Physiol Behav* 7(5):675–678, 1971.

Hart BL: Gonadal hormones and behavior of the female cat, *Feline Pract* 2(4):6–8, 1972.

Hart BL: Types of aggressive behavior, *Canine Pract* 1(1):6, 8, 1974.

Hart BL: Normal behavior and behavioral problems associated with sexual function, urination, and defecation, *Vet Clin North Am* 4(3):589–606, 1974.

Hart BL: The catnip response, *Feline Pract* 4(6):8, 12, 1974.

Hart BL: Spraying behavior, *Feline Pract* 5(4):11–13, 1975.

Hart BL: Aggression in cats, *Feline Pract* 7(2):22, 24, 28, 1977.

Hart BL: Objectionable urine spraying and urine marking in cats: evaluation of progestin treatment in gonadectomized males and females, *J Am Vet Med Assoc* 177(6):529–533, 1980.

Hart BL: *The behavior of domestic animals,* New York, 1985, WH Freeman and Company.

Hart BL, Cooper L: Factors related to urine spraying and fighting in prepubertally gonadectomized male and female cats, *J Am Vet Med Assoc* 184:1255, 1984.

Houdeshell JW, Hennessey PW: Megestrol acetate for control of estrus in the cat, *Vet Med Small Anim Clin* 72(6):1013–1017, 1977.

Houpt KA: Animal behavior as a subject for veterinary students, *Cornell Vet* 66:73–81, Jan 1976.

Jöchle W: Progress in small animal reproductive physiology, therapy of reproductive disorders, and pet population control, *Folia Vet Lat* 4:706–731, Oct/Dec 1974.

Jöchle W, Jöchle M: Reproductive and behavioral control in the male and female cat with progestins: long-term field observations in individual animals, *Theriology* 3(5):179–185, 1975.

Kavanagh AJ: The reticulo-cortical evoked response: changes correlated with behaviour and estrogen in female cats, *Diss Abstr Int* 30:995B–996B, 1969.

Kleiman DG, Eisenberg JF: Comparisons of canid and felid social systems from an evolutionary perspective, *Anim Behav* 21:637–659, Nov 1973.

Kustritz MVR: Elective gonadectomy in the cat, *Feline Pract* 24(6):36–39, 1996.

Marvin C: Hormonal influences on the development and expression of sexual behavior in animals. In Fox MW, editor: *Abnormal behavior in animals,* Philadelphia, 1968, WB Saunders.

McDonald M: Population control of feral cats using megestrol acetate, *Vet Rec* 106(6):129, 1980.

Michael RP: Neurological mechanisms and the control of sexual behaviour, *Sci Basis Med* pp 316–333, 1965.

Mosier JE: Common medical and behavioral problems in cats, *Mod Vet Pract* 56:699–703, Oct 1975.

O'Connor P, Herron MA: Estrus after ovariohysterectomy, *Feline Pract* 6(5):28, 1976.

Palen GF, Goddard GV: Catnip and oestrous behaviour in the cat, *Anim Behav* 14:372–377, 1966.

Peretz E: Estrogen dose and the duration of mating period in cats, *Physiol Behav* 3:41–43, 1968.

Pfaff DW: Interactions of steroid sex hormones with brain tissue: studies of uptake and physiological effects. In Segal SJ, editor: *The regulation of mammalian reproduction,* Springfield, Ill, 1973, Charles C Thomas Publisher.

Porter RW, Cavanaugh EB, Critchlow BV, Sawyer CH: Localized changes in electrical activity of the hypothalamus in estrous cats following vaginal stimulation, *Am J Physiol* 189:145–151, April 1957.

Remfry J: Control of feral cat populations by long-term administration of megestrol acetate, *Vet Rec* 103(18):403–404, 1978.

Romanes GJ: *Mental evolution in animals,* New York, 1969, AMS Press.

Scott JP: The analysis of social organization in animals, *Ecology* 37:213–221, April 1956.

Scott PP, Lloyd-Jacob MA: Reduction in the anoestrus period of laboratory cats by increased illumination, *Nature* 184:2022, Dec 26, 1959.

Smith BA, Jansen GR: Early undernutrition and subsequent behavior patterns in cat, *J Nutr* 103(7):29, 1973.

Smith RC: *The complete cat book,* New York, 1963, Walker & Company.

Stewart MF: Maternal behaviour in cats, *Br Vet J* 127(8):397, 1971.

Stover DG, Sokolowski JH: Estrous behavior of the domestic cat, *Feline Pract* 8(4):54–58, 1978.

Sulman FG: Suppression of estrus in cats, *Vet Med* 56(12):513–514, 1961.

Thornton DAK, Kear M: Uterine cystic hyperplasia in a Siamese cat following treatment with medroxyprogesterone, *Vet Rec* 80:380–381, March 25, 1967.

West M: Social play in the domestic cat, *Am Zool* 14:427–436, Winter 1974.

Wildt DE, Guthrie SC, Seager SWJ: Ovarian and behavioral cyclicity of the laboratory maintained cat, *Horm Behav* 10(3):251–257, 1978.

Wilkins DB: Pyometritis in a spayed cat, *Vet Rec* 91:24, July 1, 1972.

Windle WF: Induction of mating and ovulation in the cat with pregnancy urine and seminal extracts, *Endocrinology* 25:365–371, Sep 1939.

7

Feline Ingestive Behavior

The neonate generally initiates ingestive behavior within an hour after birth, usually after the completion of parturition. As maturation of the kitten progresses, numerous modifications are made in the behaviors associated with eating.

SUCKLING INGESTIVE BEHAVIOR

Early Phase

During the first 3 weeks of life, feeding sessions are initiated primarily by the queen. She arouses the usually sleeping kittens by her movements and licking and positions herself around the young, almost enclosing them with her limbs and ventrum. The rooting reflex causes the kitten to burrow into a warm object, usually its queen or littermates, and may be present up to 11 days (see Figure 2-9). Maturation of the senses, particularly vision, and of homeostatic mechanisms alters all neonatal reflexes. During the appetitive searching component of nursing behavior, the kitten's movements toward the queen are awkward, but they become progressively more coordinated as the kitten's muscular and nervous system control increases with age. Communal nests allow some queens to actually have nursing coalitions.[124]

The sucking reflex is present at birth and can be tactually stimulated over a large perioral area.[117] Such stimulation results in a head turn in the direction of the stimulus and accompanying sucking movements (see Figure 2-10). Small objects in the mouth also stimulate the reflex, which is strongest immediately after awakening. Within a few days, the sucking reflex is limited to lip contact, and foreign objects in the mouth are rejected.[117] That is probably when olfactory cues become more important in teat location than trial and error, the initial method the kitten uses. Destruction of the olfactory bulbs produces kittens that cannot initiate sucking even with previous experience, but it does not interfere with their ability to learn how to suck from a bottle.[110] This is also consistent with the finding that odor cues may be important to locate the mother, and tactile cues help locate the nipple.[118] The sucking reflex normally disappears by 23 days.[108,110] Taste and texture can be discriminated shortly after birth but are apparently of minor significance in normal sucking.[153]

The kitten's initial contact with the teat results in a withdrawal motion of the head, followed by a downward motion and perhaps another withdrawal before the teat is finally enclosed by the mouth. This random head bob decreases as the kitten's ability to discriminate the teat increases. By 4 days, kittens are relatively proficient at suckling the queen, and by 1 week, little nuzzling is necessary.

Before the end of the third day and sometimes as early as the first, a form of teat preference develops, which may become very rigid. Rear nipples are used preferentially.[52] In large litters there is an initial competitive scrambling and pushing, which decrease as the preference for specific teats develops. As many as 80% of the individuals nurse only from a specific nipple.[61,160,166] When preferences are more loosely defined, a kitten nurses from a pair of teats, usually near each other, or from a general region of the mammary surface.[160,161] Occasionally individuals do not develop any preference and will nurse randomly instead.[159,166,167] The incidence of teat preference is independent of litter size.[160] Development of teat preference may serve to minimize claw injuries among littermates, provide optimal stimulation to ensure milk production, and allow more rapid completion of nursing. Variability has developed with domestication because the behavior has not been considered in selective breeding.

If a specific teat is not sucked for about 3 days, milk production by that mammary gland stops.[65] The appearance of the mammary region of a nursing queen makes it obvious that only certain nipples are used.

Nursing positions are identified by olfactory means, and kittens seldom nurse strange teats after the first few days if normal nursing is allowed.[62,71] A kitten that takes the wrong nipple may leave it immediately or may continue to suckle until the rightful "owner" nuzzles at it. Only when nursing the preferred teat will a kitten tenaciously cling to it when challenged.[160] Unlike pigs, kittens nursing from the cranially positioned teats do not necessarily become larger than their other littermates.[61] Teat positions are maintained for approximately 1 month, at which time the preference becomes less rigid. At about the same time, kittens show less discrimination in nursing foster queens.[62,64] In cat colonies where multiple litters are housed together, kittens commonly suckle queens indiscriminately, with little or no teat preference development. When bottle feeding is necessary, repeated use of the same bottle and nipple and avoidance of noxious or unfamiliar odors on human hands are desirable.

The "milk tread," usually considered a part of the nursing behavior of kittens, consists of rhythmic alternate movements of the forepaws against the mammary gland. Initially, a somewhat similar pattern is observed as the neonate tries to steady its suckling position. Functionally the milk tread may serve to push the queen's skin away from the neonate's nose but soon becomes more important to help stimulate milk flow.[52,63,64] The behavior is primarily used when milk is not coming as fast as the kitten can drink and is usually alternated with nonrhythmic sucking.

Purring by both the queen and the kittens often accompanies nursing.[28]

The neonate initially spends a great deal of time nursing. Each session may last up to 45 minutes, totaling about 8 hours per day.[13,52,162] This amount of nursing allows most kittens to double their birth weight in 1 week, triple it in the second week, and quadruple it by the end of the third week.[13,183] Milk production does increase for large litters but not in direct proportion to litter size.[52] In addition, there is as much as a tenfold increase in subcutaneous body fat for insulation to aid in homeostasis.[183] The mean growth rate for the first 8 weeks is 7.3 g/day (kittens from litters of seven to eight) to 13.7 g/day (kittens from litters of two).[52]

Intermediate Phase

During the second phase of nursing behavior, suckling is initiated about equally by the queen and the kittens. At first, 40% of the feedings are kitten initiated, with marked increases later.[159] By 4 weeks, approximately half of the contacts are initiated by the kittens and half by the queen.[52] The intermediate phase generally lasts from the second or third week of life to the end of the fourth or fifth week, when development of vision, use of visual cues, and coordination of motor skills allow the kittens to actively approach the queen even when she is not in the nest area. She in turn lies in lateral recumbency to present the mammary region for the young to nurse (see Figure 6-9). Toward the end of this phase the kittens may initiate sucking with the female in a standing position, but she will then respond by lying down.

Avoidance Phase

Near the end of the first month, kittens are very active in initiating nursing and the queen becomes increasingly evasive of them—the avoidance phase. By 8 weeks, only 5% of the contacts are initiated by the queen, 42% by the kittens, and 42% mutually.[52] The increasing demand for milk at this time already has the mother eating twice what she normally would to keep up.[128] At first the female avoids some of the advances of the young by jumping onto objects they cannot reach, but as the kittens' motor skills develop, they become increasingly difficult to avoid. Avoidance is made even more difficult because their efforts are usually individualized rather than coordinated. Her tactics will change to making nursing progressively more difficult. The queen may lie in sternal recumbency to prevent access to the teats, and if the kittens become too persistent, she bats at them or gets up and moves away. When she does allow nursing, the queen is usually sitting or standing, with the kittens contorted into several postures. If she has only one kitten in the litter, she may not show this avoidance phase.

Weaning Phase

Weaning is a gradual, variable process that results from inaccessibility of the queen and increasing ability of the kittens to hunt. In the wild, cats do not wean their young, but if the queen is still lactating, the milk is of little nutritional value after 12 weeks.[35,169] When this decreased value is coupled with normal dispersion necessary to obtain prey, weaning simply happens. Even without increased avoidance by the female, there is a natural tendency for the young to decrease their nursing at about the time of normal weaning.[79] When kittens are confined with the queen or have ready access to her, nursing may continue for several months, although 8 to 10 weeks is most common.[71,109,160] There is an inverse correlation between litter size and length of time the female allows nursing.[13] Smaller litters nurse longer. Kittens born in the spring often continue to nurse for 3 to 5 months, until fall.[95,185] Some queens will let a kitten nurse until just before the birth of her next litter, as much as a year later, then aggressively chase it away.

The older offspring may return shortly after she queens and continue nursing, lying among the neonates.

TRANSITIONAL INGESTIVE BEHAVIOR

The transitional stage of ingestive behavior occurs while the kitten is both nursing and eating solid food. Starting near the end of the fourth week of age, this mixed nutritional period lasts until the kitten is normally weaned, at about 8 weeks. Domestic kittens begin eating solid food between 28 and 50 days of age (mean 32 days), often by following the queen to the food bowl or accidentally stepping in the food.[17,160,169] Immediately preceding the transition to solid food, kittens may be noticed to eat dirt or litter.

If the queen is a hunter, she introduces her young to solid food in the form of small, dead prey. Around 35 days, she eats it in their presence, but by 6 weeks some of the kittens start eating with her on their own. That ensures that solid food will be available to the young when they are ready. The queen apparently brings prey to the nest in response to the characteristics of kittens of an appropriate age, because a nonlactating queen may bring prey to another queen's kittens of the appropriate age.[13,63]

HUNTING BEHAVIOR

Felis catus has been described as the most perfect carnivore, because its entire body is geared to predatory life. In addition to sensory and locomotor adaptations, the cat has laterally flattened canine teeth, which permit it to sever the spinal cord of its prey without damaging the vertebral bodies. The lever action of the jaw and the scissor action of the premolars also hasten the killing and eating of prey because no molar grinding action is necessary. Thus the cat has rudimentary molars and almost no lateral jaw motion. The cat eats from the side of its mouth, using the premolars to tear flesh, rather than from the front like a grazing animal. While the cat is chewing, the ear and vibrissae on the side of the prey are noticeably flattened to the head.[75] Sharpened claws on the thoracic limbs aid in catching prey, and their retractability by means of specialized ligaments helps maintain their extreme sharpness. Padded feet allow attack by ambush, and the shortened alimentary canal permits rapid digestion so the cat does not have to carry excess weight.

Farm cats are considered primarily hunters, although in fact much of their diet is supplemented by humans. They will spend 3.9% to 25.7% of their time hunting, usually around noon and dusk, and 1.2% to 3.4% feeding.[146] Approximately 36% of cat owners report having seen their cats with prey.[157]

Developmental Hunting

Rudimentary predatory behaviors can be seen at 3 weeks of age.[143] Then, prey recognition begins toward the end of the first month, when the queen brings home dead prey for her offspring to smell and eventually taste. In another 3 or 4 weeks, the queen brings weak or wounded prey so the young can begin acquiring their own hunting skills. For each of these behaviors, the queen's own prey-killing and eating instinct must be inhibited, primarily in response to kitten-related cues. Kittens will interact with prey more quickly and for longer periods immediately after the mother's bout.[39] Between 4.5 and 7 weeks, most predatory behaviors are significantly correlated with each other.

Hunting techniques are developed by practice during play and during prey sessions with the queen. The chase and catch aspects of hunting are thought to be innate, but manipulative and positive contact responses are acquired behaviors.[13,72,158] The chasing, catching, and killing aspects of hunting may also be learned or at least perfected by learning. The nape bite is the prey-killing behavior that does not usually appear in play and must be perfected with practice on actual prey. When the kitten's hunting style fails and the mouse or other prey escapes, the kitten is given another opportunity because the queen recaptures the mouse and drags it back to the young. Kittens follow the queen on hunting trips to perfect their skills as they approach self-sufficiency. By 15 to 18 weeks, exploration and hunting take up to 68% of the young cat's time.[182]

Predatory tendencies are inherited and have probably been modified by domestication, making prey-killing cats generally less defensive and more aggressive than nonhunters.[1] These tendencies are influenced by early experience. Competency in predation is related to the presence of the queen during the kitten's exposure to prey and to experience as an adult.[23,37,38,87] Kittens hunt the same prey they observed their mother kill and bring home. Cats are better able to catch prey if they had experience with prey by approaching, manipulating, and biting them in a play context as kittens.[36] Learning to kill prey is generally limited from the sixth to approximately the twentieth week, but for the few cats that learn after that age, the process appears almost laborious.[123] If the young never observe this process, approximately half will learn hunting skills on their own. Even if a kitten is never exposed to hunting, at an appropriate age the cat responds to the squeak of a mouse by attacking it.[74] The way a kitten is raised will also be important in future hunting behavior. A young kitten raised only with a mouse or rat seldom becomes a hunter, but the approximately 17% that become hunters do not generally hunt the type of prey with which they were raised. If the kitten is raised with a mouse or rat in addition to other kittens, socialization to the natural prey is minimal.[111,112]

The Hunt

Prey capture

Although rustlings or squeaking may initially attract the cat's attention, the sight of moving prey is the primary factor initiating hunting behavior. With experience a cat can learn to recognize immobile prey.[176] Kittens can visually orient to prey as early as 9 days of age.[158] Hunger and prey killing are independent, but the former can lower the threshold for the latter.[20,122,138] After being alerted to potential prey, even prey as large as itself, a cat approaches the prey in a stalking ambush. Initially the cat will head to a particular area, and when it arrives, the gait changes to a slow walk as it looks over the area.[176] Once prey has been spotted, the cat crouches close to the ground and uses a slinking trot, stopping periodically behind cover. It lies there temporarily with forelimbs under and elbows protruding. The entire pes is on the ground under the cat. The head is stretched forward, as are the ears. Whiskers are spread. As its eyes follow the prey, the cat usually twitches its tail.[13] The stalking continues periodically until the cat nears striking range. At that time it again stops and lowers its body, proceeding at a cautious, low-profile walk (Figure 7-1). At the last available cover, there is a final pause during which its tail twitches with great intensity and the caudally positioned pelvic limbs tread, swinging its entire hindquarters to and fro.[13] Then, after a short run, if necessary, the cat springs forward to seize the prey. In this pouncing attack, its pelvic limbs usually remain on the ground and only its forefeet are used in the capture (Figure 7-2). As soon as its forelimbs leave the ground, its rear limbs spread apart to stabilize the cat and help it brake. In this way, the cat can change direction to accommodate zigzags made by the fleeing prey. If instead both thoracic and pelvic limbs were off the ground during the lunge, the cat would be committed in its direction of travel. The cat that misses its

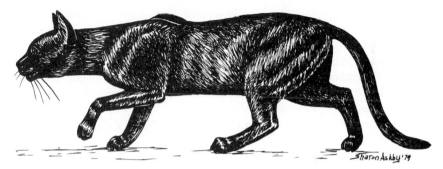

Figure 7-1 The stalking walk of prey hunting.

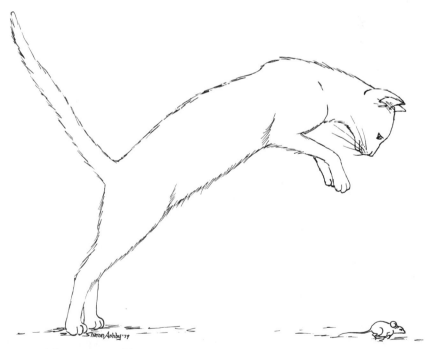

Figure 7-2 The pounce used in prey capture.

intended prey makes no attempt to correct the error. Instead it temporarily withdraws, and if conditions are still favorable, it renews its attack.[123] On average, a cat will make 3.6 pounces for each vertebrate it catches while hunting.[146] Cats have been known to leave one mouse in favor of another more active one.[13]

Nape bite

Captured prey are restrained and positioned for the kill with the forepaws and killed by the nape bite. The accomplished hunter aims this bite at the dorsal aspect of the neck, directing its canine teeth between adjacent cervical vertebrae to sever the spinal cord or into the atlantooccipital joint to pierce the medulla oblongata.[107,123] The innate directing force is governed visually by the constriction of the prey's neck and tactually by the direction of the prey's hair. The canine teeth of *F. catus* are flattened laterally so that they serve as a wedge.[64,123] In addition, there are numerous nerve receptors at the base of these teeth, probably to help direct the killing bite. Rapid contraction time for the muscles of mastication permits a rapid bite after correct placing is achieved.[64,72] A young inexperienced kitten, especially a timid one, may not initially use enough strength to kill the prey, but competition with littermates and repeated attacks increase the excitement until it eventually makes the kill. A few kittens never reach that point, and for older cats the necessary amount of excitement is very difficult to achieve. After a few successful kills, kittens appear to become less skillful as they individualize and perfect their techniques in more difficult situations, such as when the mouse is not running directly away. This may be a time when perfecting certain skills or the reorganization of the hunting behaviors means too much concentration goes to certain aspects at this time.[40] Killing of prey is related to size and hunger. The probability of a kill increases with hunger and decreases with larger prey size.[20] When these factors are in conflict, the cat is more apt to play with the prey first.[20] Diazepam used experimentally on cats that would immediately kill prey caused them to show prey play first.[116]

The learning process associated with the nape bite involves several interesting features. On occasions when the bite is not directed correctly, the kitten may secure another portion of the prey's body. The prey may turn around and bite the kitten's nose.[13] The initial kill is usually unexpected by the kitten, and it tries to continue playing with the now motionless prey. The kitten must make several kills before it associates the neck bite with its ability to transform live prey into food, and only then does hunger initiate prey-catching actions.[13,63,123] If the prey is killed by a method other than the nape bite, the cat may perform a nape bite on the dead animal, usually before eating it but occasionally after the initial stages of ingestion.[123] When not used for awhile, the skills associated with killing tend to atrophy.[123]

Prey ingestion

Eating killed prey is another behavior based on experience. If the kitten learns to eat dead prey from the queen, it will eat the prey it catches. The kitten that has eaten raw meat but not fresh prey will eat the prey it catches if the prey is cut open to release the smell of fresh tissue or if it accidentally draws blood or tears muscle during the kill. Cats raised as vegetarians will kill but usually do not eat the prey.[13]

After the kill, a cat will often groom itself and then take its dead prey to a quiet area before eating it. Farm cats will often bring prey back to their kittens, and owned cats bring it back to their owners.[95] When eating a mouse, even a young cat will begin with the head and work caudally while crouching over it. This orientation is tactile, based on the lie of the prey's hair. Some cats may try to bite the abdomen first but soon move to the head. Usually the entire animal is consumed, with the occasional exception of the tail.

Catching, killing, and eating prey are behaviors along a continuous gradient of activation.[152] Each has its own threshold level for performance. To get close enough to kill some mice, a cat must attempt to catch more than it can eat. Some mice escape, perhaps two of three.[121] A cat that is introduced to a limitless number of mice one at a time will first catch, kill, and eat the prey. In time, the animal will catch and kill but not eat the mice. With continued introduction of mice, the cat catches them but does not kill or eat. Finally, with physical fatigue, the mice are ignored.[181] Cats will catch an average of 15 mice per test.[136] Thus hunger and feeding are not necessary to maintain rodent killing by an experienced hunter.[138,154] They may serve as potentiators of hunting, particularly in naive cats.[154] Body condition and diet also do not influence the frequency of hunting.[157]

The environment probably necessitated that early felids use high-search, low-pursuit hunting techniques. Because of this evolutionary development, and because the prey is small, cats usually are solitary hunters. On occasion, two and three individuals hunt within 50 to 75 yards of each other; however, true cooperative hunting is rare and mainly restricted to courting pairs.[57,113]

As a means of rodent control, the cat is unsurpassed. Although cats are important in this control, the emigration of cats into an area without resident cats will lag the increase in the rodent populations.[150,151] Cats cannot depopulate an area of rodents completely, but they can prevent a population increase.[124] Other control methods depopulate a specific area only, but spaces within 50 yards of homes with hunting cats do not become reinfested.[59,122] In a study of recently killed, untamed cats, mice and small rats were proven the major type of food.[148] Most had 1 or 2 mice in their stomachs, but one animal had 12.[176] Seldom has a cat been seen catching more than four vertebrates per day.[146] Records that have been kept concerning ingestion of rodents show one cat killed 22,000 mice in 23 years, and another, younger than 6 months old at the time, killed 400 rats in 4 weeks.[186]

Nonrodent Prey Capture

Studies of ingested material in feral cat populations confirm that mice are the cat's primary food. Other prey varies seasonally but includes voles, bats, small reptiles, carrion, rabbits, birds, and insects. Rats weighing less than 200 g are another prey species, but half are killed and not eaten.[45] Feral cats tend to be opportunists and scavengers, so the type of prey is largely dependent on its relative abundance.[49] The availability of commercial food or table scraps does not decrease consumption of wild prey.[51,81]

Birds do not make up as much of the cat's diet as is commonly believed, with human activity being 56 times more likely to kill birds than cats.[148,149] Spring and summer hatches provide most of the supply, and cats that hunt near roads apparently kill more birds than those hunting in fields.[58,132] Most garden-type birds tend to breed at the edges of woods and in clearings where they would be preyed upon by several species of animals, not just cats.[133] Special hunting skills are required to catch flying prey, so not all cats are successful. The best hunters attack as soon as they spot the bird because ambush techniques often send the intended prey hopping or flying. The bird is usually caught with one or both forepaws and instantly brought to the mouth for the nape bite. If the bird is long necked, the nape bite may be directed close to the head or the shoulder. Instinctively, the latter is more commonly used because the size disparity is greater between body and neck than between head and neck. The best hunters do not release the catch for a better neck bite, because the bird tends to escape. Except for a few feathers, which may be plucked, the entire animal is usually eaten, beginning with the head.[13,28]

Once a cat starts hunting birds, it is almost impossible to prevent its continuation. At best, throwing things at the cat causes it to hunt on the sly. To avoid a bird-catching cat, a kitten should be selected whose mother does not hunt birds, or it should be adopted at about 6 weeks of age. In both cases, the kitten should be confined and not allowed exposure to birds, at least until after it is a year old.[27,84] Placing a bell on the cat may give birds enough of a warning.[27]

Rabbits caught are usually juveniles, probably because full-grown ones are too powerful.[176] Even then, the difficulty of the catch of such a large animal is still greater than that of other species.[176]

Another less common prey for the cat is the fish. Although most cats leave fish alone, a few are noted for pursuit of the family's goldfish. The fishing cat of Malaysia is very adept at hooking fish with its forepaws, as are certain individuals living in coastal regions or near lakes and streams. Fishing is one of the earliest skills for which selection was made in domestication. Like good bird hunters, good fishers do not let the catch go to obtain a better neck bite, because that leads to the fish's escape. Cats having no early fishing experience may actually run away from a fish flopping along a shore.

In certain parts of the world, livestock injuries from vampire bats can be significantly reduced by hunting cats.[54] Successful catches tend to occur when the bat is distracted during its hunting approach, while defending itself from the cattle, or when weighed down after feeding.

ADULT EATING BEHAVIOR

Cats continue to grow for several months after weaning. For the first 8 weeks, both sexes grow at an approximately equal rate.[52] After that, males grow faster. Females grow until about 6 months of age, and males do until 9 to 12 months.[168] A newborn needs 380 kcal/kg daily intake, and the requirements gradually decrease to a daily need of 80 kcal/kg in the adult.[168] The average mouse meal will supply approximately 30 kcal of energy, so most cats require approximately 10 mice per day.[174] Each mouse consists of 64% to 76% water, 14% to 18% protein, 6% to 18% fat, and 1% to 5% minerals.[104] These data suggest cats evolved to eat several small meals a day. The immediate ancestors of the cat also ate small prey, as frequent small meals, rather than following the "feast or famine" principle typical of their large feline cousins. If allowed to set their own schedule, domestic cats will eat 9 to 16 small, evenly sized meals a day.[*] When fed periodically, cats tend to be more aggressive and less cooperative than if fed by free choice.[66]

[*]References 24, 85, 87, 94, 104, 169, 176.

Meal-fed cats also tend to eat and drink less often, and their urine pH, magnesium, and phosphorous levels fluctuated much more than for cats fed by free choice.[66]

If the opportunity exists, a great deal of time may be spent hunting. Females spend 26% to 46% of the day hunting, compared with 5% to 34% spent by males, during bouts averaging 30 minutes (range 5 to 133 minutes).[176] As little as 1% of the waking time may be spent eating.[85] Males generally eat more, but females show more variation in body weight, primarily because of changes in eating and activity patterns related to estrous cycles. Based on high-protein body needs, a domestic cat consumes approximately 75 g of dry food or 250 g of canned food each day (each about 250 calories) or about 30 kg of dry or 90 kg of canned food per year.[47,147] Caloric intake fluctuates somewhat on a 4-month cycle along with the cyclic changes in body weight, food intake, and thyroid activity.[94,100,155]

Regulation of ingestive behavior is not completely understood. Several theories have been advanced but each has exceptions, so feeding may really be regulated by multiple factors. Environmental factors like availability and nutritional properties of the diet are major determinants of the eating pattern.[103] As caloric density decreases, cats maintain intake based on bulk, not calorie content.[103] Adult cats will also regulate intake to some extent on dry matter content. As moisture is added, consumption increases in proportion to the amount of water added.[41] As the energy and safety costs of getting food increase for a cat, the frequency of eating is reduced, and there is a compensatory increase in amount eaten per meal.[103,105] Theories on regulators of intake include palatability of food, blood levels of amino acids, and hepatic glucoreceptors.[100,163] There is no correlation of meal size and intermeal intervals,[105] and a ration is not selected because it is nutritionally balanced.[89]

Ingestive behaviors of adult cats before and after feeding have been well characterized.[30] Premeal behaviors are directed at the owner as both vocalization and directed behaviors. A cat will approach with its tail up and flicking as if to another cat. It will also rub on the owner and other objects. Postmeal behaviors are centered primarily on grooming, with much less owner interaction. As the cat starts to walk away, three fourths of the time the tail is lowered. Grooming begins with it licking its lips and progresses to body grooming with a licked "washcloth" paw. Before leaving, the cat performs some additional lip licking or head shaking.

Protocol when more than one cat approaches a food bowl is not governed by social status as in other species. Instead, cats usually adhere to the first-come, first-served principle, or they may share. Because cats do not know how to behave toward each other when eating together, the individual arriving later may choose to wait. Who eats first or how many eat at the same time depends on individuals rather than on age, sex, or other dominance factors (see Figure 4-4). One cat will occasionally take prey from another, particularly if there is a distraction.

FOOD PREFERENCES

Initial gustatory responses appear as early as the first day of life and basically involve differentiation of salty milk from regular milk.[50] By 10 days, responses are also seen to bitter, sweet, and sour.[50,178] Maturation involves changes in ingestive behavior, but environment is probably the strongest influence on food preferences. The specific prey introduced by the queen or food type fed by owners to the juvenile often determines the patterns in the adult, with food preferences generally established before 6 months of age. If the kitten was not exposed to a variety of food flavors and textures, food preferences can be so limited that the cat may even refuse to eat anything except its one or two choices. Cats tend to be extremely particular, and the assumption that the cat will eventually eat a nutritious food when it becomes hungry is not correct. They have been known to refuse a nutritionally complete, unpalatable diet for a prolonged period,[104] and they literally starve to death rather than eat an unacceptable meal. Queens have been known to eat their young while in this state, never touching the available food.[14]

Preferences can be shown behaviorally. The introduction to a food that produces a "lick/sniff food, lip lick, and groom face" response indicates it is a desirable meal.[177] A "lick/sniff food and lick nose" shows a degree of undesirability.[177] Whether the aversive food is eaten then depends to some degree on hunger. Cats that are used to a variety usually will prefer a novel diet to their regular one.[31,46,89,94] This preference is short lived, however, if the new diet is less palatable. Preferences can also change significantly over time. For cats that are not used to variety, foods should be changed gradually by mixing well 20% to 25% of the new food with the old. This first mixture should be offered until it is readily accepted, which usually takes up to 14 days. Then the mixture may be further changed by introducing another 20% to 25% of the new food. These steps should be repeated until the new diet is being fed exclusively.

Initial selection of a free-choice food depends on odor, which can provide the sole basis for dietary selection.[28,139] If the smell is acceptable, the front of the tongue brings in the next information. Undesirable odors, tastes, or textures can overrule the metabolic need for nutrition and are more important as negative factors than positive ones.[48] That explains why some cats will eat a novel diet if it is aesthetically acceptable.[85] It is related to the relatively rapid acceptance of most new foods. Rejection can also occur after a period without a particular type of food.[29] Meat is obviously the food of choice, and older cats prefer kidney.[28,178] They also choose fish and commercial cat food over rats.[94,99] Cold, dead rats are slightly more palatable than the fresh kill.[99] Ranked in decreasing order of general feline preference is flesh from sheep, cattle, horses, pigs, chicken, and fish. Whether a meat is raw or cooked is relatively unimportant; however, foods at body temperature are preferable to those at higher or lower temperatures.[28,139,178] Moisture, which may help release odors, enhances palatability, and spicy foods are usually disliked.[28,178]

The physical features of a food are involved in food selection. Cats prefer solutions with a greater density (whole versus diluted milk) but are more cautious with doughy textures.[104] As a diet becomes drier and more powdery, acceptance also decreases.[104] Fats are desirable, with tallow preferred over chicken or butter fat, and these are preferred over corn oil.[104]

Some flavors are selected against by cats. These include saccharin, cyclamate, casein, medium-chain triglycerides, caprylic acid, and certain combinations.[12,104,125] Studies conflict over a cat's ability to detect sweets.[11,12,104] That may be why sucrose does not increase palatability in cats as it does in other species.[94,100] Cats do like sweet solids like ice cream, so one could say they really find the combination of sweet, fatty, and milky texture highly palatable.[94]

Individuals can have strong preferences that are unique from other cats.[89] One cat, raised by a Jewish rabbi, observed Jewish laws by not drinking milk when eating meat, even though both were available. This illustrates that variations do occur based on individual factors and environmental influences.[114]

Prey preference can exist not only in hunting but also in consumption. Mousers generally catch all kinds of mice but refuse to eat certain types of mice, birds, moles, and shrews. Snakes, frogs, and toads are rarely eaten, although they may be hunted and caught.[13]

Food preferences are not restricted to meat, and that may again reflect the wild heritage. Grass and other vegetable matter can be found in the feces or stomachs of approximately one third of feral cats. Animals serving as normal prey for *F. catus* are primarily vegetarians, so when the prey is eaten, vegetable matter becomes part of the cat's diet. Therefore most of the vegetative matter consumed has already been partially processed by the prey's intestinal tract. Although cats can digest a small amount of fresh vegetable starch, large amounts of uncooked carbohydrate may cause vomiting or diarrhea. Because cats lack the ability to break down the beta bonds of cellulose to glucose, fresh grass remains unchanged within the gastrointestinal system and may actually become irritative.[15] Because the indoor cat is most apt to consume large quantities infrequently, grass has commonly been assigned the role of a purgative for such things as hair balls. If, however, the cat is introduced to small portions of vegetable matter early in life, it can be somewhat omnivorous. Eating grass for gastric distress may be a learned behavior, in the tradition of other species that learn self-medication.[94] Garbage is also commonly eaten, representing an opportunistic adaptation.[68]

WATER CONSUMPTION

Around the fifth week of life a young kitten begins drinking from dishes. By adulthood the average cat requires approximately 44 to 66 ml of water per kilogram of body weight per day.[168] Kittens need 66 to 88 ml/kg/day.[168] Water is available to an animal from three sources: drinking water, water in food, and water from nutrient metabolism of fat and energy.[165] A canned food diet is 74% water, making 49.8 g/kg available to the adult cat from the diet. It would supplement its intake by drinking 7.3 g/kg.[168] This means for the average cat, approximately 185 ml is available directly. About 15 ml more comes from fat metabolism. The cat may not need to drink. Dry food has only 10% water, thus supplying 7.5 ml, with another 7.5 ml available from fat metabolism.[47] In this case 185 ml of water must be ingested directly.

A kitten learns to drink by first lowering its head until the mouth touches the water. The head is then raised, and water is licked from around the mouth. The adult cat usually crouches over the water source and uses its tongue to bring water into its mouth (Figure 7-3). For this, the tip of the tongue is curled caudally, forming a ladle to lift the liquid into the mouth, and the cat usually laps four or five times before swallowing.[13] Occasionally house cats prefer to drink from the toilet bowl or a drippy faucet (Figure 7-4). Generally one of two postures is used. If possible, the cat prefers to keep both hindfeet on the floor, leaning or stretching as necessary to lap the water. If this is impossible, the cat will straddle the toilet or sink, bracing itself while it drinks. More than one cat has lost its balance, and some will then no longer use that water source.

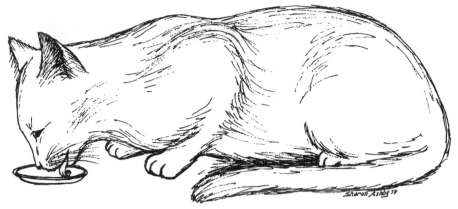

Figure 7-3 The most common drinking posture, with ladled tongue.

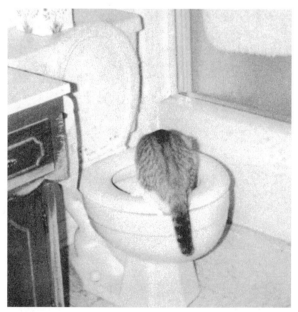

Figure 7-4 Cats often seek the freshest sources of water from toilets, sinks, or showers.

A few cats, in addition to using the regular form of drinking, have been observed to drink by dipping a paw into the water, then sucking moisture from it (Figure 7-5). If that occurs when fresh water is being added, it may represent a play behavior. However, this behavior has been seen when fresh water was not a factor. In one colony a female cat displayed the behavior, and later, so did a female kitten, a daughter of one of the first cat's littermates. Paw dipping may therefore be a genetic trait because the kitten's mother was not a dipper and observational learning could not have occurred.

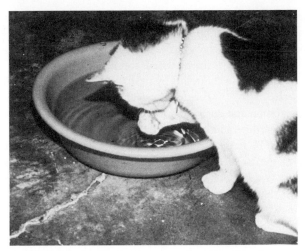

Figure 7-5 A cat drinking water by dipping its paw and sucking from it.

NEURAL AND HORMONAL REGULATION

Food Consumption

Hypothalamus

The hypothalamus is well known for its control over appetite and ingestive behavior, and specific areas control specific functions. The lateral hypothalamus is considered the "feeding center." Electrical and adrenergic stimulation of that area results in greatly increased food intake even in satiated cats. The intake increase, which occurs over a time, indicating a humoral mechanism, can be as much as 1000% greater than normal.[53] In addition, stimulation results in increased activity, which simultaneously increases the likelihood of encountering food.[6] Destruction of the lateral hypothalamus results in aphagia. Conversely, the ventromedial hypothalamus controls satiety. Stimulation of this area causes anorexia. Initially, lesions may result in reduced food intake,[88,171] but destruction of the ventromedial hypothalamus ultimately results in hyperphagia, leading to obesity. Experimentally, alterations of the lateral hypothalamus take precedence over those of the ventromedial hypothalamus, which indicates that although the lateral hypothalamus may normally control feline ingestive behavior, the ventromedial portion may exhibit inhibitory control over it.[7] Depressants of the central nervous system tend to increase the intake of food. This suggests that in the normal cat there is an active inhibition of feeding.[94] Peripheral glucoreceptors may inhibit the "satiety center" while exciting the lateral hypothalamus.[164] Stimulation of the anterior and midlateral hypothalamic areas can result in either increased eating or increased gastric acid secretion with restlessness.[188] Interestingly, it does not result in both at the same time. The anterior hypothalamus has been shown to be immediately affected by the intake of cold food, followed by peripheral vasodilation and a reduced rectal temperature.[4]

Aggression plays a significant role in food consumption because it is necessary for food capture in the wild. Specific areas of neurologic control have in the past been hard to identify because studies of affective aggression often included predatory aggression.

Most forms of aggression are controlled by the hypothalamus, but not by the same portion that controls predation. Stimulation of the lateral hypothalamus results in normal rat-hunting behaviors, from stalking through the nape bite, even in cats that have never exhibited this behavior before the experiment. These stimulated attacks are not indiscriminate, unlike most forms of aggression controlled by nearby portions of the hypothalamus; rather, specific prey is selected.[119,138,170] Postural displays are another distinguishing characteristic of predatory aggression and do not follow the pattern of affective aggression. Even the active neurotransmitters differ in the two situations.[5,19,156] Stimulation of the lateral hypothalamus is augmented by simultaneous activity of the midbrain reticular formation.[138]

Stimulation of the lateral hypothalamus has another neurologic effect related to predatory behavior. Two sensory areas around the cat's mouth become more sensitive, based primarily on the intensity of the stimulation to the brain. The perioral region becomes increasingly sensitive to touch and causes a reflex movement of the head, bringing the mouth closer to the tactile stimulus.[126] In addition, a touch reflex at the edge of the lips results in the mouth being opened.[126]

Hunger has been associated with increased excitatory changes in the hypothalamus, whereas neural activity throughout the brain decreases when the cat is satiated.[3] In this way, relative hunger may neurologically regulate stimulation of predatory behavior.[20]

Other brain areas

In cats of any age, other parts of the brain also affect ingestive behavior but to a lesser degree than the hypothalamus.[9] In fact, all parts of the brain except the cerebellum and primary sensorimotor cortical areas modify this behavior.[78] Destructive lesions of lateral positions of the amygdala may result in hyperphagia or at least increased licking and mouthing.[76,78,108] Conversely, aphagia can result from lesions of the amygdala, and hyperphagia follows amygdala stimulation.[78,135] A more specific relationship between the hypothalamus and ingestive behavior probably is related to suppressing and facilitating certain regions of the amygdala. Although ingestion is elicited by stimulation of the hypothalamus, it can be modulated via the amygdala. Physiologic differences exist in the limbic systems of predatory and nonpredatory cats. Rat killers show a significantly higher threshold for elicitation of afterdischarge (ADT) from the amygdala than nonpredatory cats, and cats with the lowest ADTs have the weakest attack tendencies.[2] That indicates neurologic differences between the two groups.

Destructive cortical lesions of the frontal and temporal lobes may increase food intake, although those of the frontal lobe have been reported to have the opposite effect.[8,78,117,135] Removal of the frontal lobes has led to the reappearance of certain portions of kittenlike sucking behavior, including the milk tread movements of the forepaws and the clumsy motions.[117] Again, these areas probably modify hypothalamic cues.[8] Complete removal of the cerebral cortex results in complete anorexia.[187]

Lesions of the brainstem can produce several abnormal behaviors, thus implicating this area in ingestive behavior. Such responses include a snap as a result of touching the lips, grabbing and swallowing small objects, overeating, holding objects that are too big to swallow, mounting and holding other animals, and chewing hair on their back or tail.[172]

Olfaction is important in eating behavior, so it stands to reason that ablation of the olfactory bulbs will result in a significant reduction in food intake.[129] Zinc sulfate treatment to the olfactory nerves can stop food consumption.[129]

Electrical stimulation of the neural septum and tegmentum can override the aphagia of hypothalamic destruction.[44,78] In the normal animal, these areas probably serve as modifiers of appetite control.[135]

The basal forebrain area integrates visceral, olfactory, and taste information used in normal eating behavior.[180] Descending pathways that facilitate swallowing from the amygdala to the brainstem pass through the lateral hypothalamus.[180]

Electroencephalographic (EEG) studies of patterns associated with ingestive behavior demonstrate different tracings for different activities. The sensorimotor rhythm is the slow-wave pattern associated with the motionless stances of hunting behavior. In contrast, ingestive reinforcement synchronization is a different type of slow-wave rhythm that appears during consumption of food. It has been described as a synchronization in the parietooccipital cortex.[42,43] Because this EEG synchronization can be prolonged by serotonin administration, eating is thought to be a pleasurable behavior.[43] Interestingly, the latter pattern is identical to that seen during drowsiness, indicating the same neural status for both satiety and drowsiness.[173] Kittens also show slow-wave patterns with food searching and satiation.[9]

Water Consumption

Water consumption is governed by an area of the lateral hypothalamus near the location that controls eating.[6,77] Onset of water consumption resulting from electrical or cholinergic stimulation of this area is delayed somewhat longer than that of food intake. However, the drinking behavior tends to have a greater duration, indicating a separate humoral mechanism related to water consumption. As expected, destruction of the lateral hypothalamus results in adipsia. Stimulation of the amygdala electrically or cholinergically can also increase water consumption, whereas stimulation of other neural areas, such as the septum, has varying effects on this behavior. Discrete areas in the dorsorostral pons are responsive to hypovolemia, and their destruction greatly increases basal water intake.[179] Cats with midbrain lesions occasionally dip their paws into water and move them about.[113]

Hormonal Control

In attempting to study feline affective aggression by observing cats attacking mice, researchers in the past were actually studying predatory aggression, and they looked at the behavioral effects of a number of hormones, drugs, and neurohormones. Those findings are valid for predatory aggression only. Hormonal influences on predatory behavior are sex dependent, probably a result of the early neonatal sex differentiation in the brain. In general the male cat has a lower threshold for elicitation of hunting behaviors than his female counterpart.[101] Castration tends to increase attack latency, whereas ovariectomy tends to have the opposite effect.[85,101] These characteristics vary with the individual however, so the results of neutering are not always predictable.

Rat studies have shown that estrogen suppresses food intake and weight gain, and progesterone has little to no effect.[94] Testosterone generally stimulates lean body growth and weight gain, with some metabolized to estrogen, which suppresses food intake. As was mentioned in Chapters 5 and 6, removal of the ovaries does tend to result in weight gain, but the effects of castration are less clear.

INGESTIVE BEHAVIOR PROBLEMS

Abnormal Nursing Behavior

Prolonged sucking

Very young kittens have an innate need to suck. Normally, nutritional sucking continues until weaning, and nonnutritional sucking decreases during this period. Kittens that are undernourished because of an inadequate milk supply from the mother, early weaning, or orphaning and that must be fed by bottle or stomach tube often develop maladaptive reactions to stress and nonnutritional sucking vices. To satisfy their natural nursing drive, these kittens suck the bodies of littermates or themselves if no littermates are available. This sucking can become a severe habit, to the point of seriously traumatizing the skin. Pendulous portions of the body, such as ears, tails, folds of the flank, vulvas, and scrotums, are most commonly sucked. A few of these deprived kittens attempt to nurse human skin, the family dog, a stuffed toy, or occasionally objects such as buttons or clothing. Sucking on other objects or maternal nursing by a kitten older than 1 year may be related to variations of normal weaning.[16] The prolonged sucking behavior may represent the feline version of thumb sucking. Although these behaviors can be seen in cats older than 2 years, variations in the behavior will occur at different ages. The kitten usually sucks during periods of relaxation, often kneading and purring at the same time.[14] Eventually the sucking stops, but the kneading and purring continue. With time, these usually disappear as well.

Because this excessive sucking can be very upsetting to owners, as well as traumatic to the skin, it is sometimes appropriate to stop the behavior. If the kitten is younger than 6 weeks, its diet should be supplemented with more protein by adding dry milk solids to a regular bottle formula. It is also better to bottle feed these kittens rather than feeding via a stomach tube (Figure 7-6). As they get older, measures can be taken to speed up

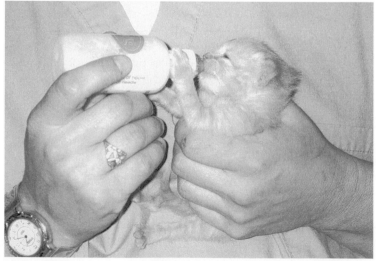

Figure 7-6 Bottle-fed kittens are less likely to have problems than tube-fed kittens.

the "weaning" process. Under natural conditions, the queen shows increasing avoidance of kittens being weaned and even displays mild aggression by batting them on the nose with her paw. Humans can separate littermates when they are sucking each other or thump them on the nose and say "no" if they try to nurse human skin. Another technique is to pick the kitten up by the nape of the neck, say "no," and put the kitten down, away from the sucked object.

Some of these kittens become very stealthy in their approaches, suddenly grabbing and sucking the skin that is being kept from them. In these situations, aversive conditioning techniques, particularly taste aversion (as described in Chapter 1), may be useful. The sucked or nursed object can be spread with a spicy sauce. If the behavior is caught early and the owner appropriately uses taste aversion, the problem can usually be broken. Encouraging exercise and play are also appropriate ways to reduce stress and get rid of excessive energy.

Medroxyprogesterone acetate and megestrol acetate have been successful in stopping self-sucking[21]; however, because of the side effects and inconsistent response, neither is currently recommended for prolonged sucking. Because cats tend to outgrow the behavior, management of the environment, perhaps with taste or smell aversion, is the preferred treatment.

Wool sucking

A second type of abnormal nursing behavior is commonly called *wool sucking;* although, in many cases *wool chewing* might be a more appropriate name. This is almost exclusively seen in Siamese, Burmese, and other Oriental breeds or their crosses, suggesting the possibility of genetic transfer of the trait.[*] Because the Siamese color pattern is recessive, the cat may not readily show its ancestry. The wool-sucking behavior usually does not begin until the cat approaches puberty,[82,83,140] even up to 4 years of age.[32] The usual owner complaint is that the cat has orally destroyed a woolen article or other piece of clothing by sucking or chewing it. Studies show 93% of the cats chose wool material, followed by cotton (64%), synthetic fabrics (53%), rubber/plastic (22%), and paper/cardboard (8%).[32,141] Twenty-four percent of the cats target a single item and three fourths of those items are wool. Another 30% go after two materials, 34% go after three materials, and 12% target four or five materials.[32,141] Food deprivation and a low-bulk diet can exacerbate the problem.[95] Occasionally a cat may even target the armpit region of a family member. The cat may be seeking the odor of lanolin or that associated with the human sweat glands, whether from the human axilla itself or from the portion of a shirt soiled by the axilla.[62,71,72] These cats sleep with, lick, suck, chew, knead, and sometimes ingest pieces of the object. Most stop the behavior by 2 years of age, but others never do.[82,83]

Several techniques have been employed to stop wool sucking, usually with limited success. Access to wool objects can be limited to one item by putting away other potential targets.[16,140] This could be one already ruined or a cheap wool item specific for this purpose. Intestinal obstructions are rare if the access is limited to wool.[140] The carnassial teeth of offending cats have been removed to prevent the objectionable damage but did not alter the behavior.[60] A lanolin-containing product may be fed to the cat in an attempt to satiate the desire for lanolin. Thyroid hormone replacement works well for

[*]References 23, 24, 32, 55, 96, 97, 115, 140, 141.

the occasional cat that shows the behavior because of hypothyroidism. It is possible to provide alternative oral stimulation such as dog chew toys or bulky dry food. These cats can sometimes be discouraged using remote punishment or taste/smell aversive conditioning.[26,115] In early stages the thump on the nose and "no" may work, if access is controlled to ensure the owner is present. Some Siamese cat breeders delay weaning until at least 12 weeks, hoping to decrease the incidence of the problem.[83] In many of these cats, wool sucking may represent an obsessive-compulsive disorder, so it would be appropriate to try treatment with serotonin-enhancing drugs like clomipramine, amitriptyline, or fluoxetine.[55,56,92,144,145]

The cats that can be challenging to manage are those that have both prolonged sucking and wool sucking. Age at onset and items targeted are helpful in determining whether the cat is showing one or both of these problems.

Hunting Behavior Problems

Approximately 10.9% of cats have some type of feeding problem.[90] Another 1.1% have problems specifically relating to hunting behavior.[90]

Atypical or abnormal variations

Some cats, primarily females, bring dead prey home and either leave it outside or present it to their owners. This may represent the cat's natural tendency to carry dead prey home or to a quiet spot before eating, or it may represent a maternal behavior—bringing prey home for phantom kittens.[13,71] These same behaviors can be represented when the cat places a toy mouse in the food bowl. Taste preference tests show cats will leave a killed rat to eat commercial food, giving rats the lowest of food preferences.[99] This unpalatability is another reason cats may bring prey home and not eat it. Presentation of live prey may again represent a much lowered maternal threshold for a seldom used normal behavior, as if a queen were bringing live prey so that phantom kittens can practice their hunting skills. The presentation may also indicate that there was enough psychologic excitement for the cat to catch prey but not enough to kill it, whether because of too many recent catches or lack of training as a kitten. Conversely, when too much excitement has been generated, the cat may have to dissipate some of it by repeatedly ambushing the corpse and tossing it into the air.[63] As the energy of excitement wears off, the prey is eaten.

Cats that attack the ankles of people walking across a room are exhibiting another form of abnormal prey killing, usually in a play connotation. This behavior is usually displayed by house cats not allowed outside and is most common between puberty and 2 years of age, during a time of "psychologic adolescence."[34] For these animals, predatory aggression has been significantly repressed, and the threshold to stalk prey is greatly lowered, so anything moving initiates prey chase and attack. The threshold can be lowered to the point that the ambush activities appear as true vacuum (spontaneous) activities.[63,186] To prevent this behavior, one must provide other methods for the release of this energy. For young kittens, another kitten playmate is very successful. For both older and younger cats, toys that move, such as a ball, or playmates, such as other pets, work well.[137] Owners should also encourage the cat to play with these toys by initiating the movement. Progestin therapy has been suggested for animals showing extremely abnormal hunting behavior,[130] but because of potential side effects and the fact that drugs do not address the cause, this is no longer considered appropriate therapy.

Undesirable prey

Cannibalism is often considered one of the least desirable of the atypical behaviors, but it is seldom truly abnormal in the cat except in stressful situations. The subject is considered in more detail in the section on maternal behavior in Chapter 6.

Cats occasionally hunt or chase nonexistent prey in a form of hallucinatory hunting behavior.[131] They have also been known to bring back inappropriate items just as they would normal prey. This usually occurs at night, so the owner awakens to socks, towels, underwear, packets of nuts and bolts, clothes from the laundry, bath mats, or rope.[25] Preventing access to these "prizes" is the most effective way of stopping these midnight excursions.

Eating birds or other prey and stealing food from counters may be considered undesirable by owners, but these behaviors are difficult to control. Aversive conditioning may deter the cat when the owner is present, but without the human's presence, cats tend to ignore their lessons. In addition, objects and verbiage hurled at cats are successful only at creating animosity between the animal and its owner. Some foods become undesirable if the food causes an unpleasant experience for the cat, such as vomiting, nausea, or foul taste. Bird corpses and partially eaten chicken legs have been tied around a cat's neck in an effort to stop the cat from eating these things.[70] A combination of smell aversion and remote punishment is probably more successful.[87] The most successful program involves finding ways to prevent access to unacceptable prey, such as keeping the cat indoors only, placing a bell on the cat, and being sure the behavior has no reward. Food should be kept off the counter.

Burying Food

Occasionally cats cover food, an uncommon behavior in the wild. In the home, covering is usually elicited by presentation of a different food. A cat may partially consume a food and then cover it as though it were fecal matter. Odors associated with defecation stimulate neural centers to induce covering, and therefore the odor of the food or prey, rather than a desire for its preservation, probably initiates the covering.[107]

Excessive Food Intake

Cats, particularly those that are nervous or have not eaten for some time, have been known to bolt food, even to the point of inducing regurgitation. Most cats reingest the food, although some are not especially interested in it. In either case, small meals fed frequently are recommended to reduce or prevent the behavior. An alternative technique is to put one or more objects that are at least 3 cm in the bowl to make it more difficult to get large quantities of food rapidly.[134]

Obesity does occur in the cat, although the rate of obesity is only about 10% and is often related to overeating as the result of certain psychologic stresses and the overabundance of a highly palatable, caloric-dense food supply[93,99,100,142] (Figure 7-7). Invasion of privacy, overcrowding, changes in routine, and postreaction to malnutrition

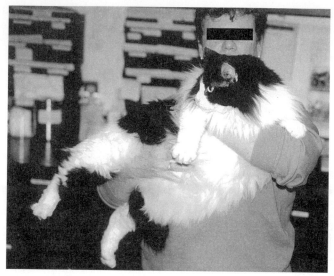

Figure 7-7 Obesity is becoming a significant problem in domestic cats. This one weighed 23 pounds.

can be initiating stresses. Food solicitation leading to obesity has also been documented as a way a cat can try for owner attention.[24] Occasionally physical conditions, such as chronic pancreatitis or brain tumors, also result in compulsive eating. Changes in metabolism such as with hyperthyroidism or hypothyroidism should be considered,[93] as should diseases like feline leukemia or feline immunodeficiency virus.

The amount of adipose tissue normally carried by a cat is regulated by several factors. Genetics is of minor importance in the overeating behavior of *F. catus* except to regulate thinness. Early dietary history; caloric concentration of food; palatability; the amount of neural activation, whether from stress or exercise; and the cat's hormonal state must be considered.[80,120] A direct correlation between lack of estrogen from an ovariohysterectomy and obesity has recently been made in the cat.[69] Under extreme conditions, cats can become as much as 74% fat.[33] Joseph, the heaviest cat on official records, weighed 48 pounds, and other cats of 40 to 46 pounds have also been reported.[10,67,186] Synthetic progestins, including megestrol acetate and medroxyprogesterone acetate; diazepam; corticosteroids; and metabolic steroids are well known for producing marked increases in appetitive behavior.

Few treatments other than the reduction of caloric intake have been highly successful in controlling obesity. Food palatability can be decreased, the bulk can be increased, or the access regulated. The reduction of food intake may result in increased irritability in the cat and is the reason it should be started very gradually. Ideally, exercise should also be increased, but this is much easier to say than to do with a cat.

Anorexia

Anorexia nervosa is one of the more serious problem behaviors encountered in cats, particularly in nervous individuals. This condition is commonly produced by emotional or physical stress, such as hospitalization, overcrowding, introduction of new people or animals, loss of a close companion, or excessive handling. Diseases impairing the sense of smell can also cause some degree of anorexia, as can approximately 95% of all cat diseases.[17] In addition to pylorospasm, vomiting, halitosis, ulcers, systemic pain, polydipsia, and adipsia, sympathetic physical signs have sometimes accompanied this condition. Generally, anorexia nervosa lasts from a few days to a week, although extended bouts are not uncommon, particularly as hepatic lipidosis sets in. Feeding meals, instead of free-choice feeding, and giving quiet space may be sufficient. One cat survived without food or water when accidentally isolated for 52 days, although that is certainly extreme.[186]

Sick and convalescing cats need full nutrition, so food intake should be strongly encouraged. Even an otherwise healthy cat deprived of food cannot exist long without starting to deplete its body's reserve. Hepatic lipidosis becomes a problem within 3 days. A dark, quiet place near food and water may provide enough security for the troubled cat. Mild tranquilization, especially with drugs of the benzodiazepine group noted for antianxiety action, is generally quite successful. Diazepam given intervenously can be useful in the anorectic cat if food is presented immediately.[127] In part, these results may be related to the antianxiety tranquilizing affects; however, diazepam has also been shown to escalate predation, probably at the lateral hypothalamus.[152] Oxazepam is another benzodiazepine particularly good in this situation.[73] In extreme cases, light anesthetization can be used, allowing the cat to recover with food nearby. Cyproheptadine has also been used to get cats to start eating again. Progestins and anabolic steroids have been used in chronic cases of partial anorexia with good results but are currently out of favor for this condition. Pharyngotomy, gastrotomy, or nasogastric tubes can be used when appropriate, particularly when lipidosis is becoming a concern, and long-term supplemental feeding is expected to be necessary.

Not all thin cats are anorectic. Some are just picky eaters. Others that have lost weight or are not gaining relative to the amount they eat may have other underlying problems like cancer or hyperthyroidism.

Pica

Occasionally cats lick, chew, or eat things that could in no way be considered food items.[22,97,106,184] Pica represents about 2.5% of the behavior problems for which owners seek help.[175] Pantyhose, phone and electric cords, and carpet pads are common and dangerous targets for pica (Figure 7-8). This list of things eaten can be extensive, but the list of differentials to consider is the same. Because the problem cat is usually younger than 1 year when the behavior starts, a genetic predisposition has been suspected but not proven. The first consideration should be to learn the feline leukemia and feline immunodeficiency virus status of the cat. Both of these diseases have been associated with abnormal behaviors for unknown reasons, and behavior therapy is unrewarding if the cat is infected. Brain tumors must also be considered and generally can be ruled out if the neurologic examination is within normal limits. Polycythemia vera has been reported to be associated with pica, such as the eating of cat litter,[106] although this condition is rare. The behavior may even be a variation of wool sucking, but there is no proof as of yet. Other differentials would include the lack of an enriched environment, attractive odors, hunger, learned behavior, teething, attention seeking, and relief of gum irritation (as with allergies).

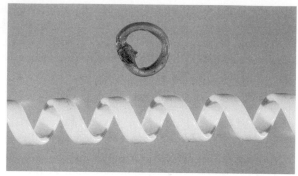

Figure 7-8 A phone cord segment recovered from a cat's stomach during foreign body surgery is shown with a regular phone cord.

The most effective treatment for pica is to prevent access to the targeted items. The owner can use a cordless phone, and lamp cords can be covered with appropriate materials. Ad libitum feeding of dry food and high-fiber levels can help,[56] particularly for cats that are hungry and those expressing an oral drive. It may become necessary to lower caloric density, however. Taste aversion, using such products as pepper sauce, commercial products, or roll-on deodorant,[22] coupled with controlled access to the target and access to appropriate oral products can be helpful.

Eating Houseplants

Eating houseplants is a common variation of ingestive behavior in cats that do not get appropriate vegetable matter in their diet. By providing a small flowerpot with grass or catnip, an owner can often eliminate the problem. For the cat that has developed a habit or preference, the owner needs to put the plant where the cat cannot get to it. Aversive taste/smell conditioning with pepper sauce or vinegar, and other forms of remote punishment, may be effective. By aiming a fine-mist water sprayer at the plant usually chewed and rigging a string to trigger the device from a distance, the owner can hide and remotely spray the cat when it disturbs the plant.[86,102] Appropriately placed mousetraps or other scare tactics that are set off by the cat's presence have also been used.

Waking Owners

Hungry cats are not happy cats. They tend to interact aggressively or noisily, pestering the owner until they are fed. Unfortunately feline activity patterns are busier at night than are most humans, so their activity often wakes the owner. The behavior is rewarded when the cat is fed. Thus begins the 4:00 AM feedings. If ignored early in this process, no problem would develop, because the cat quickly returns to its previous behavior. Nightly rewards quickly teach the cat that vocalizing will bring food on demand. Extinguishing the behavior by ignoring it means the problem will usually get worse before it gets better. Most cats will try something harder if it quits working, as if to be sure their demands are being recognized. Only after they realize the rules have changed will extinction begin. Ignoring the behavior may need to be supplemented with remote punishment, isolation away from the bedroom, or a gradual changing of the cat's internal clock. One way to do that is to gradually push back the time of the feeding each morning.

The vocalizing or aggression is also common during the day but less problematic. Cats that are used to getting a food treat at a certain time seldom tolerate the cessation of that daily ritual.

Excessive Salivation

Excessive salivation, minimization of swallowing, or both are common in the extremely relaxed cat, most commonly during petting. It probably represents parasympathetic stimulation, perhaps with decreased frequency of swallowing.

Food Allergies

Food allergies are difficult to substantiate but do occur in the cat.[136] The full ramifications of their effects are unknown but include aggression, irritableness, and seizures. The incidence of these behaviors can be related to the introduction or deletion of certain foods in the cat's diet.

Diet-Related Problems

Cats that develop strong preferences for a single food could develop problems. Several years ago there were health concerns of an all liver diet. More recently cats on an exclusive tuna diet showed behavior changes, perhaps associated with mercury levels in the fish.[98] Prevention is the best approach, by continuously varying the cat's diet and feeding quality commercial diets only.

Food Aversion

Food (taste) aversion is a conditioned response by which a cat learns to avoid a particular food or taste. This lesson can be learned very quickly, probably because taste aversions are strong reactions that represent a defense mechanism against poisoning.[18] They can be learned from various situations and involve innate aversions either to certain tastes, like bitter, or to certain foods. This can be the result of an allergy or because of an associated experience. The nausea and vomiting caused by lithium chloride will be related to the food eaten at the same time.[87] Being traumatized while eating a certain food results in the same type of aversion.

Oral Medications

Several techniques can be used for giving oral medications, but speed and dexterity are often necessary. Up to 10 ml of a liquid can be introduced at one time between the teeth and the buccal wall with an eyedropper or syringe.[35] Small amounts of liquid, gel, or paste will be ingested by a cat that is grooming if the material is placed on the hair or nose. To give medication in the food, the owner can first place a small amount of medicine on

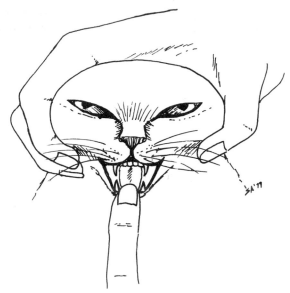

Figure 7-9 A technique used to open the cat's mouth.

the cat's nose to satiate its olfactory system. The cat will lick it off and satiate its gusta-tory system so the rest of the medication in the food will be eaten undetected.

To give tablets, minimal restraint is best, and the tablet must get into the laryn-gopharynx quickly so that it neither dissolves nor is tasted or smelled. While holding the head back, one uses the thumb and third finger to push the sides of the cat's mandible and hold it open, after the index finger of the opposite hand has opened the mouth by pushing down on the lower incisors (Figure 7-9). The cat will usually try to back away. After putting the tablet in place, one holds the mouth closed until the cat licks its nose or otherwise indicates that it has swallowed. If the animal still does not swallow, a sudden puff of air on the nose may startle it into doing so.

Another technique to administer tablets requires that the cat face the person. Using the restraining arm, one places the hand on the cat's head so that the thumb grasps one ear, the palm is near its other ear, and the fingers are at its throat. The cat's skull is rotated, without raising its head, until its nose points toward the ceiling. About 90% of the cats in this position will relax the muscles of mastication so the mouth can be eas-ily opened.[91] Again, the head is held until the cat has swallowed. The newly recognized concern of pills tending to stay in the esophagus too long means it is recommended that pill administration be followed with a small drink of water. To a cat, that represents two medications each time.

REFERENCES

1. Adamec R: The behavioral bases of prolonged suppression of predatory attack in cats, *Aggr Behav* 1:297–314, 1975.

2. Adamec RE: The neural basis of prolonged suppression of predatory attack. I. Naturally occurring physiological differences in the limbic systems of killer and non-killer cats, *Aggr Behav* 1:315–330, 1975.

3. Adamec RE: Hypothalamic and extrahypothalamic substrates of predatory attack: suppression and the influence of hunger, *Brain Res* 106:57–69, April 16, 1976.

4. Adams T: Hypothalamic temperature in the cat during feeding and sleep, *Science* 139:609–610, Feb 15, 1963.

5. Allikmets LH: Cholinergic mechanisms in aggressive behaviour, *Med Biol* 52:19–30, Feb 1974.

6. Anand BK: Nervous regulation of food intake, *Physiol Rev* 41:677–708, Oct 1961.

7. Anand BK, Brobeck JR: Hypothalamic control of food intake in rats and cats, *Yale J Biol Med* 24:123–140, Nov 1951.

8. Anand BK, Dua S, Chhina GS: Higher nervous control over food intake, *Indian J Med Res* 46:277–287, March 1958.

9. Anokhin PK, Shuleikina KV: System organization of alimentary behavior in the newborn and the developing cat, *Dev Psychobiol* 10:385–419, 1977.

10. *Austin American-Statesman,* Feb 16, 1978.

11. Bartoshuk LM, Harned MA, Parks LH: Taste of water in the cat: effects on sucrose preference, *Science* 171:699–701, Feb 19, 1971.

12. Bartoshuk LM, Jacobs HL, Nichols TL, et al: Taste rejection of nonnutritive sweeteners in cats, *J Comp Physiol Psychol* 89(8):971–975, 1975.

13. Beadle M: *The cat: history, biology, and behavior,* New York, 1977, Simon & Schuster.

14. Beaver BV: Feline behavioral problems, *Vet Clin North Am* 6(3):333–340, 1976.

15. Beaver BV: Grass eating by carnivores, *Vet Med Small Anim Clin* 76(7):968–969, 1981.

16. Beaver BV: Disorders of behavior. In Sherding RG, editor: *The cat: diseases and clinical management,* New York, 1989, Churchill Livingstone.

17. Berkson G: Maturation defects in kittens, *Am J Ment Defic* 72:757–777, 1959.

18. Bernstein IL: Taste aversion learning: a contemporary perspective, *Nutrition* 15(3):229–234, 1999.

19. Berntson GG, Leibowitz SF: Biting attack in cats: evidence for central muscarinic mediation, *Brain Res* 51:366–370, 1973.

20. Biben M: Predation and predatory play behaviour of domestic cats, *Anim Behav* 27(1):81–94, 1979.

21. Bigbee HG: Personal communication, 1977.

22. Bixby DE, Beaver B, Hart BL: Chewing behavior, *Feline Pract* 16(1):12, 1986.

23. Blackshaw JK: Abnormal behaviour in cats, *Aust Vet J* 65(12):395–396, 1988.

24. Blackshaw JK: Management of orally based problems and aggression in cats, *Aust Vet Practit* 21(3):122–125, 1991.

25. Blackshaw JK: Management of behavioral problems in cats, *Feline Pract* 22(3):25–29, 1994.

26. Bloxham JC: Replies to dialog, *Feline Pract* 3(2):6, 1973.

27. Borchelt PL, Voith VL: Aggressive behavior in cats, *Compend Contin Educ Pract Vet* 9(1):49–57, 1987.

28. Boudreau JC, Tsuchitani C: *Sensory neurophysiology,* New York, 1973, Van Nostrand Reinhold.

29. Bradshaw JWS: Mere exposure reduces cat's neophobia to unfamiliar food, *Anim Behav* 34(2):613–614, 1986.

30. Bradshaw JWS, Cook SE: Patterns of pet cat behaviour at feeding occasions, *Appl Anim Behav Sci* 47(1,2):61–74, 1996.

31. Bradshaw JWS, Healey LM, Thorne CJ, et al: Differences in food preferences between individuals and populations of domestic cats *Felis silvestris catus, Appl Anim Behav Sci* 68(3):257–268, 2000.

32. Bradshaw JWS, Neville PF, Sawyer D: Factors affecting pica in the domestic cat, *Appl Anim Behav Sci* 52(3,4):373–379, 1997.

33. Brobeck JR: Mechanism of the development of obesity in animals with hypothalamic lesions, *Physiol Rev* 26(4):541–559, 1946.

34. Brunner F: The application of behavior studies in small animal practice. In Fox MW, editor: *Abnormal behavior in animals,* Philadelphia, 1968, WB Saunders.

35. Bryant D: *The care and handling of cats,* New York, 1944, Ives Washburn.

36. Caro T: Relations between kitten behaviour and adult predation, *Z Tierpsychol* 51:158–168, 1979.

37. Caro TM: The effects of experience on the predatory patterns of cats, *Behav Neural Biol* 29(1):1–28, 1980.

38. Caro TM: Effects of the mother, object play, and adult experience on predation in cats, *Behav Neural Biol* 29(1):29–51, 1980.

39. Caro TM: Predatory behaviour in domestic cat mothers, *Behaviour* 74(1–2):128–148, 1980.

40. Caro TM: Predatory behaviour and social play in kittens, *Behaviour* 76:1–24, 1981.

41. Castonguay TW: Dietary dilution and intake in the cat, *Physiol Behav* 27(3):547–549, 1981.

42. Cervantes M, De La Torre L, Beyer C: Analysis of various factors involved in EEG synchronization during milk drinking in the cat, *Brain Res* 91(1):89–98, 1975.

43. Cervantes M, Ruelas R, Beyer C: Serotonergic influences on EEG synchronization induced by milk drinking in the cat, *Pharmacol Biochem Behav* 18(6):851–855, 1983.

44. Chase MH, Wyrwicka W: Facilitation of feeding in aphagic. In Novin D, Wyrwicka W, Bray GA, editors: *Hunger: basic mechanisms and clinical implications,* New York, 1976, Raven Press.

45. Childs JE: Size-dependent predation on rats *(Rattus norvegicus)* by house cats *(Felis catus)* in an urban setting, *J Mammal* 67(1):196–199, 1986.

46. Church SC, Allen JA, Bradshaw JWS: Anti-apostatic food selection by the domestic cat, *Anim Behav* 48(3):747–749, 1994.

47. Collins DR: Drinking water requirements of cats, *Mod Vet Pract* 51:27, Oct 1970.

48. Collins DR: Feline anorexia: the veterinarian's enigma, *Feline Pract* 2(1):17–21, 1972.

49. Coman BJ, Brunner H: Food habits of the feral house cat in Victoria, *J Wildl Manage* 36:848–853, 1972.

50. Cruickshank RM: Animal infancy. In Carmichael L, editor: *Manual of child psychology,* New York, 1946, John Wiley and Sons.

51. Davis DE: The use of food as a buffer in a predator-prey system, *J Mammal* 38:466–472, Nov 1957.

52. Deag JM, Manning A, Lawrence CE: Factors influencing the mother-kitten relationship. In Turner DC, Bateson PPG, editors: *The domestic cat: the biology of its behavior,* Cambridge, 1988, Cambridge University Press.

53. Delgado JMR, Anand BK: Increase of food intake induced by electrical stimulation of the lateral hypothalamus, *Am J Physiol* 172(1):162–168, 1953.

54. Delpietro H, Konolsaisen F, Marchevsky N, Russo G: Domestic cat predation on vampire bats *(Desmodus rotundus)* while foraging on goats, pigs, cows and human beings, *Appl Anim Behav Sci* 39(2):141–150, 1994.

55. Dodman NH: Pharmacological treatment of behavioral problems in cats, *Vet Forum* 62–65, 71, April 1995.

56. Dodman NH, Shuster L: Pharmacologic approaches to managing behavior problems in small animals, *Vet Med* 89(10):960–969, 1994.

57. Eaton RL: The evolution of sociality in the Felidae. In Eaton RL, editor: *The world's cats,* ed 3, Seattle, 1976, Carnivore Research Institute.

58. Eberhard T: Food habits of Pennsylvania house cats, *J Wildl Manage* 18:284–286, April 1954.

59. Elton CS: The use of cats in farm rat control, *Br J Anim Behav* 1:151–155, Oct 1953.

60. Eschenroeder HC, Coughlin BE, Clarke AP: Wool-eating cats, *Feline Pract* 6(6):5–6, 1976.
61. Ewer RF: Sucking behaviour in kittens, *Behaviour* 15:146–162, 1959.
62. Ewer RF: Further observations on suckling behaviour in kittens, together with some general considerations of the interrelations of innate and acquired responses, *Behaviour* 17:247–260, 1961.
63. Ewer RF: *Ethology of mammals,* London, 1968, Paul Elek.
64. Ewer RF: *The carnivores,* Ithaca, NY, 1973, Cornell University Press.
65. Ewer RF: Viverrid behavior and the evolution of reproductive behavior in the Felidae. In Eaton RL, editor: *The world's cats,* Seattle, 1974, Feline Research Group.
66. Finco DR, Adams DD, Crowell WA, et al: Food and water intake and urine composition in cats: influence of continuous versus periodic feeding, *Am J Vet Res* 47(7):1638–1642, 1986.
67. Fireman J: *Cat catalog,* New York, 1976, Workman Publishing.
68. Fitzgerald BM: Diet of domestic cats and their impact on prey populations. In Turner DC, Bateson P, editors: *The domestic cat: the biology of its behaviour,* Cambridge, 1988, Cambridge University Press.
69. Flynn MF, Hardie EM, Armstrong PJ: Effect of ovariohysterectomy on maintenance energy requirement in cats, *J Am Vet Med Assoc* 209(9):1572–1581, 1996.
70. Forbush EH: *The domestic cat: bird killer, mouser, and destroyer of wild life, means of utilizing and controlling it,* Boston, 1916, Wright & Potter Printing.
71. Fox MW: *Understanding your cat,* New York, 1974, Coward, McCann & Geoghegan.
72. Fox MW: The behaviour of cats. In Hafez ESE, editor: *The behaviour of domestic animals,* ed 3, Baltimore, 1975, Williams & Wilkins.
73. Fratta W, Mereu G, Chess P, et al: Benzodiazepine-induced voraciousness in cats and inhibition of amphetamine-anorexia, *Life Sci* 18(10):1157–1165, 1976.
74. Galambos R: Processing of auditory information. In Brazier MAB, editor: *Brain and behavior,* vol 1, Washington, DC, 1961, American Institute of Biological Sciences.
75. Glasofer S: Practice pointers, *Vet Med Small Anim Clin* 67(7):718, 1972.
76. Green JD, Clemente CD, DeGroot J: Rhinencephalic lesions and behavior in cats, *J Comp Neurol* 108:505–545, Dec 1957.
77. Grossman SP: Eating or drinking elicited by direct adrenergic or cholinergic stimulation of hypothalamus, *Science* 132:301–302, July 29, 1960.
78. Grossman SP: Neurophysiologic aspects: extrahypothalamic factors in the regulation of food intake, *Adv Psychosom Med* 7:49–72, 1972.
79. Hart BL: Maternal behavior. II. The nursing-suckling relationship and the effects of maternal deprivation, *Feline Pract* 2(6):6, 7, 10, 1972.
80. Hart BL: Feeding behavior, *Feline Pract* 4(1):8, 1974.
81. Hart BL: Predatory behavior, *Feline Pract* 4(2):8–9, 1974.
82. Hart BL: Quiz on feline behavior, *Feline Pract* 6(3):10, 13, 1976.
83. Hart BL: Behavioral aspects of selecting a new cat, *Feline Pract* 6(5):8, 10, 14, 1976.
84. Hart BL: Behavioral aspects of raising kittens, *Feline Pract* 6(6):8, 10, 20, 1976.
85. Hart BL: Appetite and feeding: problems with too much or too little, *Feline Pract* 8(5):10–12, 1978.
86. Hart BL: Water sprayer therapy, *Feline Pract* 8(6):13, 15, 16, 1978.
87. Hart BL, Hart LA: *Canine and feline behavioral therapy,* Philadelphia, 1985, Lea & Febiger.
88. Hart BL, Voith VL: Changes in urine spraying. Feeding and sleep behavior of cats following medial preoptic-anterior hypothalamic lesions, *Brain Res* 145:406–409, 1978.
89. Hegsted DM, Gershoff SN, Lentini E: The development of palatability tests for cats, *Am J Vet Res* 17:733–737, 1956.
90. Heidenberger E: Housing conditions and behavioural problems of indoor cats as assessed by their owners, *Appl Anim Behav Sci* 52(3,4):345–364, 1997.

91. Hilton FE: Medicating a cat: "the Hilton modification," *Feline Pract* 6(6):44–45, 1976.

92. Horwitz DF: Compulsive disorders in cats. Available at www.avma.org/noah/members/convention/conv01/notes/04010101.asp.

93. Houpt K: Ingestive behavior problems of dogs and cats, *Vet Clin North Am Small Anim Pract* 12(4):683–692, 1982.

94. Houpt KA: What the technician should know about feeding behavior of dogs and cats, *Compend Contin Educ Anim Health Tech* 1(1):43–50, 1980.

95. Houpt KA: Companion animal behavior: a review of dog and cat behavior in the field, the laboratory and the clinic, *Cornell Vet* 75:248–261, 1985.

96. Houpt KA: Feeding and drinking behavior problems, *Vet Clin North Am Small Anim Pract* 21:281–298, March 1991.

97. Houpt KA: Behavioral genetics of cats and dogs. Available at www.avma.org/noah/members/convention/conv01/notes/04010101.asp.

98. Houpt KA, Essick LA, Shaw EB, et al: A tuna fish diet influences cat behavior, *J Toxicol Environ Health* 24:161–172, 1988.

99. Houpt KA, Smith SL: Taste preferences and their relation to obesity in dogs and cats, *Can Vet J* 22(4):77–81, 1981.

100. Houpt KA, Wolski TR: *Domestic animal behavior for veterinarians and animal scientists,* Ames, 1982, Iowa State University Press.

101. Inselman-Temkin BR, Flynn JP: Sex-dependent effects of gonadal and gonadotropic hormones on centrally-elicited attack in cats, *Brain Res* 60:393–409, Oct 12, 1973.

102. Jacobs DL: Behavior modification technique, *Feline Pract* 8(2):6, 1978.

103. Kanarek RB: Availability and caloric density of the diet as determinants of meal patterns in cats, *Physiol Behav* 15(5):611–618, 1975.

104. Kane E: Texture, odor, and flavor important in determining feline food preference, *DVM* 18(6):46, 47, 54, 1987.

105. Kaufman LW, Collier G, Hill WL, Collins K: Meal cost and meal patterns in an uncaged domestic cat, *Physiol Behav* 25(1):135–137, 1980.

106. Khanna C, Bienzle D: Polycythemia vera in a cat: bone marrow culture in erythropoietin-deficient medium, *J Am Anim Hosp Assoc* 30(1):45–49, 1994.

107. Kleiman DG, Eisenberg JF: Comparisons of canid and felid social systems from an evolutionary perspective, *Anim Behav* 21:637–659, Nov 1973.

108. Kling A, Kovach JK, Tucker TJ: The behaviour of cats. In Hafez ESE, editor: *The behaviour of domestic animals,* ed 2, Baltimore, 1969, Williams & Wilkins.

109. Koepke JE, Pribram KH: Effect of milk on the maintenance of sucking behavior in kittens from birth to six months, *J Comp Physiol Psychol* 75:363–377, June 1971.

110. Kovach JK, Kling A: Mechanisms of neonate sucking behavior in the kitten, *Anim Behav* 15(1):91–101, 1967.

111. Kuo ZY: The genesis of the cat behavior toward the rat, *J Comp Psychol* 11:1–35, 1930.

112. Kuo ZY: Further study on the behavior of the cat toward the rat, *J Comp Psychol* 25(1):1–8, 1938.

113. Lakso V, Randall W: Fishing behavior after lateral midbrain lesions in cats, *J Comp Physiol Psychol* 68(4):467–475, 1969.

114. Landers A: Cat, dog follow kosher household rules, *The Bryan Eagle* 102:6A, Aug 1978.

115. Landsberg G: Feline behavior and welfare, *J Am Vet Med Assoc* 208(4):502–505, 1996.

116. Langfeldt T: Diazepam-induced play behavior in cats during prey killing, *Psychopharmacologia* 36:181–184, 1974.

117. Langworthy OR: Behavioral disturbances related to the decomposition of reflex activity caused by cerebral injury: an experimental study of the cat, *J Neuropathol Exp Neurol* 3:87–100, 1944.

118. Larson MA, Stein BE: The use of tactile and olfactory cues in neonatal orientation and localization of the nipple, *Dev Psychobiol* 17(4):423–436, 1984.

119. Levinson PK, Flynn JP: The objects attacked by cats during stimulation of the hypothalamus, *Anim Behav* 13(2,3):217–220, 1965.

120. Levitsky DA: Obesity and the behavior of eating, *Gaines Dog Res Prog* pp 4–5, Winter 1972.

121. Leyhausen P: *Cat behavior: the predatory and social behavior of domestic and wild cats,* New York, 1978, Garland STPM Press.

122. Liberg O: Predation and social behaviour in a population of domestic cat. An evolutionary perspective, Dissertation, Lund, Sweden, 1981, Department of Animal Ecology, University of Lund.

123. Lorenz K, Leyhausen P: *Motivation of human and animal behavior,* New York, 1973, Van Nostrand Reinhold.

124. Macdonald DW, Apps PJ, Carr GM, Kerby G: *Social dynamics, nursing coalitions, and infanticide among farm cats,* Felis catus, Berlin, 1987, Paul Parey Scientific Publishers.

125. MacDonald ML, Rogers QR, Morris JG: Aversion of the cat to dietary medium-chain triglycerides and caprylic acid, *Physiol Behav* 35(3):371–375, 1985.

126. MacDonnell MF, Flynn JP: Control of sensory fields by stimulation of hypothalamus, *Science* 152:1406–1408, June 3, 1966.

127. Macy DW, Gasper PW: Diazepam-induced eating in anorexic cats, *J Am Anim Hosp Assoc* 21(1):17–20, 1985.

128. Martin P: An experimental study of weaning in the domestic cat, *Behaviour* 99:221–249, 1986.

129. May K: Association between anosmia and anorexia in cats, *Ann N Y Acad Sci* 510:480–482, 1988.

130. McFarland CA, Hart BL: Aggressive behavior, *Feline Pract* 8(4):13,1978.

131. McKeown DB, Luescher UA, Halip J: Stereotypies in companion animals and obsessive-compulsive disorder, *Purina Specialty Review* pp 30–35, 1992.

132. McMurry FB, Sperry CC: Food of feral house cats in Oklahoma, a progress report, *J Mammal* 22:185–190, May 1941.

133. Mead DJ: Ringed birds killed by cats, *Mammal Rev* 12(4):183–186, 1982.

134. Morganti T, Norsworthy GD: Slowing down the "wolfing" cat, *Vet Forum* p 33, Sep 2001.

135. Morgenson GJ, Huang YH: The neurobiology of motivated behavior, *Prog Neurobiol* 1:55–83, 1973.

136. Morris ML, Teeter SM: *Allergy: a commentary on nutritional management of small animals,* Topeka, Kan, 1977, Mark Morris Associates.

137. Mosier JE: Common medical and behavioral problems in cats, *Mod Vet Pract* 56(10):699–703, 1975.

138. Moyer KE: Kinds of aggression and their physiological basis, *Commun Behav Biol A* 2:65–87, 1968.

139. Mugford RA: Comparative and developmental studies of feeding behaviour in dogs and cats, *Br Vet J* 133:98, 1977.

140. Nagle AC, Houpt KA, Niebuhr BR, et al: Depraved appetite, *Feline Pract* 15(5):28–29, 1985.

141. Neville PF, Bradshaw JWS: Fabric eating in cats, *Vet Pract Staff* 6(5):26–29, 1994.

142. Norris MP, Beaver BV: Application of behavior therapy techniques to the treatment of obesity in companion animals, *J Am Vet Med Assoc* 202(5):728–730, 1993.

143. Overall KL: Preventing behavior problems: early prevention and recognition in puppies and kittens, *Purina Specialty Review* pp 13–29, 1992.

144. Overall KL: Recognition, diagnosis, and management of obsessive-compulsive disorders. Part 1: A rational approach, *Canine Pract* 17(2):40–44, 1992.

145. Overall KL: Management related problems in feline behavior, *Feline Pract* 22(1):13–15, 1994.

146. Panaman R: Behaviour and ecology of free-ranging female farm cats (*Felis catus* L.), *Z Tierpsychol* 56:59–73, 1981.

147. Papurt ML: Exaggerated cost of feeding a Great Dane, *Vet Med Small Anim Clin* 2(4):513, 1977.

148. Parmalee PW: Food habits of the feral house cat in east-central Texas, *J Wildl Manage* 17(3):375–376, 1953.

149. Patronek GJ: Free-roaming and feral cats-their impact on wildlife and human beings, *J Am Vet Med Assoc* 212(2):218–226, 1998.

150. Pearson OP: Carnivore-mouse predation: an example of its intensity and bioenergetics, *J Mammal* 45(2):177–188, 1964.

151. Pearson OP: The prey of carnivores during one cycle of mouse abundance, *J Anim Ecol* 35:217–233, Feb 1966.

152. Pellis SM, O'Brien DP, Pellis VC, et al: Escalation of feline predation along a gradient from avoidance through "play" to killing, *Behav Neurosci* 102:760–777, 1988.

153. Pfaffmann C: Differential responses of the new-born cat to gustatory stimuli, *J Genet Psychol* 49:61–67, 1936.

154. Polsky RH: Hunger, prey feeding, and predatory aggression, *Behav Biol* 13:81–93, 1975.

155. Randall WL, Parsons VL: The concomitancy in the rhythms of caloric intake and behavior in cats: a replication, *Psychon Sci* 15:35–36, 1969.

156. Reis DJ: Central neurotransmitters in aggression, *Res Publ Assoc Res Nerv Ment Dis* 52:119–147, 1974.

157. Robertson ID: Survey of predation by domestic cats, *Aust Vet J* 76(8):551–554, 1998.

158. Rogers WW: Controlled observations on the behavior of kittens toward rats from birth to five months of age, *J Comp Psychol* 13:107–125, 1932.

159 Rosenblatt JS: Suckling and home orientation in the kitten: a comparative developmental study. In Tobach E, Aronson LR, Shaw E, editors: *The biopsychology of development*, New York, 1971, Academic Press.

160. Rosenblatt JS: Learning in newborn kittens, *Sci Am* 227:18–25, 1972.

161. Rosenblatt JS, Turkewitz G, Schneirla TC: Early socialization in the domestic cat as based on feeding and other relationships between female and young. In Foss BM, editor: *Determinants of infant behaviour*, New York, 1961, John Wiley and Sons.

162. Rosenblatt JS, Turkewitz G, Schneirla TC: Development of suckling and related behavior in neonate kittens. In Bliss EL, editor: *Roots of behavior*, New York, 1962, Harper & Row.

163. Russek M: Hepatic receptors and the neurophysiological mechanisms controlling feeding behavior, *Neurosci Res* 4:213–282, 1971.

164. Russek M, Morgane PJ: Anorexic effect of intraperitoneal glucose in the hypothalamic hyperphagic cat, *Nature* 199:1004–1005, Sep 7, 1963.

165. Sauer LS, Hamar D, Lewis LD: Effect of diet composition on water intake and excretion by the cat, *Feline Pract* 15(4):16–21, 1985.

166. Schneirla TC, Rosenblatt JS: Behavioral organization and genesis of the social bond in insects and animals, *Am J Orthopsychiatry* 31(2):223–253, 1961.

167. Schneirla TC, Rosenblatt JS, Tobach E: Maternal behavior in the cat. In Rheingold HL, editor: *Maternal behavior in mammals*, New York, 1963, John Wiley and Sons.

168. Scott PP: Nutrition and disease. In Catcott EJ, editor: *Feline medicine and surgery*, ed 2, Santa Barbara, Calif, 1975, American Veterinary Publications.

169. Scott PP: Diet and other factors affecting the development of young felids. In Eaton RL, editor: *The world's cats*, ed 3, Seattle, 1976, Carnivore Research Institute.

170. Siegel A, Edinger H: Neural control of aggression and rage behavior. In Morgane PJ, Panksepp J, editors: *Behavioral studies of the hypothalamus,* vol 3, pt B, New York, 1981, Marcel Dekker.

171. Skultety FM: Changes in caloric intake following brain stem lesions in cats. II. Effects of lesions in medial hypothalamic region, *Arch Neurol* 14:541–552, May 1966.

172. Sprague JM, Chambers WW, Stellar E: Attentive, affective, and adaptive behavior in the cat, *Science* 133(3447):165–173, 1961.

173. Sterman MB, Wyrwicka W, Roth S: Electrophysiological correlates and neural substrates of alimentary behavior in the cat, *Ann N Y Acad Sci* 157:723–739, May 15, 1969.

174. Timmins R: Personal communication, Jan 1994.

175. Turner D, Appleby D, Magnus E: The Association of Pet Behaviour Counsellors: annual review of cases, 2000. Available at www.apbc.org.uk/2000/report.htm.

176. Turner DC, Meister O: Hunting behaviour of the domestic cat. In Turner DC, Bateson P, editors: *The domestic cat: the biology of its behaviour,* Cambridge, 1988, Cambridge University Press.

177. van den Bos R, Meijer MK, Spruijt BM: Taste reactivity patterns in domestic cats *(Felis silvestris catus), Appl Anim Behav Sci* 69(2):149–168, 2000.

178. Walker AD: Taste preferences in the domestic dog and cat, *Gaines Dog Res Prog* pp 1, 6, Summer 1975.

179. Ward DG, Ward JH: Control of water intake: evidence for the role of a hemodynamic pontine pathway, *Brain Res* 262(2):314–318, 1983.

180. Weerasuriya A, Bieger D, Hockman CH: Basal forebrain facilitation of reflex swallowing in the cat, *Brain Res* 174(1):119–133, 1979.

181. Weigel I: Small cats and clouded leopards. In Grzimek HCB, editor: *Grzimek's animal life encyclopedia,* vol 12, New York, 1975, Van Nostrand Reinhold.

182. West M: Social play in the domestic cat, *Am Zool* 14:427–436, Winter 1974.

183. Widdowson EM: Food, growth, and development in the suckling period. In Graham-Jones O, editor: *Canine and feline nutritional requirements,* New York, 1965, Pergamon Press.

184. Wilkins R, Bicks J, Thompson A, Beaver B: Unusual eating behavior, *Feline Pract* 16(6):14–15, 1986.

185. Wolski TR: Feline behavioral problems: Social causes and practical solutions, *Cornell Feline Health Cent News* 3:1, 2, 4–6, May 1981.

186. Wood GL: *Animal facts and feats,* Garden City, NJ, 1972, Doubleday.

187. Worden AN: Abnormal behaviour in the dog and cat, *Vet Rec* 71:966–978, Dec 26, 1959.

188. Wyrwicka W: Effects of electrical stimulation within the hypothalamus on gastric acid secretion and food intake in cats, *Exp Neurol* 60:286–303, 1978.

ADDITIONAL READINGS

Adamec R: Behavioral and epileptic determinants of predatory attack behavior in the cat, *Can J Neurol Sci* 2:457–466, Nov 1975.

Adamec RE: The interaction of hunger and preying in the domestic cat *(Felis catus);* an adaptive hierarchy? *Behav Biol* 18:263–272, Oct 1976.

Anand BK, Dua S: Feeding responses induced by electrical stimulation of the hypothalamus in cat, *Indian J Med Res* 43:113–122, Jan 1955.

Anand BK, Dua S, Shoenberg K: Hypothalamic control of food intake in cats and monkeys, *J Physiol* 127:143–152, Jan 28, 1955.

Bado A, Lewin MJM, Dubrasquet M: Effects of bombesin on food intake and gastric acid secretion in cats, *Am J Physiol* 256:R181–R186, 1989.

Bado A, Rodriguez M, Lewin MJM, et al: Cholecystokinin suppresses food intake in cats: structure-activity characterization, *Pharmacol Biochem Behav* 31(2):297–303, 1988.

Ballarini G: Animal psychodietetics, *J Small Anim Pract* 31(10):523–532, 1990.

Bandler R, Flynn JP: Visual patterned reflex present during hypothalamically elicited attack, *Science* 171:817–818, 1971.

Beaver BV: Reflex development in the kitten, *Appl Anim Ethol* 4(1):93, 1978.

Berntson GG, Hughes HC, Beattie MS: A comparison of hypothalamically induced biting attack with natural predatory behavior in the cat, *J Comp Physiol Psychol* 90(2):167–178, 1976.

Berry CS: An experimental study of imitation in cats, *J Comp Neurol Psychol* 18:1–26, Jan 1908.

Brown JL, Hunsperger RW: Neurothology and motivation of agonistic behaviour, *Anim Behav* 11:439–448, Oct 1963.

Chertok L, Fontaine M: Psychosomatics in veterinary medicine, *J Psychosom Res* 7:229–235, 1963.

Chi CC, Flynn JP: Neural pathways associated with hypothalamically elicited attack behavior in cats, *Science* 171:703–706, Feb 19, 1971.

Cooper JB: A description of parturition in the domestic cat, *J Comp Psychol* 37:71–79, 1944.

Courthial AS: The persistence of infantile behavior in a cat, *J Genet Psychol* 36:349–350, 1929.

Egger MD, Flynn JP: Effects of electrical stimulation of the amygdala on hypothalamically elicited attack behavior in cats, *J Neurophysiol* 26(5):705–720, 1963.

Eleftheriou BE, Scott JP: *The physiology of aggression and defeat,* New York, 1971, Plenum Publishing.

Errington PL: Notes on food habits of the southern Wisconsin house cats, *J Mammal* 17(1):64–65, 1936.

Everett GM: The pharmacology of aggressive behavior in animals and man, *Psychopharmacol Bull* 13(1):15–17, 1977.

Ewert JP: *Neuroethology,* New York, 1980, Springer-Verlag.

Fitzgerald BM, Karl BJ: Food of feral house cats (*Felis catus* L.) in forest of the Orongorongo Valley, Wellington, *N Z J Zool* 6:107–126, 1979.

Fox MW: New information on feline behavior, *Mod Vet Pract* 56(4):50–52, 1965.

Fox MW: Psychomotor disturbances. In Fox MW, editor: *Abnormal behavior in animals,* Philadelphia, 1968, WB Saunders.

Fox MW: Psychopathology in man and lower animals, *J Am Vet Med Assoc* 159(1):66–77, 1971.

Fraser AF: Behavior disorders in domestic animals. In Fox MW, editor: *Abnormal behavior in animals,* Philadelphia, 1968, WB Saunders.

Gonyea W, Ashworth R: The form and function of retractile claws in the Felidae and other representative carnivorans, *J Morphol* 145(2):229–238, 1975.

Hart BL: The brain and behavior, *Feline Pract* 3(5):4, 6, 1973.

Hart BL: Disease processes and behavior, *Feline Pract* 3(6):6–7, 1973.

Hart BL: Behavior of the litter runt, *Feline Pract* 4(5):14–15, 1974.

Hart BL: A quiz on feline behavior, *Feline Pract* 5(3):12, 14, 1975.

Hart BL: Psychosomatic aspects of feline medicine, *Feline Pract* 8(4):8, 10, 12, 1978.

Hirsch E, Dubose C, Jacobs HL: Dietary control of food intake in cats, *Physiol Behav* 20(3):287–295, 1978.

Houdeshell JW, Hennessey PW: Megestrol acetate for control of estrus in the cat, *Vet Med Small Anim Clin* 72(6):1013–1017, 1977.

Houpt KA: Animal behavior as a subject for veterinary students, *Cornell Vet* 66:73–81, Jan 1976.

Hubbs EL: Food habits of feral house cats in the Sacramento Valley, *California Fish and Game* 37:177–189, April 27, 1951.

Huidekopper RS: *The cat,* New York, 1895, D Appleton & Company.

Hutchinson RR, Renfrew JW: Stalking attack and eating behaviors elicited from the same sites in the hypothalamus, *J Comp Physiol Psychol* 61(3):360–367, 1966.

Jackson WB: Food habits of Baltimore, Maryland, cats in relation to rat populations, *J Mammal* 32:458–461, 1951.

Jalowiec JE, Panksepp J, Shabshelowitz H, et al: Suppression of feeding in cats following 2-deoxy-D-glucose, *Physiol Behav* 10(4):805–807, 1973.

Jenkins TW: *Functional mammalian neuroanatomy,* Philadelphia, 1972, Lea & Febiger.

Jones RJ: Hyperthyroidism in the cat, *Pulse South Calif Vet Med Assoc* 22:14, Nov 1980.

Joshua JO: Abnormal behavior in cats. In Fox MW, editor: *Abnormal behavior in animals,* Philadelphia, 1968, WB Saunders.

Kalber LA: Dog and cat food trends, *J Am Vet Med Assoc* 161(12):1678, 1972.

Katz RJ, Thomas E: Effects of scopolamine and α-methylparatyrosine upon predatory attack in cats, *Psychopharmacologia* 42:153–157, May 28, 1975.

Katz RJ, Thomas E: Effects of a novel anti-aggressive agent upon two types of brain stimulated emotional behavior, *Psychopharmacology (Berlin)* 48:79–82, July 9, 1976.

Kremer K: Pilling a cat not so routine, *DVM* 1S, Oct 2001.

Kuo ZY: Studies on the basic factors in animal fighting. VII. Inter-species coexistence in mammals, *J Genet Psychol* 97:211–225, 1960.

Kuo ZY: *The dynamics of behavior development,* New York, 1976, Plenum Publishing.

Landry SM, Van Kruiningen HJ: Food habits of feral carnivores: a review of stomach content analysis, *J Am Anim Hosp Assoc* 15(6):775–782, 1979.

Levinson BM: Man and his feline pet, *Mod Vet Pract* 53:35–39, Nov 1972.

Leyhausen P: The communal organization of solitary mammals, *Symp Zool Soc Lond* 14:249–263, 1965.

Lubar JF, Numan R: Behavioral and physiological studies of septal function and related medial cortical structures, *Behav Biol* 8(1):1–25, 1973.

MacDonnell MF: Some effects of ethanol, amphetamine, disulfiram and *p*-CPA on seizing of prey in feline predatory attack and on associated motor pathways, *Q J Stud Alcohol* 33:437–450, June 1972.

MacDonnell MF, Fessock L, Brown SH: Ethanol and the neural substrate for affective defense in the cat, *Q J Stud Alcohol* 32(2):406–419, 1971.

MacDonnell MF, Fessock L, Brown SH: Aggression and associated neural events in cats. Effects of *p*-chlorophenylalanine compared with alcohol, *Q J Stud Alcohol* 32:748–763, Sep 1971.

Maxwell JC Jr: Cats trigger pet-food gains, *AAIIA Trends* II(1):42 44, 1986.

McDougall W, McDougall KD: Notes on instinct and intelligence in rats and cats, *J Comp Psychol* 7:145–175, 1927.

McMurry FB: Three shrews, *Cryptotis parva,* eaten by a feral housecat, *J Mammal* 26:94, 1945.

Mereu GP, Fratta W, Chessa P, Gessa GL: Voraciousness induced in cats by benzodiazepines, *Psychopharmacologia* 47:101–103, May 5, 1976.

Morgane PJ, Kosman AJ: Alterations in feline behaviour following bilateral amygdalectomy, *Nature* 180:598–600, Sep 21, 1957.

Pearson OP: Additional measurements of the impact of carnivores on California voles *(Microtus californicus),* *J Mammal* 52:41–49, 1971.

Polsky RH: Developmental factors in mammalian predation, *Behav Biol* 15:353–382, Nov 1975.

Roberts WW, Bergquist EH: Attack elicited by hypothalamic stimulation in cats raised in social isolation, *J Comp Physiol Psychol* 66(3):590–595, 1968.

Roberts WW, Keiss HO: Motivational properties of hypothalamic aggression in cats, *J Comp Physiol Psychol* 58(2):187–193, 1964.

Satinder KP: Reactions of selectively bred strains of rats to a cat, *Anim Learn Behav* 4(2):172–176, 1976.

Schmidt JP: Psychosomatics in veterinary medicine. In Fox MW, editor: *Abnormal behavior in animals,* Philadelphia, 1968, WB Saunders.

Shaikh MB, Steinberg A, Siegel A: Evidence that substance P is utilized in medial amygdaloid facilitation of defensive rage behavior in the cat, *Brain Res* 625(2):283–294, 1993.

Sharp JC, Nielson HC, Porter PB: The effect of amphetamines upon cats with lesions in the ventromedial hypothalamus, *J Comp Physiol Psychol* 55(2):198–200, 1962.

Sheard MH: Behavioral effects of *p*-chlorophenylalanine: inhibition by lithium, *Commun Behav Biol* 5(pt A):71–73, 1970.

Starer E: Effects of frustration of the nursing process on kittens, *J Genet Psychol* 105:113–117, Sep 1964.

Toner GC: House cat predation on small animals, *J Mammal* 37:119, Feb 1956.

Voith VL, Marder AR: Feline behavioral disorders. In Morgan RV, editor: *Handbook of small animal practice,* New York, 1988, Churchill Livingstone.

Wemmer C, Scow K: Communication in the Felidae with emphasis on scent marking and contact patterns. In Sebeok TA, editor: *How animals communicate,* Bloomington, 1977, Indiana University Press.

Wyrwicka W: Lateral hypothalamic "feeding" sites and gastric acid secretion, *Experientia* 32(10):1287–1289, 1976.

Wyrwicka W: The problem of motivation in feeding behavior. In Novin D, Wyrwicka W, Bray GA, editors: *Hunger: basic mechanisms and clinical implications,* New York, 1976, Raven Press.

Wyrwicka W: Changes in gastric acid secretion in aphagic or hyperphagic cats after hypothalamic lesions, *Exp Neurol* 63(2):293–303, 1979.

Wyrwicka W, Doty RW: Feeding induced in cats by electrical stimulation of the brain stem, *Exp Brain Res* 1:152–160, 1966.

8

Feline Eliminative Behavior

ELIMINATIVE BEHAVIOR DEVELOPMENT

Infantile Patterns

The neonate cannot voluntarily urinate and defecate. Instead, eliminative behaviors are controlled for several weeks by the urogenital reflex. Stroking of the kitten's perineal region or caudal abdomen, as a queen would do while cleaning her young, results in urination and defecation. When the young are not mobile enough to leave the nest, it is critical to their survival in the wild that the nest be reasonably undetectable, which requires that it have relatively little odor. Because the kittens can eliminate only when the queen is present to tactually stimulate them, the urogenital reflex ensures that she can consume their wastes and prevent their soiling the nest. Even after this period of relative kitten immobility, the queen continues to stimulate this reflex because the home nest remains the center of activity until the kittens are about 6 weeks of age, when it begins to share significance with other sites specific for feeding, playing, and eliminating.[113] The anogenital reflex disappears between 23 and 39 days of age; however, kittens can voluntarily eliminate by 3 weeks of age.

Initially most of the queen's grooming and ingestion of waste occur during nursing or shortly thereafter; however, as the kittens get older the queen may directly approach certain individuals. Commonly the kitten assumes dorsal recumbency with the limbs abducted. Younger kittens are passive until the grooming-toilet session is completed, and older ones tend to squirm.

Kittens have a natural tendency to "earth-rake" loose sand and dirt as a prelude to the use of this behavior in elimination. Around 30 days of age, a kitten begins to spend time in a litterbox or in soft dirt, moving the particles one way and then another. Ingestion of litter or dirt as a form of oral exploration is also common at this time. Because this can be expected, clumping litters are not appropriate for young kittens.[89] Absorbent plastic pellets should not be used either. This oral behavior is usually followed within a few days by the species' behaviors of eliminating in a certain area and covering the elimination.

The neural mechanism for eliminative behavior can be demonstrated to be functional by electrical stimulation of the hypothalamus at 2 weeks of age. Thus neurologic maturation of these pathways has occurred as long as 2 weeks before the actual onset of the behavior.[34,76] The kittens learn the specific toilet area by observing the queen and by olfactory cues.

Litter Training

Because kittens naturally complement innate behaviors, such as burying wastes, with learned patterns, such as where to eliminate, a newly acquired kitten generally does not have to be "litter trained." However, occasionally individuals such as orphans or outdoor cats do not have the opportunity to learn, and the owner must educate them. Young cats also learn surface and location preferences[12] and should not be considered "trained" until at least 6 months of age.

It is initially important that any cat be confined to a small area to take advantage of the fastidious feline nature. This makes the litter readily accessible. It is not realistic to expect a kitten that spends most of its time in the living room to reliably use a litterbox kept in a back bedroom on the second floor.[2] The owner should place the untrained kitten in the litter pan shortly after each meal and manipulate its forepaws to make digging motions. The kitten is allowed to jump out, so this process can be repeated one or two times.[73] For the older outdoor cat that is becoming an indoor pet, the same procedures can be used, but it is often desirable to use dirt or sand initially and gradually change to litter. With these older individuals, particular care must be taken to keep potted plants out of the area so that the cat does not use the dirt in the pot for its toilet area. The plant could instead be protected by various forms of remote punishment or by putting decorative stones, pine bark chips, moth balls, or aluminum foil on the surface.[2,80]

Litter training may at first require leaving small traces of excretions in the box so that the smell can be used as a cue. If the kitten uses the area of the litterbox but not the box specifically, the owner can place the droppings in the tray to give it the appropriate odor and show the cat where the preferred area is. The litterbox location should be easily accessible yet afford some privacy and be relatively nearby. Cats prefer open large areas over the small covered box. Litter should not be scented and preferred types are fine grained. Although the cat instinctively eliminates in soft loose dirt, it can learn to use other locations either by itself or by special learning techniques. Litterbox substance is relatively easily changed from dirt or clay, typical of outdoor substances, to other loose material such as sand, commercial litter, wood shavings, or shredded newspaper. Most litters are 6 mm or less in particle diameter and all particles should feel similar in size to the cat.[10] Preferences seem to go to clumping products and Ever Clean, the recycled paper product,[10] over sand, which is more preferred than clay litter.[49] Unshredded newspapers may even be acceptable to the cat. In fact, cats often choose to use whole newspaper lying around the home instead of a litterbox. It is also important to have a size appropriate for the size of the cats and at least one litterbox per cat.[22,58,80,89,98] These should be available in multiple locations and various styles and sizes.[102] Litterboxes should have urine and feces removed at least daily with some fresh litter added to keep litter depth at 2 to 3 inches. The box needs to be completely dumped every 2 to 7 days or whenever the odor gets strong to the cat. Clumping litter can be changed less often, unless there is a rapid accumulation of small pieces of feces, as happens with soft feces. It is important to remember that odor at 6 inches from the litter is stronger than that at 3 feet. Boxes should be washed each week with a mild detergent and discarded when they are old.

Certain individuals, particularly of popular breeds such as the Persian, may be exceptionally difficult for either the queen or the owner to litter train.[13] It may indicate a genetic problem resulting from the popularity of the breed and consequent indiscriminate breeding. Perhaps "house trainability" was not considered in genetic selection, neurologic or learning deficiencies have been bred into the population, or cat domestication in general has created the difficulty.

ADULT URINATION

Eliminative Urination

Urinary postures and associated behaviors are ordinarily quite similar between the sexes. The cat usually digs a small hole in soft dirt or litter with its forepaws and then positions itself so that the urine is expressed into this area. The cat assumes a posture almost like that of sitting, except that the pelvic limbs are slightly abducted and the tail is held more rigidly, usually pointed caudally (Figure 8-1). Urine is forcefully ejected in a stream, probably because of abdominal pressure and urinary bladder contraction. When finished, the cat stands and moves dirt or litter over the urine with its forepaws (Figure 8-2). This happens 2.3 ± 2.1 times a day,[107] usually as short litterbox visits. Of these trips, 73% occur in the morning.[60]

Cats often learn on their own to urinate in a sink, bathtub, or toilet. Because some of the larger felids eliminate over streams, the domestic cat may adopt a more urban version to remove waste products. If this practice is undesirable, the owner can fill the tub with a few inches of water for several days and place a litterbox next to the tub. The water technique will not work if the cat straddles the sink when it urinates. In this case, an object like a cactus can be placed in the sink, with the litterbox nearby. For the cat that continues this behavior or that urinates in the toilet, the sink or toilet seat is lined

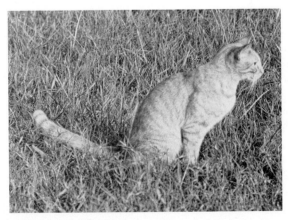

Figure 8-1 The urination posture of a cat.

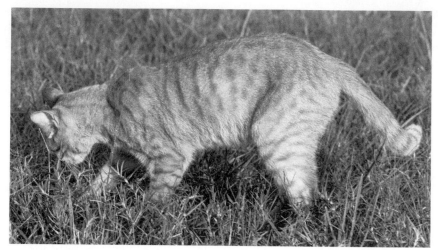

Figure 8-2 Earth-raking to cover fresh urine.

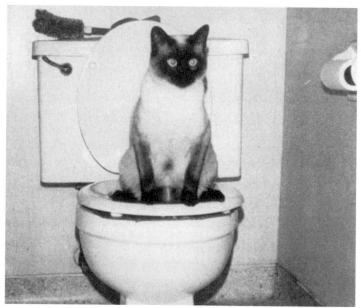

Figure 8-3 A toilet-trained cat. (*From Hart BL:* Feline Pract *5(5):12, 1975.*)

with aluminum foil or plastic wrap and then filled with litter. Once the cat learns to use the litter, the owner moves the litter to a box beside the sink or toilet.[11,54] The owner can gradually, as it is used, move the box short distances at a time until it is located in the preferred spot. The reverse technique can be used to train a cat to urinate in the toilet (Figure 8-3). The owner gradually brings the litterbox next to the toilet and then fastens plastic wrap to the toilet seat securely enough to hold quite a bit of litter, thus creating a litterbox. After a few days, the cat will accept a decrease in the amount of litter.

As the plastic becomes visible, the owner puts some holes in it to drain the urine. The last stage is the removal of the plastic and litter. Because this posture is somewhat awkward for the cat, the animal may occasionally slip off the toilet seat, and repetition of some of the procedures may be necessary to retrain it.[42,54]

Because of the incidence of urethral obstruction and feline lower urinary tract disease, the relationship between eating and urination has been investigated. The frequency of urination was not different between cats fed by free choice and those fed twice daily.[33] Those fed periodically did produce less urine and their urine pH level was lower in the morning and higher in the afternoon compared with cats fed ad libitum.[33]

Marking Urination

Spraying urination is used by cats, particularly intact males, to mark the edges of its territory, mark an activating landmark, communicate familiarity for reassurance, and signal its presence, thus minimizing the frequency and severity of encounters with intruders.[29,38] The odors of sprayed urine do not frighten other cats away,[39,75,107] indicating they are more for informational purposes. Both sexes can distinguish urine from strange versus familiar males, with males tending to investigate urine odors longer.[75] Because several cats may share a hunting area at different times, scents may be useful for avoidance.[75] To spray urine, the cat stands with its tail erect and quivering, although a few flex their elbows to lower the forequarters[132] (see Figure 3-17). Urine is ejected onto a vertical object in spurts that cover a relatively larger surface than normal urination, at a level 1 to 2 feet high. Earth raking afterward is rare.[119]

Because this marking behavior is sexually dimorphic, it is used primarily by intact tomcats and occasionally by females and castrated males when environmental situations become excessively stressful. Breeding males will spray two to four times more often than females or other males.[75,82] This averages 22.0 times per hour for breeding males, 12.9 times per hour for nonbreeding males, and 3.6 times per hour for females.[75] More spraying occurs near favorite hunting locations, by cats with larger home ranges, and when traveling.[75] Only 14.8% of the episodes follow agonistic encounters.[75] Male spraying peaks in the spring and then gradually decreases until late fall.[82] No seasonal variation is reported for females.[82] There is a genetic component to urine marking, making it more likely to occur in certain lines of cats.[39]

Emotional states affect renal circulation and thus urine formation. Excitatory states result in vasoconstriction, as in the intestinal vessels, because of neurogenic factors and a humoral component. During natural sleep there is renal vasodilation, probably resulting from vascular autoregulation.[84] These physiologic factors result in decreased urine output during excitement and increased output during sleep.

ADULT DEFECATION

Outdoor cats defecate 3.2 ± 1.5 times in a 24-hour period,[72,107] although there is quite a bit of variation depending on the diet. Newer concentrated foods can reduce the number of defecations to fewer than 1 a day. Behaviors associated with defecation resemble those used for normal urination. Posturing is similar, but the back is slightly more

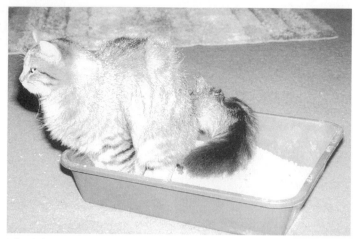

Figure 8-4 The defecation posture of a cat.

rounded and the perineum slightly higher off the ground (Figure 8-4). Cats may not dig as much before defecating as they do before urinating.[107] Burying feces is uncommon outside the cat's core area. Away from a home location, cats will bury feces only 45% of the time.[82] This could apply to indoor cats living in a large home. When feces is not covered, it tends to be along hunting paths or on elevated sites, with two or three scats accumulating per site.[75] Territorial males are more likely to use these prominent sites,[22] but the consensus is that cats do not mark with feces.[7,34,37,40]

The earth raking associated with burying feces is initiated by the odor of fecal matter, so most cats will sniff the feces before covering.[107] Feces that is not sniffed is seldom covered and not all feces that is sniffed is covered. Cats that miss the litterbox may perform earth raking on the floor, even though they move only air.[74] Odors from other sources, including some foods, can also stimulate this behavior. The artificial selections of domestication have changed some of the genetic factors of this behavior, and consequently some cats do not bury their feces even in their core area. Conversely, some cats are so fastidious that they cover not only their feces, but any other cat's exposed feces.

There is no one toilet area for the free-roaming cat, so feces are widely spread. This dispersal, along with the covering behavior, serves as a form of parasite control. Because the concentrated odor of fecal matter may actually inhibit the use of a certain area, litterboxes must be frequently cleaned.

ELIMINATIVE BEHAVIOR PROBLEMS: HOUSESOILING

Housesoiling is the most common problem in cats.[3,98] In cat owner surveys, researchers found that 47% to 55% of owners have a behavior problem with their cat, and 10% to 24% of pet cats will show an elimination problem at some time in their life.[10,12,31,57,98] Specialists dealing with behavior problems may have 45% to 65% of their cat cases related to eliminative problems.[83,98] Cats that have at least weekly elimination problems are at the highest risk to be surrendered to an animal shelter.[108] To work effectively with these cats, history taking is the most important part of the workup, because the most common reason for failures to use a litterbox are directly related to the litterbox, its contents, or its location.[65] A number of methods can be used, including a taxonomy.[3] Regardless of the specific approach, one must determine which cat is soiling, what specific type of elimination is occurring, where the cat is eliminating, and how long the behavior has been occurring. The history of litterbox use by the cat and box maintenance by the owner is also necessary. In multicat households, an owner may assume a particular cat has been housesoiling because it "looks guilty" or they do not particularly like the animal. Because treatment of the wrong cat is not successful, the true problem animal must be found. Isolation of individuals may indicate which cat is soiling. Other options are to give salicylates and test for their presence in serum or urine with ferric chloride.[114] Fluorescein can be given orally or subcutaneously to a single cat and fresh urine spots checked with an ultraviolet light[47,54,55,119]; however, owners should be cautioned that carpet or clothing can be stained by the fluorescein. The injection is 0.3 ml of a 10% solution, and the oral preparation is 0.5 ml of the 10% solution or six large animal ophthalmic strips (9 mg of fluorescein per strip) in two no. 4 gelatin capsules.[22,97,121] Check the urine in 1 or 2 days. A washout period of 24 to 48 hours is recommended between cats.[119]

The specific type of eliminative problem must be determined. Differentiate feces from urine and spraying from urination. If the owner has not seen the cat eliminate outside the litterbox, determine whether the wet spots are on vertical surfaces such as a wall or drape or whether a specific item or person is targeted such as the owner's pillow, dirty clothes, or favorite chair. A positive answer to questions regarding any of these indicate spraying (or urine marking) is the problem.

Where the housesoiling occurs may also indicate why or suggest an appropriate course of action. Owners may indicate the cat is soiling all over the house when the actual problem may be confined to one or two rooms or even spots. Areas near windows and doors or where cats can see outside are favorite targets for spraying when strange cats roam, especially during the mating season. When items belonging to a certain person are urinated on, there is a disturbance with that individual that bothers the cat. If the problem is confined to a single room, it can be closed off and the problem easily stopped.

Litterbox maintenance requires several questions.[99] The number, size, and location of the boxes should be determined. Also, information about the type of litter used; recent changes; and the frequency of removing feces, removing urine, and complete litter changes are needed. When and how is the box cleaned and how often is the box replaced?

Another important piece of information needed is how long the housesoiling behavior has been occurring. A single episode of missing the litterbox rarely requires intervention, but a 5-year history of not using the box at all is very difficult to change. If the cat never learned to use a litterbox, it is not reasonable to expect that it will begin just because it moves to a new home or the owners get new carpet. Factors that contributed to the onset of housesoiling can be different from those maintaining it,[66] so early and current factors may need to be considered.

A thorough physical examination should be part of the evaluation of housesoiling cats. Palpable abnormalities such as urinary calculi, abnormal kidney size, joint crepitus, or visible evidence of poor body or hair coat condition can point to medical causes of behavior problems.

Laboratory evaluation of most of these cats is also indicated. This is particularly true for geriatric animals because of the increased likelihood of several conditions.[64,97] Anatomic abnormalities, calculi, constipation, crystalluria, cystitis, diabetes mellitus, diarrhea, feline immunodeficiency virus (FIV), feline infectious peritonitis (FIP), feline leukemia (FeLV), feline lower urinary tract disease (FLUTD), food allergies, hyperthyroidism, incontinence, inflammatory bowel disease, internal parasites, interstitial cystitis, maldigestion/malabsorption, metabolic encephalopathies, pain, and pyelonephritis can cause housesoiling problems that require medical intervention. One study of spraying cats found 38% had abnormalities of the urogenital tract.[35,36] Because FLUTDs are a very common cause of inappropriate urination, it is important to learn where the cat is soiling; bathtub, sink, bath mat, and laundry are often used with this problem.[115,121] Dietary information should also be obtained because of the link between diet and FLUTDs.[15] Diet information is also important for constipation-related inappropriate defecation, particularly where the history may suggest occasional running in pain.[115] FeLV- and FIV-positive cats can show behavior changes such as the loss of housetraining, so testing for these diseases is appropriate.[32] In addition, if drug therapy is going to be used, a minimum database of a complete blood cell count, blood chemistry, urinalysis, and thyroid screen should be done.

The failure to use a litterbox can be classified in several ways. The method used here is to determine the type of housesoiling. It divides inappropriate elimination into defecation and urination. Marking can be urine marking, including spraying, or feces marking, which is extremely rare in cats. Another classification technique is to look at etiology such as litter aversion, surface preference, location preference, or location aversions.[*]

The prognosis for any of these problems depends on many factors, not all of which apply to any given situation. Included are (1) duration of the problem—the longer the problem, the more difficult it is to stop; (2) sex of the cat—males have an increased tendency to spray; (3) neutered status—intact cats are more likely to spray; (4) number of other cats in the home—multicat households have more problems; (5) number of areas soiled—more locations are more complicated; (6) ability to control stimuli—keeping the cat indoors or cleaning a box daily instead of weekly are relatively easy for most owners, whereas minimizing cats roaming nearby probably is not; (7) previous history of litterbox use—cats who have used a litterbox are significantly more likely to use the box again compared with a cat that never used one; (8) temperament of the cat—innately nervous individuals are more difficult; (9) ability to use drug therapy—drug therapy can be helpful in certain cases if owners can/will use medication; (10) coexisting medical problems, which can exacerbate problems or complicate treatment; and (11) owner commitment—magic cures are rare. Owner expectations, information about what has already been tried, and willingness to try different things are important pieces of information.[6] It is constantly amazing how many owners have lived with a housesoiling cat for several years and want the problem instantly stopped because their new carpet has arrived. Others get a cat from the shelter with a history of three previous owners having surrendered it for housesoiling but who cannot believe the cat would soil in their home too.

[*]References 11, 12, 27, 28, 86, 129, 130.

Many owners will have partial success with their own therapies, but more than 80% need professional interventions.[57] First, owners must not punish a cat for housesoiling. Doing so only increases the level of the cat's stress, which may aggravate things further, and it does not change the original motivation.[61]

Urine Marking

Urine marking is a common behavior problem, constituting up to 44% of the housesoiling complaints.[*] This number is probably low as well, because urine marking on horizontal surfaces is commonly diagnosed as inappropriate elimination unless specific horizontal targets can be identified. Urine spraying is generally related to sexual behavior and is commonly described as a problem of tomcats during the mating season. Male-female differences in response to lesions in the medial preoptic-anterior hypothalamic region support the concept of spraying as a sexually dimorphic behavior. Lesions usually stop spraying by males but have no effect in females.[56] Urine spraying is a behavior that is mainly territorial or anxiety based. The resident cat may spray to scent mark whenever it becomes uncomfortable with its surroundings, such as when there is decreased attention, punishment, owner absences, changes in routine, changes in surroundings, overcrowding, cat aggression, competition, introduction of a new cat, smell of another cat, or other stressors. The incidence of spraying is directly proportional to the number of cats in the household, increasing from 25% in single-cat households to 100% in households with more than 10 cats.[11,66,71,101] However, when spraying does occur, the severity of the problem is generally worse in single-cat homes. One study showed the incidence of spraying to be 16.1 marks per week compared with 7.4 marks per week in multicat homes.[68] About 5% of females and 10% of neutered males may also mark, but the behavior for them usually requires a higher threshold than for tomcats. Estrous females will spontaneously mark too. Some cats seem to be more easily upset by changes, so it is likely that individual temperaments also influence the tendency to urine mark.

Because male cats (77%) and cats from multicat households (89%) are the most likely to have urine-marking problems,[110] one must understand and address the social causes of urine marking.[102,103] Causes likely to result in urine marking include agonistic interactions with outside cats (49%), aggressive interactions with other cats in the home (28%), limiting outdoor access (26%), moving into a new home (9%), new inanimate objects in the home (6%), and interactions with the owner (6%).[110] Items most commonly targeted include (1) furniture, (2) walls or windows where the cat sees outside cats, (3) other walls, (4) appliances, and (5) novel items.[110] The remedy basically consists of altering either the cat's normal response or the stimulus. These may be accomplished by eliminating the environmental source of the problem, isolating the resident cat from the offending environment, altering the perception of stress, or minimizing the hormonal influence of the situation. The owner needs to have multiple feeding areas, multiple litterboxes, and several single-cat perches of different heights scattered throughout the house.[97]

*References 3, 5, 9, 20, 83, 98.

Certain episodes of urine marking seem to involve vindictiveness on the cat's part, almost as though the cat were punishing its owner for some slight. "Spiteful" eliminations probably do occur, such as when the cat urinates on the owner's bed or clothes immediately after a scolding, a trip out of town, or the introduction of a new cat, but definite proof of spitefulness is extremely difficult. When the resident cat deposits urine on objects belonging to a specific person, it may indicate the cat has singled out that relationship as less than desirable. When the objects targeted are more horizontal than vertical, the owner will describe a squatting posture. This makes it difficult to determine whether the cat is marking the object or housesoiling on an absorbable surface. Historical information about location and timing of the event relative to potential stressors is particularly important. When several objects are urinated on and they all belong to a particular individual with multiple people around, there is a good probability the cat is urine marking. Additional history may show the person is not fond of cats, and of course, the cat's behavior does not help. The simplest solution usually involves having the targeted person feed the cat. It is best if the cat can be given one or two small meals of canned food so that it has a strong desire to approach. Other people in the household should minimize their interaction with the cat during this time.

The treatment protocols for marking behavior usually involve several approaches at the same time. The first is the most obvious, because castration eliminates spraying behavior in 87% of tomcats. Testosterone will reach levels typical for a castrate (less than 50 ng/dl) within 8 to 16 hours after surgery,[49] so a fairly rapid change in behavior should be expected. Of those that respond, 78% exhibit a rapid postsurgical change, and the remaining 9% change gradually over a few months.[50] Approximately 10% of prepubertally gonadectomized cats will start spraying later in life, indicating learning and testosterone are not always factors.[51,54,116] Males are also more apt to spray if there are female cats in the household[51,54] or if they detect an estrous female in the presence of urine odors of other males.[106] About 5% of spayed females spray.[52,53,91]

Drug therapy is helpful and often necessary to get urine marking under control (Figure 8-5). A number of different drugs can be used, although success is somewhat mixed. Good comparative studies have yet to be done. The progestins used to be the drugs of choice, particularly medroxyprogesterone acetate and megestrol acetate. These products are effective in approximately one third of the cases, working better in male, single-cat households.[23,44,47] Males responded positively 50.0% of the time in multicat homes and 85.7% of the time if they were the only cat.[23] This compares with a success rate for females of 16.7% in multicat environments and 37.5% in single-cat households.[23] The progestins will also depress spermatogenesis and stimulate the appetite, in addition to having some serious side effects if used long term.[77,109,112] Other hormones, such as repository stilbestrol, ethylestrenol, and progesterone, have been used occasionally to control spraying, but their side effects can also be serious.[7,96,122] Currently anxiolytics are the most helpful. The benzodiazepine tranquilizers, particularly diazepam, are useful if stress is the precipitating factor in housesoiling.[2,61] They help in social facilitation and make cats less reactive to stimuli and surroundings.[103] These drugs are more helpful than hormone therapy when the problem involves females and/or multicat households.[85,87] In studies, diazepam eliminated or reduced spraying 55% to 74% of the time.[23,92,119] Male cats in multicat homes were positively affected 63.6% of the time, and those in single-cat homes were positively affected 33.3% of the time.[23]

	Multicat		Single cat		Overall		Combined
	Male	Female	Male	Female	Male	Female	
Progestins	48%-50%	17%-18%	86%	38%	50%	10%-15%	30%
Diazepam	64%	60%	33%	33%	52%-84%	25%-60%	55%
Buspirone	55%	75%			55%	75%[†]	55%-58%
Clomipramine							69%-80%
Facial pheromone							52%-96.7%

*References 23, 29, 35, 36, 48, 49, 52, 53, 67, 92, 105.
† 50% after 2 years.

Figure 8-5 Comparison of drug therapies for urine spraying in cats.*

Females in multicat environments were positively affected 60.0%.[23] There is a high probability of reoccurrence when medication is stopped, perhaps because of dependancy to the drug.[23,92] For this reason, gradual reduction of the dose by 10% to 25% per week is recommended.[119]

Tricyclic antidepressants (TCAs), selected serotonin reuptake inhibitors (SSRIs), and azaperones are other categories of drugs currently being used for spraying cats, although it can take 2 to 4 weeks before their effects are noticed. Clomipramine, a TCA, has been reported helpful in 69.2% to 100% of cats, even though some of the cats had been unsuccessfully treated with other drugs.[29,81,90,120] Fluoxetine, an SSRI, can significantly reduce the frequency of urine spraying in approximately 2 weeks.[111] The fact that most return to pretreatment levels of spraying when treatment stops in 8 weeks emphasizes the need for long-term drug therapy and environmental management for this drug and for other drugs. Buspirone, an azaperone, is a dopamine receptor antagonist and partial serotonin agonist, which in combination may result in less concern about perceived threats and increased capabilities to interact in an appropriate way socially.[104] Thus it can be used to reduce anxiety, with the added benefit of helping shy cats become more assertive and reducing their need to mark.[105] Statistically, this has about the same effectiveness as diazepam, with 55% to 58% of the patients from multicat homes responding, compared with none in single-cat homes.[30,52,53,104,105] The success rate was approximately equal for males and females.[53] Recurrence of spraying after medication is stopped is about 50%,[53] although this is not statistically different from that for diazepam.[104]

Cyproheptadine has been successfully used in a few cases of spraying.[116,117] Bromocriptine, an ergot alkaloid acting on dopamine agonists, is another drug that has had limited trials. The overall success rate against spraying is 78% to 85% for males and 40% for females.[118]

Feliway is a synthetic analog of the F_3 fraction of the feline facial pheromone that is now commercially available. It has been tested in homes with spraying cats and shown to significantly reduce the incidence of spraying.[68,97] The problem stopped completely in 33.3% of the homes and failed to result in any change in 9.3%.[68] The overall success rate reported was 51.5% to 96.7%.[35,36,67,131] The success rate does not seem to be particularly related to chronicity of the problem.[131] In all cases, best results can be expected if the initiating factors are removed at the time treatment begins and if the drugs are used only initially to decrease stress levels, because none are without occasional serious side effects (see Chapter 1).

In addition to drug therapy, environmental changes and behavior modification have to be used to eliminate spraying. Removal or confinement away from environmental stimuli, particularly other cats, and good litterbox hygiene can markedly reduce the incidence of spraying, almost to the point of resolving the problem.[110] These often change the significance of the sprayed site.[128] If the cat can be constantly observed, aversive conditioning or punishment might be successful. Timing is critical and should start each time just as the behavior starts.[127] A water pistol, plant sprayer, noise, light flash, or thrown object can deter spraying if used consistently at the moment the cat begins to spray. Strips of aluminum foil can be hung on the object usually sprayed so that the noise, the reflected spray, or both inhibits the cat.[41,125,126] The idea is interesting and the technique has been successful in a few cases, not because it was aversive, but because the cat was distracted by playing with the foil. Thus the procedure should probably not be considered dependable.[125] Shock mats, sticky surfaces, or irregular objects like bubble wrap may discourage cats from certain locations. Other things that can be tried include commercial repellants, moth balls, blocking the windows, more time outside, or no time outside.[61,128] The presence of other cats outside needs to be discouraged, so bird feeders and outdoor food should be eliminated.[71] Food bowls or litter pans have been placed near the area that is usually sprayed with some success. A cat can be fitted with a diaper, held in place by cloth.[62] The diaper will confine the wetness and may be aversive to the cat. Isolation in a small room with food, water, and a litter pan may help alleviate the problem by minimizing some environmental stresses.

New cats should be confined to a single room when first introduced into a home. This allows resident cats to get used to the new smells and noise first, and the new cat can get comfortable in a small territory before spending more time investigating the rest of the house with a gradual introduction. Moving an older cat to a new home should also involve confinement to a small area. This allows the cat to establish a territory, leaving hair and dander as the territorial odor rather than urine. Gradual access to the rest of the house lets the cat explore in a nonthreatening way.

For the chronic, refractory spraying cat, neurosurgical procedures could be tried but are rarely performed. Placing lesions in the medial preoptic area reduced or stopped spraying in six of six male cats; however, side effects made it undesirable as a clinical procedure.[12,56,126] Olfactory tractotomy was approximately 50% successful and was not associated with significant side effects.[12,45–47,54,61] Cutting the ischiocavernosus muscles has also been reported to significantly reduce the incidence of chronic spraying in castrated male cats.[61,78,87]

Inappropriate Elimination

The most common complaint related to feline urinary behavior is urination out of the box (50%), and defecation is a problem 10% to 29% of the time.[3,20,57,98] Causative factors are similar for both, so they are covered together. Owners will often try various therapies before seeking help, but fewer than 20% say they were successful with what they tried.[57] In addition, 55% of cats that display inappropriate urination have medical problems.[93] Careful questioning of the owner is necessary to be sure the cat's posture while urinating is typical of normal urination. In studying cats with inappropriate elimination, researchers have found that a high percentage are Persians (23%) and declawed (23%).[93] Although most urination problems occur in multicat homes, the numbers are evenly divided between multicat and single-cat households for defecation problems.[98] The presenting problem 32% to 38% of the time is urination.[93,98] Defecation is a problem 17% to 20% of the time, and both urination and defecation occur in 19% to 42% of the cases.[93,98]

In taking the history, the veterinarian should ascertain whether the cat has ever been litter trained. Only if it has used the litterbox correctly at some time should specific causes for housesoiling be sought. The cat that has never used the litterbox or has not used it for several years should be considered untrained instead. Approaches for this cat are mentioned later.

Problem cats behave differently from nonproblem cats relative to their litterbox use. Although a normal cat spends 60% of its litterbox time covering excreta, problem cats spend only 30% of their time earth raking.[123] Normal cats also spend significantly more time in the litterbox in covering, digging, sniffing, and total time.[123] In addition, declawed cats spend significantly more time earth raking air or floor (not litter) compared with cats with claws.[123] When the litter or box is unacceptable, some problem cats will not cover, rarely scratch after elimination, paw air or the floor instead of litter, or shake their paws.[10,61,102,121,128]

Litterbox issues

A general approach to inappropriate elimination is to look at the accessibility and desirability of the current litterbox(es) compared with the accessibility and desirability of the new location (Figure 8-6). Evaluating the litterbox can be very beneficial because the source of the problem of housesoiling is often near the litterbox. Litterbox avoidance can develop quickly from a particularly bad experience or gradually from a series of undesirable experiences.[24,102] The fastidious nature of some cats demands that the litter be changed frequently, sometimes more frequently than the owners care to change it.

A: Things that make a litterbox undesirable[80,83,88,102]
  Bad experiences at the box
  Busy locations
  Deodorized litter
  Difficult to get to
  Hooded litterbox
  Illness
  Inaccessible
  Insufficient cleaning
  Lack of privacy
  Liners
  Near food
  Noise
  Noisy litters
  Old plastic boxes
  Pain
  Remote location
  Repeatedly being caught at the box
  Strong disinfectants or detergents
  Unacceptable litter texture
B: Things to make a litterbox more desirable (leave one regular box)[80,102]
  Covered litterbox
  Larger litterbox
  Litter texture options
    Clumping litter
    Sandy litter
    Softer litter

Figure 8-6 Factors that affect the cat's relationship with a litterbox.

There may be too few litterboxes for the number of cats, or the box may to too small. The average household does nothing to a litterbox except dump it completely every 5 to 7 days. A dirty box to a cat probably resembles our reaction to the portable toilets used at outdoor sporting events. Simply by removing feces once or twice daily, the owner may be able to stop the soiling out of the box.[25,100] This is even more important if several cats use the same box. Ideally, there should be one litterbox for each cat and at least one extra if the house is large.[59] Litter should be completely replaced frequently because trapped odors are more obvious to the cat than to the owner. Cats usually prefer a certain amount of privacy, which an improperly placed litterbox may not provide. Covered litterboxes may offer privacy, but they can allow odors to build up, hide the view of a potential ambusher, or be too confining. In the wild, cats do not seek out caves or covered spots for toilet areas.[24] Also, access to the litterbox is sometimes accidentally blocked, or the box is moved. Kittens should not be trusted completely until about 6 months of age, and boxes placed in a third-floor back bedroom might just as well be in Siberia to the little one. New cats brought into a home should be isolated in a single room until its toilet habits stabilize and anxieties decrease.[14]

Odors associated with certain litters, such as chlorophyll, may prove undesirable to the cat, and the history will often connect a litter change with the change in elimination behaviors.[10,26,54] Cats tend to prefer a specific type of litter; therefore changes, when necessary, should be gradual. Odor can also serve as a deterrent when excessive amounts of cleaning solutions are used to clean litterboxes. Plastic litterboxes should be replaced periodically because urine reacts with them over time to change their basic odor.

A few cats have come to associate an unpleasant experience with the litterbox and prefer to avoid it. Experiences such as painful defecations, fearful events, raking after a declaw, or being repeatedly caught at that site and given a pill can adversely condition these cats. Retraining the animal to use the litterbox is often necessary and is best started in a different, isolated location. Once correct habits are reestablished, increased access to the house can be allowed. The owner can gradually move the litterbox to a more desirable location.

If the cat attempts to use the litterbox but misses, other measures must be taken. The box itself should be evaluated. It may be too small or the cat may position itself too near the edge. The solution usually involves supplying a larger litterbox or one with higher sides. Plastic storage boxes offer 25% to 100% more space than conventional litterboxes.[24]

Cats apparently associate pain with location, so any housesoiling cat should be examined to ensure no medical basis for the problem exists.[1,2,4] When a cat is urinating frequently, not using the litterbox as usual, or both, physical evaluation and a good history are important. Recurrent cystitis, often with small calculi, and interstitial cystitis present the same signs. Routine diagnostic procedures may not indicate a medical problem even though one exists, because a normal urine pH level may not be acceptable for a few individuals. Urinary acidifiers may be sufficient to control the problem. A dietary change, ammonium chloride, apple cider vinegar, or even tomato juice on the food have been used successfully.[2,19,124] If the animal continues to have a serious problem, however, the possibility of urinary calculi should be strongly considered. Vinegar has been successful as an oral therapy for atypical urination or spraying, probably because the underlying condition was medical rather than behavioral. Clinical and subclinical constipation can result in painful defecations and the cat choosing to eliminate in a different location. Many of these cats are on special low-residue diets. If the feces can be picked up with a tissue and not cling, the stool is probably too firm. Changing the diet, increasing water consumption, or adding a stool softener such as psyllium or canned pumpkin can correct the underlying problem. An additional litterbox should then be placed at the chosen defecation spot. After relearning has occurred, the new box can be gradually moved. Anal sacs should also be checked.

In the very old cat, there may be changes in eliminative behavior related to age. Certainly there can be loss of sphincter control and associated incontinence, but other painful conditions, such as arthritis, can decrease the animal's desire to move to the litterbox, which results in more accidents.[43,70] It can also mean that previously accessible locations have become functionally inaccessible, as for the 10-year-old cat expected to hurdle a child gate each time it needs to get into the room containing the litterbox.

Chosen location issues

A cat may choose a new elimination location for many reasons, and they often start because something is undesirable about the old litterbox site. There are also many ways to make that location unattractive when problems with the litterbox have been addressed (Figure 8-7). First, assess the desirability of the chosen location from the cat's perspective. If the urine or feces is deposited near the litterbox, it is generally an indication that the box itself is not aversive to the cat, but that it may be too dirty, too small, have an unacceptable litter, or not have sides high enough for the whole cat to get inside. Second, recently declawed cats may find the texture of the litter painful, trying to stand on the edge of the box instead. Third, cats that urinate or defecate remotely from the litterbox select locations because they are more quiet, cleaner, safer, or more accessible. Drawings of the house are helpful to identify potential feline concerns. As an example, one home might have the litterbox in the utility room, but to get to it the cat would have to jump over a Dutch door into a hallway where the dogs stay and then have to hurdle a child gate into the utility room. The question becomes why bother at all? Although this might be an extreme, it does point out the value of looking at the positional settings of problem spots to the environment. Carpet wicks urine away and owners are usually very diligent about picking up feces from the carpet. This means the chosen location remains clean. Kitchens, utility rooms, and second bathrooms are common locations for litterboxes. In a kitchen, a box can be too near the cat's food, in too noisy a location, or in too busy a location. The noises of the washer and dryer can make a utility room unacceptable. Bathroom doors are easily closed accidentally or guarded by other cats, and their tight space can limit litterbox size.

Because the cat has chosen a location it wants to use, the owner can try placing a litterbox on that favorite spot. If the cat will consistently use the box for a prolonged period to reestablish its acceptance of litter, the owner can eventually move the box to a nearby location, an inch a day. It is important to emphasize that it should be moved gradually and that the final location needs to be near the chosen spot.

A chosen location must be made less desirable or accessible at the same time litterbox issues are corrected. Confining the cat to a second bathroom gives it ready access to the litterbox and a smorgasbord of litters can be tried to see which the cat likes best. The chosen area should also be blocked off so that the cat cannot get back to the favorite spot.

A: Things that make a new location desirable[102]
   Accessibility
   Frequent cleaning
   Low-traffic area
   Not frequented by other cats
   Open areas
   Quiet locations
   Soft substrates
   Wicking substrates
B: Things to make an unacceptable location less desirable[*]
   Change the texture
      Aluminum foil
      Electric shock mats
      Marble chips (for potted plants)
      Pine cones (for potted plants)
      Plastic
      Sticky surfaces
   Cover the spot
      Food
      Furniture
      Potted plants
   Electric beam to activate blowing air
   Inaccessibility
      Block access
      Close doors
   Odor neutralizers
   Unacceptable odors
      Moth balls
      Room air fresheners
   Upside-down mousetraps
   Water in the bathtub or sink

[*]*References 49, 80, 88, 95, 102, 121, 128.*

Figure 8-7 Factors that affect the cat's relationship with a particular toilet area.

If that is not possible, it should at least be made undesirable. Plastic covering the carpet, sticky coverings, overturned plastic carpet runners, furniture on the spot, or electrified mats change the feel or accessibility. Certain odors can repel cats, particularly mothballs, pine-scented cleaners, citronella, or citrus-scented commercial air fresheners in containers that can be set on the spot. Mothballs can be crushed, with $\frac{1}{4}$ teaspoon put on the spot once a week.[83] Electric eye devices that activate an alarm or blast of air can scare many cats. If the sink or tub is the chosen site, a few inches of water discourage most cats. In all cases, it is also important to remove deep sources of odor too.

    Longstanding housesoiling problems give a cat time to learn that the new texture is acceptable and perhaps even favored over litter. Therefore correcting this problem brings a special set of considerations. Confinement is necessary so that the cat has ready access to the litterbox, but this will need to be done for an extended period so the cat can unlearn the new texture and relearn acceptable litterbox usage. After a month or so, the cat can be in the remainder of the house immediately after it uses the litterbox, provided the owner can actually watch the pet. Then the cat can be out during those times when it normally does not eliminate, and finally out all the time, again as it proves it will consistently use the box. The second option for the chronically housesoiling cat is to create a cat room with a tile floor and a litterbox smorgasbord to find which litter is most attractive to it. This way if the cat chooses not to use the litterbox at all, the soiling is confined to one room and that room can be easily cleaned. Encourage owners to schedule time in the room to interact with the cat, even if it is while watching television.

When an outdoor cat is to become an indoor one, owners should have at least two litterboxes per cat, use an unscented litter, and keep the box immaculately clean. It may be necessary to top the litter with soil initially and gradually reduce the amount over time.[63]

Cats that never used the litterbox or have not used it for a long time are difficult to manage. They can either be very gradually made into an indoor-outdoor cat or retrained to use litter. If making it an indoor-outdoor cat is an option, the owner should continue to feed it at specific times so that it stays around. After it learns and prefers to eliminate outside, it can gradually be allowed back inside for longer periods. With the transition being gradual, even declawed cats learn to manage very well. This technique also works well for spraying cats when the owners cannot stand to have the cat indoors any longer. If this is not an option, or if the owners really want to keep the cat indoors, they may train a cat to use a litterbox. The process is not easy, the technique is messy, and it takes time, so the owners should be warned. The cat is confined to a small room or large carrier and the entire floor is covered with a thin layer of litter. Each week the amount of floor covered by litter is reduced, provided the cat uses the litter area for elimination and not the bare floor. Eventually the litterbox is the only litter area. If it is used appropriately for an additional week, gradual access can be given to the rest of the house.[2] If at any time the cat soils on the floor instead of the litter, the amount of floor covered by litter is increased.

Substrate issues

Some cats develop definite litter preferences. Even without this preference, if the type of litter is abruptly changed, 50% will stop using the litterbox. Half of those will start again, but many owners remain unhappy. Thus abrupt changes of litter type are not recommended. To owners, carpet is the most common undesirable substrate preference.[24] The cat must be confined away from its preferred substrate, even for a couple of months. After the initial 2 to 3 weeks, the cat can have controlled access to a problem spot for a few minutes at a time, but only under the direct supervision of the owner. Sometimes it is necessary to create a cat room without carpet.

Drug therapy

The use of drugs for inappropriate elimination problems is generally not indicated because the cat is showing a normal behavior, but in an unacceptable location. There is an exception to this statement, because occasionally it is stress that drives the cat away from the litterbox. This could be a social stress where one cat guards the box, or stresses associated with medical conditions like interstitial cystitis. Use of the facial pheromone is helpful in approximately half of the housesoiling–urination cases.[69] Interstitial cystitis is often associated with some blood in a urinalysis. In one study, 73.4% of cats presented for stranguria, hematuria, pollakiuria, or housesoiling–urination had no anatomic defect, urolith, or tumor.[17] Of these, 73.4% to 87.5% were eventually diagnosed with interstitial (idiopathic) cystitis, with the rest having a primary behavior problem.[17] In humans, the condition often has an on-again/off-again history and stress is a significant factor in recurrences.[16] This suggests blood will not always be present in the urine. Amitriptyline has become the treatment of choice.[16,18,21] The anxiolytic properties help control the perception of stress, both external and internal, and the antihistaminic and analgesic properties help clinically if interstitial cystitis is present. Actual diagnosis of interstitial cystitis must be confirmed by cystoscopic examination.

Prognosis

The prognosis is best if the problem is caught early, with 83% to 100% cured or significantly better if the duration is 6 months or less.[93] Housesoiling–urination has a 91% improvement rate, compared with 50% for housesoiling–defecation and 60% if both are problems.[93] The overall improvement rate is 77%, being higher for indoor-outdoor cats (88%) and lower for indoor-only cats (67%), Persians/Himalayans (57%), and declawed cats (62%).[93]

Miscellaneous Behavioral Changes

Emotional states and attention seeking may result in urine marking, breaking of house-training, or other problems. Short-term stress, fear, or tension can result in nonburial of feces, psychologic incontinence, vomiting, and diarrhea within 2 or 3 days. If these conditions are prolonged and suppressed, the gastrointestinal tract decreases its activity, which results in constipation and urine retention. Emotional changes can affect the stomach and small intestine. In house cats that normally eliminate outside, owners who notice frequent trips in and out may not see the cat actually eliminate, complicating history taking and actual acknowledgment of a problem.

Cats with upper respiratory tract infections may develop secondary diarrhea or stop using the litter pan. This secondary diarrhea is associated with mucous ingestion but may possibly be related to emotional stresses of disease, treatment, or hospitalization. It has been suggested that the anosmia associated with upper respiratory tract disease may be a contributing factor, but experimental destruction of olfactory epithelium is not usually associated with changes in litterbox use.[94]

Once a mild odor of urine or feces becomes associated with an area, that area becomes attractive; therefore thoroughly cleaning soiled spots is a must. Several products have been used, from carbonated soda water to soapy water with a vinegar-water rinse to various commercial products[8,43,73,95] (Figure 8-8). Other products cover the odor or actually combine to form worse odors. Products containing ammonia should be avoided because of their similarity to urine.[43] To prevent recurrence, small food bowls or additional litterboxes can be placed where inappropriate urination or defecation occurs.

AOE/KOE
Anti-Icky-Poo
Arm & Hammer Carpet and Room Deodorizer
Cat-Off
Elimin-odor
FON
Nature's Miracle
Odorzout
Outright
Oxyfresh
Petzorb
PON
The Equalizer
X-O
Woolite spray foam rug cleaner

Figure 8-8 Commercial products that work well at eliminating cat urine odors (it is important to neutralize all of the source).[8,95,99,100]

Cats that eliminate in a neighbor's garden, flower bed, or sandbox present a serious challenge and can be a zoonotic hazard. Discouraging their presence is difficult unless the areas can be physically blocked off when humans are not present, as with chicken wire or plastic ground covers. A number of commercial cat repellants have an aversive odor or emit sounds that are not tolerated by cats. Other techniques that may work include placing more readily available products in the problem area, like citrus peels or red pepper. Fine-screen squares covered with a thin layer of dirt will catch claws of digging cats, or buried popsicle sticks that have only 2 or 3 inches exposed make walking and sitting difficult. A cat tends to be repelled by the shine or reflection of a glass jar filled with water laying on its side.[79]

REFERENCES

1. Beaver B: Therapy of behavior problems. In Kirk RW, editor: *Current veterinary therapy VIII: Small animal practice,* Philadelphia, 1983, WB Saunders.
2. Beaver BV: Disorders of behavior. In Sherding RG, editor: *The cat: diseases and clinical management,* New York, 1989, Churchill Livingstone.
3. Beaver BV: Housesoiling by cats: a retrospective study of 120 cases, *J Am Anim Hosp Assoc* 25(6):631–637, 1989.
4. Beaver BV: *Taxonomy for feline housesoiling,* St Louis, 1989, Sci Proc Am Anim Hospital Assoc.
5. Beaver BV: Psychogenic manifestations of environmental disturbances. In August JR, editor: *Consultations in feline medicine,* Philadelphia, 1991, WB Saunders.
6. Beaver BV: Differential approach to house-soiling dogs and cats, *Vet Q* 16(suppl 1):47S, April 1994.
7. Beaver BV, Terry ML, LaSagna CL: Effectiveness of products in eliminating cat urine odor from carpet, *J Am Vet Med Assoc* 194(11):1589–1591, 1989.

8. Beaver BVG: Feline behavioral problems, *Vet Clin North Am* 6(3):333–340, 1976.

9. Blackshaw JK: Abnormal behaviour in cats, *Aust Vet J* 65(12):395–396, 1988.

10. Borchelt PL: Cat elimination behavior problems, *Vet Clin North Am Small Anim Pract* 21(2):257–264, 1991.

11. Borchelt PL, Voith VL: Diagnosis and treatment of elimination behavior problems in cats, *Vet Clin North Am Small Anim Pract* 12(4):673–681, 1982.

12. Borchelt PL, Voith VL: Elimination behavior problems in cats, *Compend Contin Educ* 8(3):197–205, 1986.

13. Brunner F: The application of behavior studies in small animal practice. In Fox MW, editor: *Abnormal behavior in animals,* Philadelphia, 1968, WB Saunders.

14. Bryant D: *The care and handling of cats,* New York, 1944, Ives Washburn.

15. Buffington CAT: Lower urinary tract disease in cats—new problems, new paradigms, *J Nutr* 124:2643S–2651S, 1994.

16. Buffington CAT, Chew DJ, DiBartola SP: Interstitial cystitis in cats, *Vet Clin North Am Small Anim Pract* 26(2):317–326, 1996.

17. Buffington CAT, Chew DJ, Kendall MS, et al: Clinical evaluation of cats with nonobstructive urinary tract diseases, *J Am Vet Med Assoc* 210(1):46–50, 1997.

18. Buffington CAT, Chew DJ, Woodworth BE: Feline interstitial cystitis, *J Am Vet Med Assoc* 215(5):682–687, 1999.

19. Campbell WE: Correcting house-soiling problems in cats, *Clin Insight* 3(11):528, 1988.

20. Chapman B, Voith VL: Geriatric behavior problems not always related to age, *DVM* 18(3):32, 33, 38, 39, 1987.

21. Chew DJ, Buffington CAT, Kendall MS, et al: Amitriptyline treatment for severe recurrent idiopathic cystitis in cats, *J Am Vet Med Assoc* 213(9):1282–1286, 1998.

22. Cooper LL: Feline inappropriate elimination, *Vet Clin North Am Small Anim Pract* 27(3):569–600, 1997.

23. Cooper LL, Hart BL: Comparison of diazepam with progestins for effectiveness in suppression of urine spraying behavior in cats, *J Am Vet Med Assoc* 200(6):797–801, 1992.

24. Crowell-Davis S: Elimination behavior problems in cats. Proceedings of the American Animal Hospital Association, March 10–14, 2001.

25. Crowell-Davis SL: Elimination behavior problems in cats: I. *Vet Forum* p 10, Nov 1986.

26. Crowell-Davis SL: Elimination behavior problems in cats: II. *Vet Forum* pp 14–15, Dec 1986.

27. Crowell-Davis SL: Elimination behavior problems in cats: III. *Vet Forum* p 16, Jan 1987.

28. Crowell-Davis SL: Elimination behavior problems in cats: IV. *Vet Forum* p 20, Feb 1987.

29. Dehasse J: Feline urine spraying, *Appl Anim Behav Sci* 52(3,4):365–372, 1, 1997.

30. Dodman NH: Pharmacological treatment of behavioral problems in cats, *Vet Forum* pp 62–65, 71, April 1995.

31. Doherty O: Behaviour problems: inappropriate elimination in cats, *Irish Vet J* 50(5):311–314, 1997.

32. Dow SW, Dreitz MJ, Hoover EA: Exploring the link between feline immunodeficiency virus infection and neurologic disease in cats, *Vet Med* 87(12):1181–1184, 1992.

33. Finco DR, Adams DD, Crowell WA, et al: Food and water intake and urine composition in cats: influence of continuous versus periodic feeding, *Am J Vet Res* 47(7):1638–1642, 1986.

34. Fox MW: The behaviour of cats. In Hafez ESE, editor: *The behaviour of domestic animals,* ed 3, Baltimore, 1975, Williams & Williams.

35. Frank D: Feliway clinical trial. Paper presented at the American Veterinary Society Animal Behavior meeting, New Orleans, July 12, 1999.

36. Frank DF, Erb HN, Houpt KA: Urine spraying in cats: presence of concurrent disease and effects of a pheromone treatment, *Appl Anim Behav Sci* 61(3):263–272, 1999.

37. Gorman ML, Trowbridge BJ: The role of odor in the social lives of carnivores. In Gittleman JL, editor: *Carnivore behavior, ecology, and evolution,* Ithaca, NY, 1989, Cornell University Press.

38. Gosling LM: A reassessment of the function of scent marking in territories, *Z Tierpsychol* 60:89–118, 1982.

39. Halip JW, Luescher UA, McKeown DB: Inappropriate elimination in cats, part 1, *Feline Pract* 20(3):17–21, 1992.

40. Hart BL: Normal behavior and behavioral problems associated with sexual function, urination, and defecation, *Vet Clin North Am* 4(3):589–606, 1974.

41. Hart BL: Spraying behavior, *Feline Pract* 5(4):11–13, 1975.

42. Hart BL: Learning ability in cats, *Feline Pract* 5(5):10, 12, 1975.

43. Hart BL: Inappropriate urination and defecation, *Feline Pract* 6(2):6–7, 1976.

44. Hart BL: Objectionable urine spraying and urine marking in cats: evaluation of progestin treatment in gonadectomized males and females, *J Am Vet Med Assoc* 177(6):529–533, 1980.

45. Hart BL: Olfactory tractotomy for control of objectionable urine spraying and urine marking in cats, *J Am Vet Med Assoc* 179(3):231–234, 1981.

46. Hart BL: Neurosurgery for behavioral problems: a curiosity or the new wave? *Vet Clin North Am Small Anim Pract* 12(4):707–714, 1982.

47. Hart BL: Urine spraying and marking in cats. In Slatter DH, editor: *Textbook of small animal surgery,* Philadelphia, 1985, WB Saunders.

48. Hart BL: New perspectives in spraying behavior in cats. Paper presented at the American Veterinary Medical Association meeting, Minneapolis, Minn, July 18, 1993.

49. Hart BL: Feline behavior problems, *Friskies Symposium on Behavior* pp 28–39, 1994.

50. Hart BL, Barrett RE: Effects of castration on fighting, roaming, and urine spraying in adult male cats, *J Am Vet Med Assoc* 163(3):290–292, 1973.

51. Hart BL, Cooper L: Factors relating to urine spraying and fighting in prepubertally gonadectomized cats, *J Am Vet Med Assoc* 184(10):1255–1258, 1984.

52. Hart BL, Eckstein RA: The role of gonadal hormones in the occurrence of objectionable behaviours in dogs and cats, *Appl Anim Behav Sci* 52(3,4):331–344, 1997.

53. Hart BL, Eckstein RA, Powell KL, Dodman NH: Effectiveness of buspirone on urine spraying and inappropriate urination in cats, *J Am Vet Med Assoc* 203(2):254–258, 1993.

54. Hart BL, Hart LA: *Canine and feline behavioral therapy,* Philadelphia, 1985, Lea & Febiger.

55. Hart BL, Leedy M: Identification of source of urine stains in multi-cat households, *J Am Vet Med Assoc* 180(1):77–78, 1982.

56. Hart BL, Voith VL: Changes in urine spraying, feeding and sleep behavior of cats following medial preoptic-anterior hypothalamic lesions, *Brain Res* 145:406–409, 1978.

57. Heidenberger E: Housing conditions and behavioural problems of indoor cats as assessed by their owners, *Appl Anim Behav Sci* 52(3,4):345–364, 1997.

58. Hetts S, Estep DQ: Behavior management: preventing elimination and destructive behavior problems, *Vet Forum* pp 60–61, Nov 1994.

59. Houpt KA: Companion animal behavior: a review of dog and cat behavior in the field, the laboratory and the clinic, *Cornell Vet* 75:248–261, 1985.

60. Houpt KA: Personal communication, 1988.

61. Houpt KA: Housesoiling: treatment of a common feline problem, *Vet Med* 86(10):1000, 1002–1006, 1991.

62. Houpt KA: Sexual behavior problems in dogs and cats, *Vet Clin North Am Small Anim Pract* 27(3):601–615, 1997.

63. Houpt KA: Transforming an outdoor cat into an indoor cat, *Vet Med* 95(11):830, 2000.

64. Houpt KA: Cognitive dysfunction in geriatric cats. In August JR, editor: *Consultations in feline internal medicine,* vol 4, Philadelphia, 2001, WB Saunders.

65. Houpt KA, Honig SU, Reisner IR: Breaking the human-companion animal bond, *J Am Vet Med Assoc* 209(10):1653–1659, 1996.

66. Hunthausen W: Feline housesoiling problems, *Friskies PetCare Small Anim Behav* pp 25–32, 1997.

67. Hunthausen W: Evaluation of the use of a pheromone analogue (Feliway) to control urine marking in cats. Paper presented at the American Veterinary Society of Animal Behavior meeting, Baltimore, July 27, 1998.

68. Hunthausen W: Evaluating a feline facial pheromone analogue to control urine spraying, *Vet Med* 95(2):151–155, 2000.

69. Hunthausen W: Use of Feliway for urine voiding, Internet: AVSAB-L, March 28, 2000.

70. Hunthausen WL: Rule out medical etiologies first in geriatric behavior problems, *DVM* 22(7):24, 38, 1991.

71. Hunthausen WL: Dealing with feline housesoiling: a practitioner's guide, *Vet Med* 88(8):726–735, 1993.

72. Jackson WB: Food habits of Baltimore, Maryland, cats in relation to rat populations, *J Mammal* 32(4):458–461, 1951.

73. Kahn B: Out of the frying pan-into the litter pan, *Cat Fancy* 15:18–21, Nov/Dec 1972.

74. Kleiman DG, Eisenberg JF: Comparisons of canid and felid social systems from an evolutionary perspective, *Anim Behav* 21:637–659, Nov 1973.

75. Kerby G, Macdonald DW: Cat society and the consequences of colony size. In Turner DC, Bateson PPG, editors: *The domestic cat: the biology of its behaviour,* Cambridge, 1988, Cambridge University Press.

76. Kling A, Kovach JK, Tucker TJ: The behaviour of cats. In Hafez ESE, editor: *The behaviour of domestic animals,* ed 2, Baltimore, 1969, Williams & Williams.

77. Knubley PF, Hart BL: Inappropriate urination, *Feline Pract* 16(2):28, 1986.

78. Komtebedde J, Hauptman J: Bilateral ischiocavernosus myectomy for chronic urine spraying in castrated male cats, *Vet Surg* 19(4):293–296, 1990.

79. Landers A: Gardens can be "cat-proofed" humanely, *The Bryan-College Station Eagle* p A7, July 17, 2000.

80. Landsberg G: Feline behavior and welfare, *J Am Vet Med Assoc* 208(4):502–505, 1996.

81. Landsberg GM: Clomipramine –beyond separation anxiety, *J Am Anim Hosp Assoc* 37(4):313–318, 2001.

82. Liberg O: Spacing patterns in a population of rural free roaming domestic cats, *Oikos* 35(3):336–349, 1980.

83. Luescher AU: Inappropriate elimination in cats. Paper presented at Friskies PetCare Symposium on Small Animal Behavior, Austin, Tex, Oct 4, 1998.

84. Mancia G, Baccelli G, Zanchetti A: Regulation of renal circulation during behavioral changes in the cat, *Am J Physiol* 227:536–542, Sep 1974.

85. Marder A: Personal communication, July 20, 1987.

86. Marder A: House soiling in cats. Paper presented at American Veterinary Medical Association meeting, Orlando, Fla, July 16, 1989.

87. Marder A: Personal communication, July 22, 1990.

88. Marder A: House soiling, *Pet Vet* 4(4):6, 7, 10–12, 1992.

89. Marder A: Managing behavioural problems in puppies and kittens, *Friskies PetCare Small Animal Behavior* pp 15–24, 1997.

90. Marder A: Clomipramine for the treatment of spraying and urine marking in cats, *Newslett Am Vet Soc Anim Behav* 19(2):3, 1997.

91. Marder AR: Animal behavior problems. Paper presented at American Veterinary Medical Association meeting, Las Vegas, July 24, 1985.

92. Marder AR: Psychotropic drugs and behavioral therapy, *Vet Clin North Am Small Anim Pract* 21(2):329–342, 1991.

93. Marder AR, Friedman L: Long-term follow-up on feline elimination problems. Paper presented at American Veterinary Society of Animal Behavior meeting, Baltimore, July 27, 1998.

94. McClung AW, Hart BL: Olfactory loss affecting behavior? *Feline Pract* 8(3):17, 1978.

95. Melese P: New techniques in detection and neutralization of urine contamination. Paper presented at American Veterinary Medical Association meeting, San Francisco, July 10, 1994.

96. Mosier JE.: Common medical and behavioral problems in cats, *Mod Vet Pract* 56(10):699–703, 1975.

97. Neilson JC: Thinking inside the box: feline elimination problems, American Veterinary Medical Association. Available at www.avma.org/noah/members/convention/conv01/notes/04010105.1sp.

98. Olm DD, Houpt KA: Feline house-soiling problems, *Appl Anim Behav Sci* 20(3–4):335–346, 1988.

99. Overall K: Obtaining thorough history critical in curbing inappropriate feline elimination problems, *DVM* 26(6):20S, 22S, 1995.

100. Overall K: An accurate diagnosis critical to treating behavioral disorders, *DVM* 27(5):1S, 4S, 1996.

101. Overall KL: Preventing behavior problems: early prevention and recognition in puppies and kittens, *Behav Probl Small Anim Purina Spec Rev* pp 13–29, 1992.

102. Overall KL: Diagnosing and treating undesirable feline elimination behavior, *Feline Pract* 21(2):11–15, 1993.

103. Overall KL: Drug therapy for spraying cats, *Feline Pract* 24(6):40–42, 1996.

104. Overall KL: Feline elimination disorders complex; use caution when prescribing, *DVM* 27(2):13S, 17S, 20S, 1996.

105. Overall KL: Animal behavior case of the month, *J Am Vet Med Assoc* 211(11):1376–1378, 1997.

106. Pageat P: Experimental evaluation of the efficacy of a synthetic analogue of cats' facial pheromones (Feliway) in inhibiting urine marking of sexual origin in adult tom-cats, *J Vet Pharmacol Ther* 20(suppl 1):169, July 8, 1997.

107. Pannaman R: Behaviour and ecology of free-ranging female farm cats (*Felis catus* L.), *Z Tierpsychol* 56:59–73, 1981.

108. Patronek GJ, Glickman LT, Beck AM, et al: Risk factors for relinquishment of cats to an animal shelter, *J Am Vet Med Assoc* 209(3):582–588, 1996.

109. Pemberton PL: Canine and feline behavior control: progestin therapy. In Kirk RW, editor: *Current veterinary therapy,* vol 8, *Small animal practice,* Philadelphia, 1983, WB Saunders.

110. Pryor PA, Hart BL, Bain MJ, Cliff KD: Causes of urine marking in cats and effects of environmental management on frequency of marking, *J Am Vet Med Assoc* 219(12):1709–1713, 2001.

111. Pryor PA, Hart BL, Cliff KD, Bain MJ: Effects of a selective serotonin reuptake inhibitor on urine spraying behavior in cats, *J Am Vet Med Assoc* 219(11):1557–1561, 2001.

112. Romatowski J: Use of megestrol acetate in cats, *J Am Vet Med Assoc* 194(5):700–702, 1989.

113. Rosenblatt JS: Suckling and home orientation in the kitten: a comparative developmental study. In Tobach E, Aronson LR, Shaw E, editors: *The biopsychology of development,* New York, 1971, Academic Press.

114. Rubin J: Urine marker. Available at Internet-subscribers@tvma.org-A Texvetmed Post, 2000.

115. Schomacker IE: Inappropriate litterbox behavior: what are your patients trying to tell you? *Vet Forum* p 58, July 1994.

116. Schwartz S: Use of cyproheptadine to control urine spraying and masturbation in a cat, *J Am Vet Med Assoc* 214(3):369–371, 1999.

117. Schwartz S: Use of cyproheptadine to control urine spraying in a castrated male domestic cat, *J Am Vet Med Assoc* 215(4):501–502, 1999.

118. Seksel K: Use of bromocriptine in spraying, *Appl Anim Behav Sci* 46(1–2):132, 1995.

119. Seksel K: Feline urine spraying. In Houpt KA, editor: *Recent advances in companion animal behavior problems,* International Veterinary Information Service. Available at www.ivis.org.

120. Seksel K, Lindeman MJ: Use of clomipramine in the treatment of anxiety-related and obsessive-compulsive disorders in cats, *Aust Vet J* 76(5):317–321, 1998.

121. Simpson BS: Feline housesoiling, part I: inappropriate elimination, *Compend Contin Educ Small Anim* 20(12):1319–1328, 1998.

122. Spraying by castrated tomcats, *Mod Vet Pract* 56(10):729–731, 1975.

123. Sung W, Crowell-Davis S: The elimination behavior patterns of domestic cats *(Felis catus)* with and without elimination behavior problems. Paper presented at American Veterinary Society on Animal Behavior meeting, New Orleans, July 12, 1999.

124. Taton GF, Hamar DW, Lewis LD: Evaluation of ammonium chloride as a urinary acidifier in the cat, *J Am Vet Med Assoc* 184(4):433–436, 1984.

125. Voith VL: Personal communication, 1978.

126. Voith VL: Therapeutic approaches to feline urinary behavior problems, *Mod Vet Pract* 61(6):539–542, 1980.

127. Voith VL: Treating elimination behavior problems in dogs and cats: the role of punishment, *Mod Vet Pract* 62(12):951–953, 1981.

128. Voith VL: Elimination behavior problems in cats, *Kal Kan Forum* 3(3):60–64, 1984.

129. Voith VL: Behavior disorders. In Davis LE, editor: *Handbook of small animal therapeutics,* New York, 1985, Churchill Livingstone.

130. Voith VL, Marder AR: Feline behavioral disorders. In Morgan R, editor: *Handbook of small animal practice,* New York, 1988, Churchill Livingstone.

131. White JC, Mills DS: Efficacy of synthetic feline facial pheromone analogue for the treatment of chronic non-sexual urine spraying by the domestic cat, *Newslett Am Vet Soc Anim Behav* 19(2):7, 1997.

132. Whitehead JE: Tomcat spraying, *Mod Vet Pract* 46(2):68, 1965.

ADDITIONAL READINGS

Abdel-Rahman M, Galeano C, Elhilali M: New approach to study of voicing cycle in cat. Preliminary report on pharmacologic studies, *Urology* 22:91–97, July 1983.

Beadle M: *The cat: history, biology, and behavior,* New York, 1977, Simon & Schuster, Inc.

Bernstein KS: A physiological reason for defecating outside the litterbox, *Vet Med Small Anim Clin* 72(10):1549, 1977.

Boudreau JC, Tsuchitani C: *Sensory neurophysiology,* New York, 1973, Van Nostrand Reinhold.

Campbell WE: Correcting house-soiling problems in cats, *Mod Vet Pract* 66(1):53–54, 1985.

Chalifoux A, Gosselin Y: The use of megestrol acetate to stop urine spraying in castrated male cats, *Can Vet J* 22(7):211–212, 1981.

Chertok L, Fontaine M: Psychosomatics in veterinary medicine, *J Psychosom Res* 7:229–235, 1963.

Davidson MG, Baty KT: Anaphylaxis associated with intravenous sodium fluorescein administration in a cat, *Prog Vet Comp Ophthalmol* 1:127–128, 1991.

Ewer RF: *The carnivores,* Ithaca, NY, 1973, Cornell University Press.

Fox MW: New information on feline behavior, *Mod Vet Pract* 56(4):50–52, 1965.

Fox MW: Aggression: its adaptive and maladaptive significance in man and animals. In Fox MW, editor: *Abnormal behavior in animals,* Philadelphia, 1968, WB Saunders.

Fox MW: Psychomotor disturbances. In Fox MW, editor: *Abnormal behavior in animals,* Philadelphia, 1968, WB Saunders.

Fox MW: Psychopathology in man and lower animals, *J Am Vet Med Assoc* 153(1):66–77, 1971.

Fox MW: *Understanding your cat,* New York, 1974, Coward, McCann & Geoghegan.

Greaves JP, Scott PP: Urinary amino acid pattern of cats on diets of varying protein content, *Nature* 187:242, July 16, 1960.

Hart BL: Behavioral effects of castration, *Feline Pract* 3(2):10–12, 1973.

Hart BL: Psychopharmacology in feline practice, *Feline Pract* 3(3):6, 8, 1973.

Hart BL: Behavioral effects of long-acting progestins, *Feline Pract* 4(4):8, 11, 1974.

Hart BL: Quiz on feline behavior, *Feline Pract* 6(3):10, 13, 1976.

Hart BL: Behavioral aspects of raising kittens, *Feline Pract* 6(6): 8, 10, 20, 1976.

Hart BL: Medication for control of spraying, *Feline Pract* 7(3):16, 1977.

Hart BL: The client asks you: a quiz on feline behavior, *Feline Pract* 8(2):10–13, 1978.

Hart BL: Feline behavior problems, *Friskies Symposium on Behavior* pp 28–39, 1994.

Heath S: Commonly encountered feline problems, *Vet Q* 16(S1):51S, April 1994.

Jones RM, Baldwin CJ: Inappropriate feline elimination behavior, *Iowa State Univ Vet* 55(1):24–30, 1993.

Joshua JO: Abnormal behavior in cats. In Fox MW, editor: *Abnormal behavior in animals,* Philadelphia, 1968, WB Saunders.

Levinson BM: Man and his feline pet, *Mod Vet Pract* 53:35–39, Nov 1972.

Levy JK, Cullen JM, Bunch SE, et al: Adverse reaction to diazepam in cats, *J Am Vet Med Assoc* 205(2):156–157, 1994.

McCrory RG: Urine spraying, *Feline Pract* 3(2):6, 1973.

Overall KL: Rational behavior pharmacology, *Friskies Symposium on Behavior* pp 18–28, 1996.

Northway RB: Manual stimulation of micturition, *Med Vet Pract* 56(12):832, 1975.

Podberscek AL, Blackshaw JK, Beattie AW: The behaviour of laboratory colony cats and their reactions to a familiar and unfamiliar person, *Appl Anim Behav Sci* 31(1–2):119–130, 1991.

Riddle BL, Deats PH, Meyer H, Gilbride AP: Solution to spraying cats, *Feline Pract* 5(1):6–7, 1975.

Schmidt JP: Psychosomatics in veterinary medicine. In Fox MW, editor: *Abnormal behavior in animals,* Philadelphia, 1968, WB Saunders.

Turner D, Appleby D, Magnus E: The Association of Pet Behaviour Counsellors: annual review of cases. Available at www.apbc.org.uk/2000/report.htm.

Vollmer PJ: Can a cat be retrained to use a litterbox? *Vet Med Small Anim Clin* 72(7):1161–1162, 1977.

Vollmer PJ: Feline inappropriate elimination. Part 1, *Vet Med Small Anim Clin* 74(6):796, 798, 1979.

Vollmer PJ: Feline inappropriate elimination. Part 2, *Vet Med Small Anim Clin* 74(7):928, 930, 1979.

Vollmer PJ: Feline inappropriate elimination. Part 3, *Vet Med Small Anim Clin* 74(8):1101–1102, 1979.

Vollmer PJ: Feline inappropriate elimination. Part 4—marking, *Vet Med Small Anim Clin* 74(9):1241, 1979.

Vollmer PJ: Feline inappropriate elimination. Part 5—conclusion, *Vet Med Small Anim Clin* 74:1419, 1421, Oct 1979.

Vollmer PJ: Feline inappropriate elimination—some aspects of diagnosis and treatment, *Calif Vet* 33(7):13–17, 1979.

Wemmer C, Scow K: Communication in the Felidae with emphasis on scent marking and contact patterns. In Sebeok TA, editor: *How animals communicate,* Bloomington, 1977, Indiana University Press.

Wolski TR: Feline behavioral problems: social causes and practical solutions, *Cornell Feline Health Center News* 3:1, 2, 4–6, May 1981.

Worden AN: Abnormal behavior in the dog and cat, *Vet Rec* 71:966–978, Dec 26, 1959.

9

Feline Locomotive Behavior

The life of a cat is basically one revolving around eating, sleeping, and reproducing. Because of this, the ability to ambulate at various speeds is an absolute necessity. In this regard, the locomotor patterns and their reciprocal sleep patterns have been specialized to allow successful hunting and survival, as well as adequate rest. The comparative development of these patterns is shown in Appendix C.

FETAL GROWTH AND MOVEMENTS

The kitten begins in utero the development of movement patterns that will be necessary in the adult, and these patterns, as with sensory systems, parallel the development of the nervous system.[77] Neuronal pathways become myelinated in their phylogenetic order of development.[78]

Approximately 25 days after conception, the 15- to 16-mm fetal kitten shows its first spontaneous movement as a unilateral flexion of its head and passive flexion of its shoulder. After growth of a few more millimeters, spontaneous neck mobility increases and local response to touch develops, along with ventral neck flexion, bilateral flexion of the head and upper neck, and rotation of the head. By 20-mm crown to rump length, the embryo will begin to show flexion of the lumbar and sacral vertebral column and active flexion of the shoulder joint.[150,151]

During the twenty-sixth day after conception (21 to 22 mm), rotation of the trunk first occurs, as does flexion of the elbow. In another 2 days flexion of the hips is seen, probably in passive response to the waves of muscular movements along the body. Motor responses continue to develop, so by day 30 (27 to 30 mm), flexion of the carpus and slight activation of the masticatory muscles occur. Flexion of the tail can be observed at 33 days (38 mm), as can adduction of the forelimb. During this time of completion of facial and forelimb muscular development, there is also flexion of the stifle, extension of the vertebral column and manus, and withdrawal by flexion from a touch sensation. By 36 days (50 mm), the abdominal and intercostal muscles begin to function.[150,151]

Sometime between 38 and 40 days after conception (60 mm), flexion of the tarsus begins and tongue muscles begin to function. By 42 days (75 to 80 mm) the pes flexes and the diaphragm starts functioning; however, breathing movements are not regular for another 7 days. After an additional 8 days of growth (100 mm), most motor responses have been shown. The pelvic limb is capable of adduction and digital flexion, and the muscles of facial expression and those of the larynx associated with phonation become active.[150]

Spontaneous body-righting capabilities are initially present at about 50 days (100 mm), although they are by no means adultlike and are probably not vestibular in origin.[41,149,150] Vestibular righting does not appear until approximately 4 days (15 mm) later.[149] Several sensory reflexes develop about the same time as the spontaneous body righting, including the scratch, sucking, light blink, and forelimb crossed-extensor reflexes. The ear-scratch reflex develops at this time also, as does ipsilateral flexion and contralateral extension of the forelimb.[38,150] The coordinated action of the limbs necessary for progressive forward movement occurs near term, indicating that the coordination involved in walking is innate, not learned.[41]

INFANT GROWTH AND MOVEMENTS

Prewalking Movements

At birth the motor skills continue to mature in conjunction with the central nervous system, but additional motor behaviors can be learned. Movements initially involve the whole limb, but with time and maturation, discrete segmental movements are employed.[22] Neonatal movements toward the queen are the stiff paddling-like motion of the forelimbs that matured shortly before birth, and these movements are sufficiently coordinated within 8 minutes of birth to pull the suckling for the short distances it must travel. The limbs still lack a great deal of motor coordination and strength because they are unable to bear weight and the claws are not retractable. The poorly developed motor coordination at this stage functions to prevent the young from wandering. Thermoregulation is also poorly developed until approximately 2 weeks of age and further serves to keep the kittens close to one another and to the queen. A strong rooting response, the burrowing into warm objects, is present for up to 16 days, giving an indication about the progression of homeostatic mechanisms (see Figure 2-9).

The body-righting response that occurs when kittens are accidentally pushed over by the queen is also continued from the prenatal behaviors and is fully mature by 1 month.[89] The righting response of cats dropped from a height does not appear until 35 days.[134] Vestibular function develops slowly during the first few days of life. Nystagmus associated with rotatory stimulation appears experimentally at the end of the first week, although it has been associated with deviation of the eyes and oscillating eye movements during this early appearance. Vestibular nystagmus becomes adultlike by the end of the third week.[34]

Flexor and extensor dominance of the vertebral musculature, caused by an imbalance of the nervous innervation to them, is not highly consistent among kittens. Flexor dominance is present in most kittens from birth into adolescence (Figure 9-1). After approximately the first month, the curled-up posture may modify so that the neck is extended, but the rest of the body position is similar to what it had been. Extensor dominance is much more variable. Starting as early as day 1, this activated vertebral extensor stage can also last into adolescence (Figure 9-2). Kittens may initially exhibit extensor dominance and then within a few seconds progress into a more prolonged flexor dominant stage. This dual sequence is especially noticeable between days 15 and 40. Other kittens show neither dominance at birth, and others exhibit a great deal of squirming when suspended from the neck.

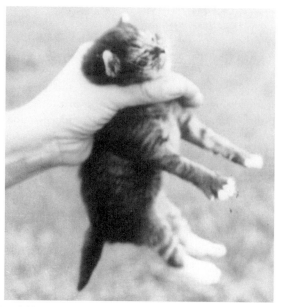

Figure 9-1 A 14-day-old kitten exhibiting flexor dominance.

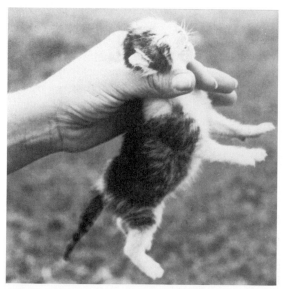

Figure 9-2 A 7-day-old kitten exhibiting extensor dominance.

Nonvisual placing of a limb onto a surface in response to its touching the edge of the surface occurs consistently for the thoracic limbs first, sometime during the first 5 days of life (mean 2.3 days; see Figure 2-12). Development of nonvisual placing of the pelvic limbs is much less uniform and may initially appear during the first 12 days (mean 3.6 days), although not consistently until sometime during the first 19 days (mean 11.3 days).

When a young kitten is suspended by the ventral midline while still in a normal dorsoventral relationship, the Landau reflex may be activated. In this reflex, the forelimbs and hindlimbs are extended in response to the positioning. Although the reflex can last up to 19 days, the mean ending age is 6.8 days.

The forelimb crossed-extensor reflex is acquired by some individuals before birth. For others, this reflex and the hindlimb crossed-extensor reflex may appear up to the third day of life (mean 1.4 days), although either or both may never develop (Figure 9-3). The crossed-extensor reflex will end between days 2 and 17 (mean 8.1 days).

Body support by the limbs develops in four stages shortly after birth. In the first stage, when the kitten is held by the lumbar and pelvic areas and lowered to a table, its forelimbs will start to support weight between 1 and 10 days of age (mean 3.5 days). Direct forelimb support of the body weight, the second stage, also appears during the first 10 days, but the mean is 5.7 days (Figure 9-4). Pelvic limb support, the third stage, begins to be demonstrated during the first 16 days (mean 14.3 days) when the kitten is suspended by the thorax and the pelvic limbs are allowed to touch the table (Figure 9-5). Finally, the ability to completely elevate the body off the ground by the additional strength in the rear limbs begins between days 5 and 25 (mean 10 days).

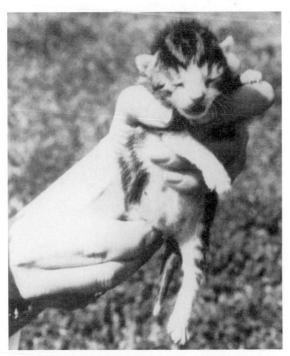

Figure 9-3 The crossed-extensor reflex of the pelvic limbs in a 7-day-old kitten.

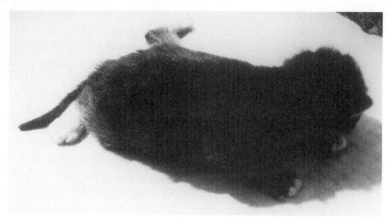

Figure 9-4 This 14-day-old kitten is supporting body weight with the thoracic limbs but not yet with the pelvic limbs.

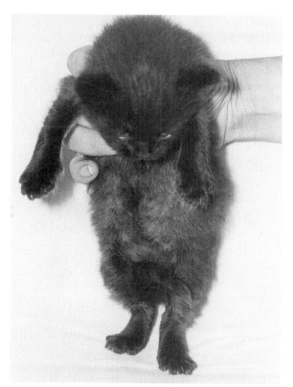

Figure 9-5 The pelvic limbs are supporting weight when this 2-week-old kitten is lowered to a solid surface.

Walking and Other Later Movements

Locomotor functions continue to mature, and by 20 days the kitten is sitting. It is unsteadily walking in another day or two. With early body support and standing, or with infant handling, the process can be speeded so that the kitten is actually walking at about 15 days.

Once walking has begun, several behaviors change. The avoidance reaction progresses from a primitive stage, in which the kitten vocalizes and squirms, to one more typical of an adult, in which it backs away from the stimulus. This latter type of avoidance appears about the twenty-fifth day.[130] Kittens actively approach specific people and littermates as early as 18 days of age, especially if the earlier experience has been enriched by handling, and they become good followers, a necessity so that they can undergo visual learning from the queen's examples.[37,116] Running first appears toward the end of the third or fourth week, and it is accompanied by the onset of active social play. Shortly thereafter the kitten has matured enough for the air-righting reflex to have developed, and all gaits in adult locomotion are in use by 7 weeks.[22,89]

Within a few days of walking, generally between 23 and 40 days of age (mean 31 days), the kitten will start climbing, usually in an attempt to escape from the nesting box. At first these escapes are brief, but within 5 days, 68% of the young one's time is spent out of the box.[107] By 8 weeks of age, 82% of the time is spent out, an increase that coincides with the time the kitten changes its orientation from the home area to the queen.[107,110,111] Once out of the box, the kitten's climbing attempts will then be made on other environmental obstacles. Success in climbing is related to another factor: control of the claws. During the first 2 weeks of life, the young cat does not have the ability to retract its claws. Through a gradual process, control is gained over the retractability, and by 3 weeks the kitten has reasonable control over its distal phalanges.

Sensorimotor Coordination

The sense of vision plays a significant role in the development of certain aspects of locomotion. Kittens raised experimentally without being able to see their forelimbs are not able to place their feet accurately at a later age. In addition, batting at dangling objects, reaching for objects, or avoidance stepping is not very successful for these individuals, because the controlled placing response requires a certain amount of integration of the visual and motor systems.[50,52] Kittens allowed to watch one paw but not the other will permanently be unable to guide the unseen paw.[50,51] Similar studies have been conducted under conditions of light deprivation. After a minimum of 4 weeks of darkness, visual depth discrimination is affected. However, minimal stimulation, such as 1 hr/day of exercise on a patterned surface, with exercise being the key factor, results in normal movement discrimination.[108,137] Time to develop this ability in older kittens who have been deprived is somewhat similar to that required for visually normal neonates to acquire it after birth.[133] For the kitten that has visual stimulation but is experimentally never allowed to propel itself, with locomotion supplied by others, visually guided behavior is severely affected.[53] Therefore both factors are necessary for sensorimotor coordination.

Eye-paw coordination is necessary for locomotor play with inanimate objects. This type of play increases sharply around 7 to 8 weeks with the maturation of both sensory and motor systems.[89] More complex tasks such as walking and turning on a narrow plank are not seen until 10 or 11 weeks of age.[89]

Weight Gains

In addition to developing locomotor skills, kittens are growing in size. In general a kitten will double in size each week, from a birth weight of 85 to 140 g, until the eighth week. This weight increase is significant not only because the youngster is growing larger, but also because it necessitates growing stronger at a much faster rate. Rapid cerebellar growth is also necessary, and any or all of these processes can be severely impaired by malnutrition.

ADULT MOVEMENTS

Adult cats are active throughout a 24-hour period, with two peak activities that are apparently influenced by environmental factors.[101] In farm cats, 62.6% of the active behavior occurs during daylight hours.[101] In suburban cats, most occurred between 6 PM and 4 AM.[8] This type of activity pattern is also reflected on the circadian pattern of cortisol production, with the highest endogenous production in the evening and the lowest in the morning.[103] Free-roaming farm cats will travel between 24.5 and 53.3 minutes in this time, not counting the additional 3.6 hours they spend hunting.[101] While roaming the cat will cover 1765 ± 765 m, and not counting meandering, the distance covered in any 1 hour does not exceed 750 m.[101] House cats will normally spend 3% of their time standing, 3% walking, and 0.2% highly active.[4] Most of the time they are on the ground, but 20% of time will be spent at a height up to 1 m, and 4% of time will be spent at a location higher than 1 m.[4]

Active movement for adult cats involves several gaits, and these patterns of movement can be described as alternative or in-phase locomotion.[92] A gait has been described as an accustomed, cyclic manner of moving in terrestrial locomotion.[59] In animals, there are at least 13 named gait sequences, many of which are used by cats. In alternative gaits (walk, amble, trot), the ipsilateral limbs strike at alternate halves of stride. In-phase gaits (pace, gallop) are characterized by limbs on the same side of the body moving forward during the same part of the stride. Because gaits differ between ground and treadmills,[9] natural movement should be used to describe cat locomotion.

Walking

The walk is a four-beat gait, meaning that each of the cat's paws contacts the ground at a separate time during the stride. During any one phase of this gait, there are at least two feet having ground contact. In a slow walk, such as the stalking walk, there are usually three and occasionally four contacting feet (Figure 9-6). The rapid walk has two or three feet on the ground at a time (Figure 9-7). The walk has also been described as symmetric, because the left limbs repeat the position of the right, one half stride later. The forward speed is approximately 0.9 m/sec; however, a rapid walk will almost double the rate.[39,42]

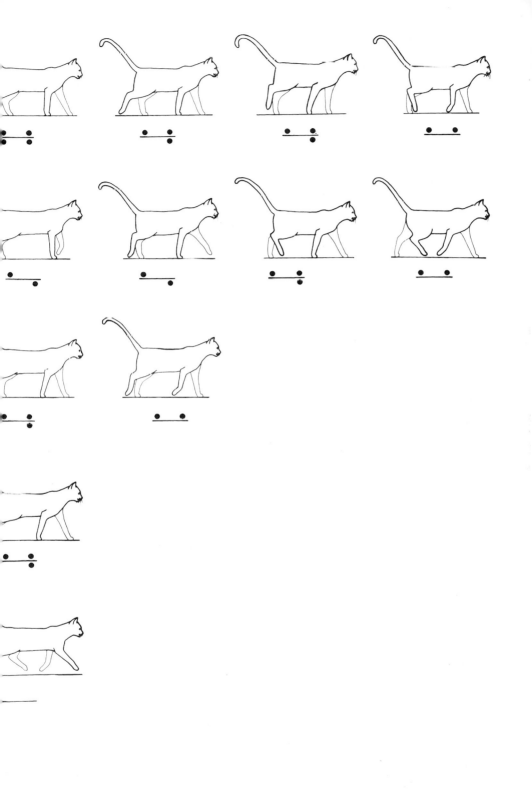

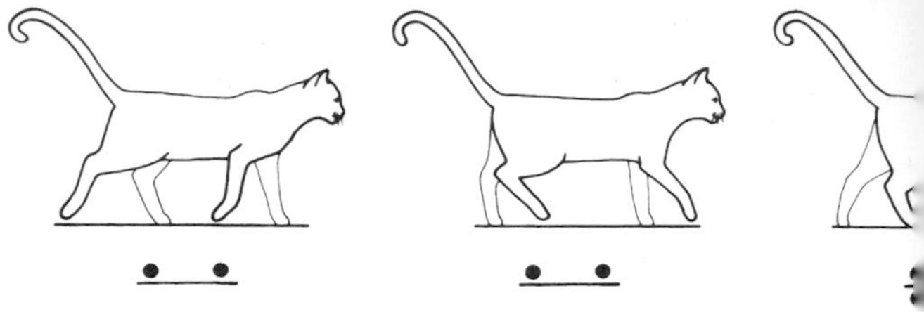

Fig. 9-12.
Slow pace.

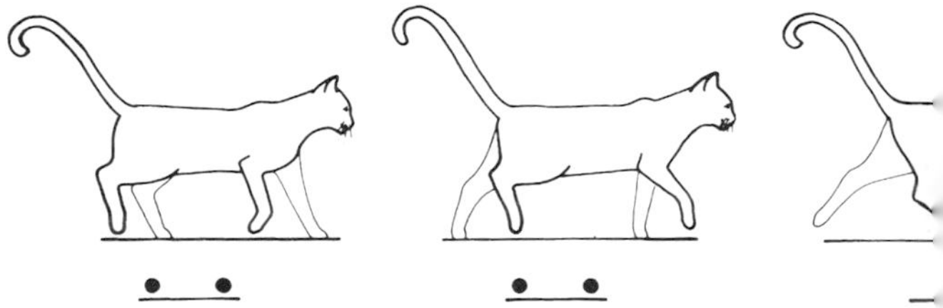

Fig. 9-13.
Fast pace.

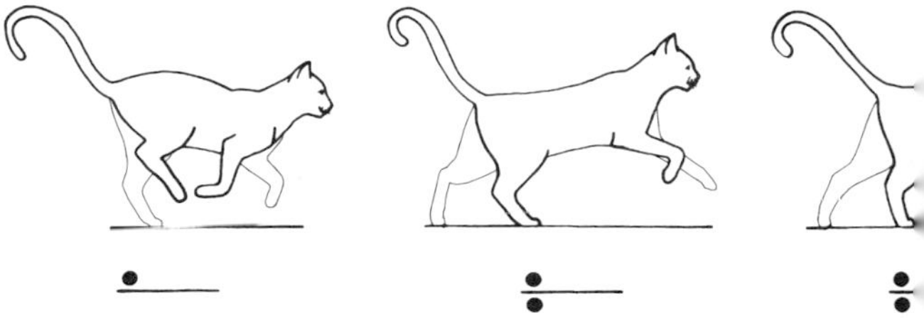

Fig. 9-14.
Slow gallop.

The cat is leading with both the right forefoot and hindfoot.

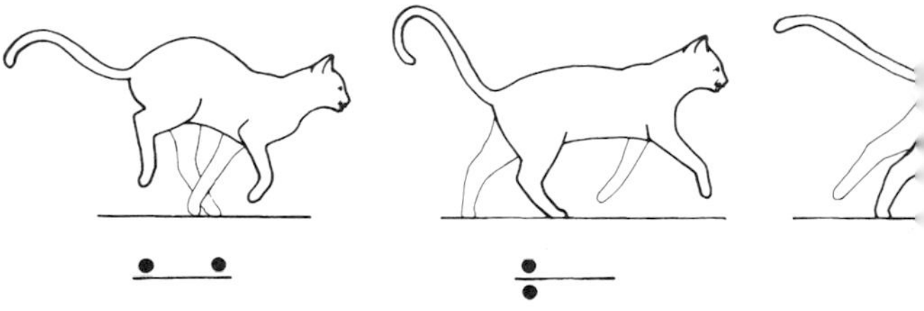

Fig. 9-15.
Single suspension
form of the gallop.

The cat is leading with the left forefoot and right hindfoot.

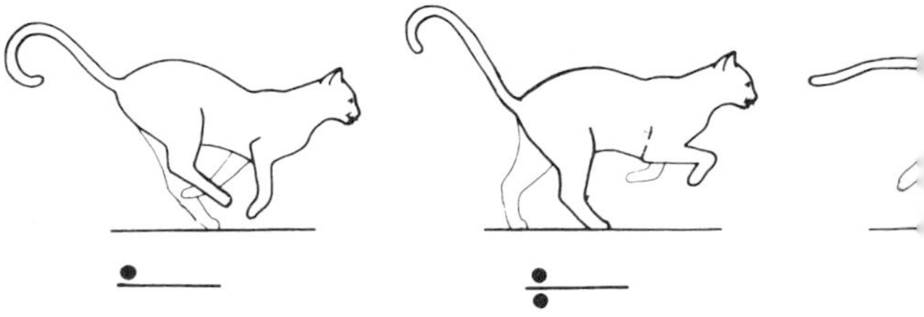

Fig. 9-16.
Fast, double suspension
form of the gallop.

The cat is leading with the left forefoot and right hindfoot.

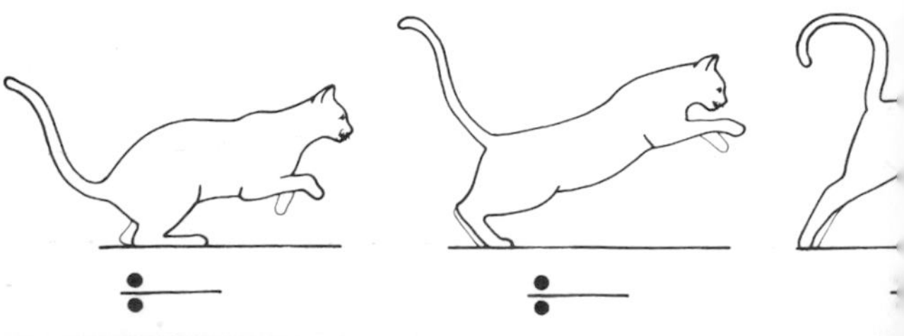

Fig. 9-17.
Half-bound variation
of the gallop.

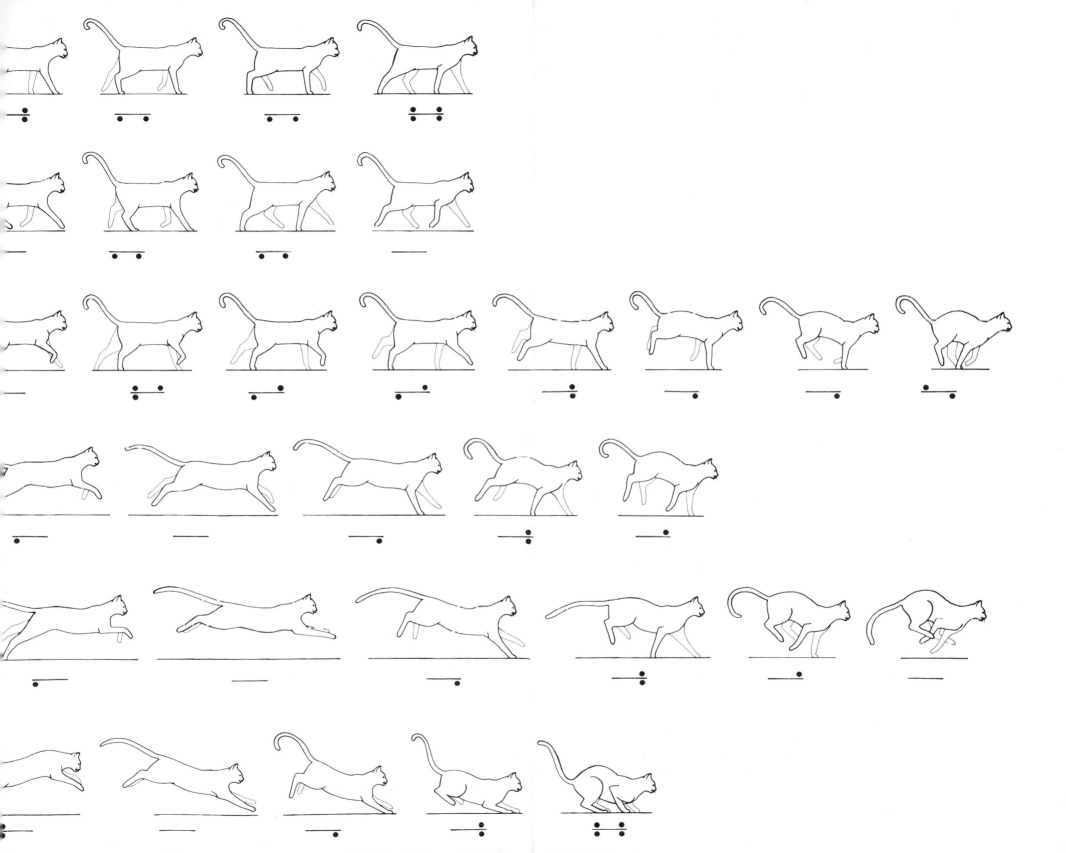

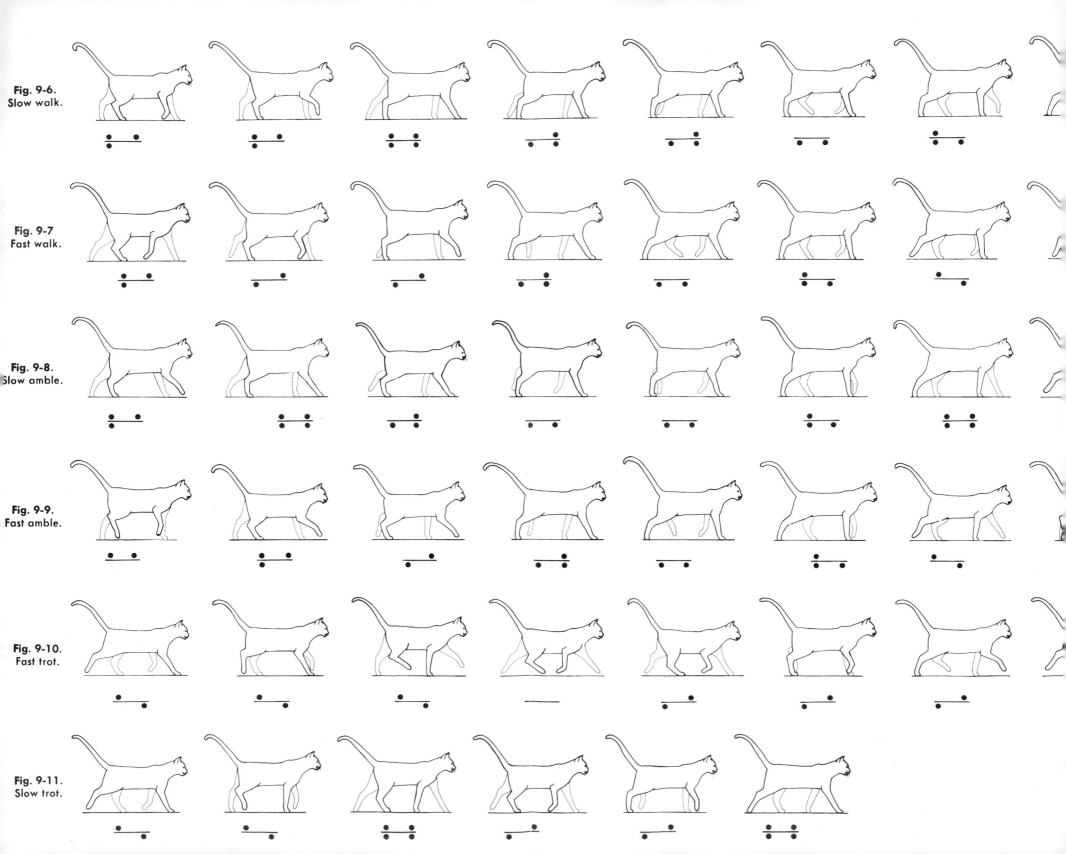

Fig. 9-6.
Slow walk.

Fig. 9-7
Fast walk.

Fig. 9-8.
Slow amble.

Fig. 9-9.
Fast amble.

Fig. 9-10.
Fast trot.

Fig. 9-11.
Slow trot.

About 60% of the body weight load is carried by the thoracic limbs, primarily because the center of gravity is closer to them. As the cat moves from four legs on the ground to three, the majority of weight will be supported by the diagonally opposing limb pair. The center of gravity also shifts toward those limbs, ending up within a triangular area determined by the three supporting limbs.[21]

Vertical and horizontal forces are associated with walking, with the vertical thrust fluctuating between a high of approximately 4000 g to a low of approximately 2600 g twice during each complete cycle. At normal speed, the maximal vertical thrust is realized during the three-foot support phase, and minimal thrust occurs when only two paws are on the ground. Individual horizontal forces are greater for the thoracic limbs than for the pelvic limb counterparts. Both the period of forward propulsion and that of negative, retarding propulsion, when the forelimb is being returned to a cranial position, provide greater calculated values than corresponding values for the pelvic limbs. Because of the vertical thrust of the forelimbs, however, the net longitudinal force is a small forward impulse, much less than for the hindlimbs.[42,88] In forward movement, the primary function of the thoracic limbs is to produce the upward acceleration of the body, and that of the pelvic limbs is for forward progress. Force changes associated with each limb are consistent for that animal but will differ between individuals.[21] If an obstacle hinders the forward swing of a foot, the cat will quickly respond by lifting the foot over the obstacle, possibly indicating spinal rather than cortical control.[139] Neural and electromyographic aspects of locomotion have also been studied.[30,145,146]

Cats often will submit to and almost appear to enjoy going for walks on lead. However, cats generally prefer to choose the course. Resistance may be shown by the cat when the cat and the owner do not want to go in the same direction.

Ambling

Another four-beat gait used by the cat has been referred to by a number of terms, including the *amble, slow pace, running walk,* and *walk.* The footfall pattern is the same as for the walk, but the timing of the placement of the limbs differs (Figures 9-8 and 9-9). At this gait, the cat has the appearance of moving the limbs on one side of the body forward at almost the same time. Whether the cat uses the walk, amble, or a sequence somewhat in between is an individual factor.

Trotting

For traveling long distances at fair speed, the trot is most often used. This two-beat gait is less tiring than other gaits because there is less body movement over the center of gravity. An added feature, as a result of steadying the shift of gravity, is that the gait then provides more stability of footing. To achieve this symmetric gait, the contralateral forefeet and hindfeet are on the ground simultaneously. At normal or fast speeds, one pair of contralateral paws propels the body forward, leaving a brief suspended interval when no limbs are supporting the body (Figure 9-10). The alternate pair of limbs then lands and pushes off to complete the cycle. At a slow rate of speed, the suspension stage does not occur, because the third and fourth paws contact the ground before the first and second leave it (Figure 9-11).

Pacing

Another two-beat gait of fair speed, the pace, is not commonly used by cats. Except that ipsilateral limbs move forward and back as a unit, the ground contact and suspension phases are the same as those described for the trot (Figures 9-12 and 9-13).

Galloping

When speed is needed to chase prey or escape enemies, the gallop is used. This four-beat, asymmetric gait has several variations, depending on the speed needed and the individual performing it. At a slow rate (a gait that is also called a *canter*), there is at least one paw on the ground at all times or as many as three during certain phases (Figure 9-14). As the caudal paws touch the ground, the foot contacting the ground last is positioned in advance of the other. The same positioning occurs when the cranial paws land. The foot that lands last and ahead of its counterpart may be termed the *lead foot,* and if these were the right forelimb and the right hindlimb, the cat could be said to have the right lead in front and the right lead behind.

When its speed increases, the cat has a suspension phase after the push with the pelvic limbs (Figure 9-15). At great speed, a second suspension phase occurs after the push by the thoracic limbs (Figure 9-16). About 80% of a stride is spent in extended flight, almost 20% in forelimb ground contact, and a very minimal amount in ground time for the pelvic limbs.[39] Generally, at faster speeds, the cat will lead with opposite feet, fore and rear, to allow for overreaching as a result of the great amount of flexion in its back. The supple spine can increase the speed and length of each stride by several inches. If the vertebral column extends just before the last limb leaves the ground, before the suspended phase, and does not flex until the next limb touches the ground, the effect is that of adding several inches to the length of the animal and thus of adding length to its stride. If the extension occurs after the cat is airborne, the effect on the stride and speed is nullified.[58] Faster speeds require more energy to obtain the suspension phase and therefore are seldom maintained for prolonged distances.

A very short, fast chase has also been termed *dashing* and is generally thought to use the half-bound variation of the gallop[23,39] (Figure 9-17). At this gait, the cat pushes off with both hindfeet at the same time, although they are usually not positioned adjacent to each other. When landing on the forepaws, the cat has a timing sequence that is the same for the gallop: One limb lands first and will be caudal to the second.

Climbing

A general concept associated with cats is that they climb trees. Some individual cats, notably Siamese, will spend a considerable amount of time on tall objects, including ceiling beams, roofs, and people, as well as trees, but prefer to find these new or odd places themselves. Thus climbing is an important part of the cat's locomotor behavior. Cats that like to climb people often learn this behavior as a kitten from owners who do not discourage it or, in some cases, actually encourage this "cute" kitten behavior. For the adult animal, climbing may represent an attempt to get close to the person's face, as in the facial approach of social greeting, or it may be an attempt to get to a higher location, especially if the shoulder or head is the final destination. The movement of limbs in climbing follows the same sequence as that used for walking: It is a four-beat rhythm. If the cat is in a hurry, however, a form of gallop pattern is used. The presence of claws is not required for climbing all objects, although claws are used if they are present. The removal of these ungual processes may necessitate a feline relearning experience.

Climbing down is generally difficult, and a kitten needs time to perfect the technique. At first the kitten backs down but later learns to come down head first in a rather haphazard fashion. Upon reaching a certain height, it will jump the remainder of the distance. Unless the cat is in a state of shock, it will eventually come down from any object it climbs if given enough time and motivation. In most cases it is the owner's lack of time and patience that result in attempts to "rescue" the cat, rather than there being a real need by the animal.

Air Righting

Cats have the ability to alter their position in midair so that they can land feet first after a fall. Air righting develops over time and will be seen first as a head rotation, which is shortly followed by the beginning of a rotation of the trunk. The reflex appears between 21 and 30 days of age (mean 23.5 days), with complete righting abilities being perfected between 33 and 48 days (mean 40 days).[16,22,140] Deaf cats will develop this reflex because their vestibular apparatus is seldom defective. Sight is required to perfect the righting reflex, the development of which correlates with that of visual acuity; however, once righting abilities are perfected, blindfolding the cat does not greatly hinder the process.

A cat that is dropped with its feet generally higher than its body responds by turning so that it will land on its feet. The basic occurrences that result in this air righting begin when the vertebral column flexes so that the cranial half of the body is at an approximate right angle from the initial starting position (Figure 9-18). The thoracic limbs are held close to the body while the pelvic limbs and tail are held away from the trunk (Figure 9-19). The cranial half is then rotated 180 degrees about its axis while this motion is offset by a 5-degree counterrotation of the caudal body (Figure 9-20). The thoracic limbs now are extended and vertical, and the pelvic limbs retain their relationship with the caudal part of the body, although they are flexed slightly (Figure 9-21). Then the caudal body rotates to line up with the front of the body (Figure 9-22). Occasionally cats may overrotate the caudal body by as much as 30 degrees, but a counterrotation by the tail and other body muscles usually corrects this problem rapidly. The original flexion of the vertebral column is maintained during the turn so that when the cat lands the back is arched with the four limbs extended[65,90] (Figure 9-23).

When falling, a cat can turn in a distance equal to that of its standing height and in a time span between 0.125 and 0.5 second.[65,90] Because it takes 0.4 second to fall 5 feet, most cats are capable of making the turn.[65,120]

Many remarkable falls have been survived by cats, some even without physical damage. The free-fall record was 129 feet, or 11 stories, by a London cat in 1965.[152] Later reports have taken into account the surface landed on, and survival records for those have been established. When the landing is a hard surface, 18 stories have been the maximal distance survived; 20 stories are the maximal for shrubbery; and 28 stories is the

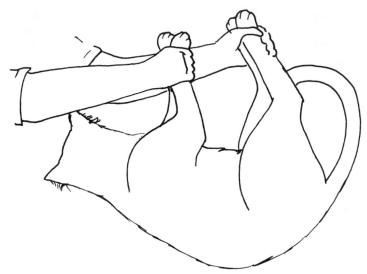

Figure 9-18 Air righting begins with vertebral flexion.

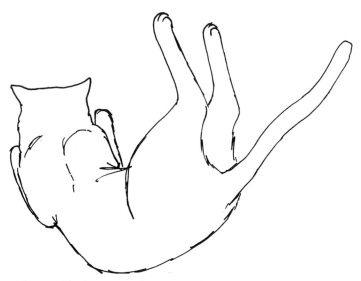

Figure 9-19 The initial limb positions during air righting.

maximal for a canopy or awning.[109] When falling, a cat reaches a terminal velocity approaching 40 mph in 60 feet.[90] Theoretically then, if a cat can survive a fall of 60 feet, it should be able to withstand a fall from any height.

Most cats have an excellent sense of balance, but when they do slip from a precarious perch or fall out of an unexpectedly open window, medical reports of the "highrise syndrome" reflect the cat's unique righting behavior. Of all traumatic occurrences to cats, 13.9% are the result of a fall. Of these reported injuries, 31% to 57% occur to the head, usually the mandible, 31% to 68% occur to the thorax, and 39% to 43%

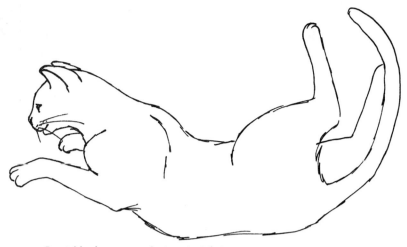

Figure 9-20 Cranial body rotation during air righting.

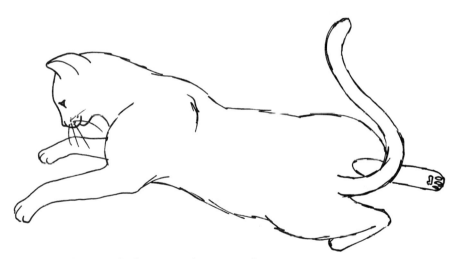

Figure 9-21 Changes in limb positions during air righting.

occur to the limbs.[75,147] In falls from 2 to 32 stories, 90% of cats survive and 60% need relatively minor care.[62]

To show the air-righting reflex, the cat must be dropped so that its limbs are in approximately the same horizontal plane. When dropped with the cranial or caudal end first, the cat cannot correct its position until one pair of limbs touches the ground[90] (Figure 9-24).

Jumping

Several behavioral series participated in by cats involve a leaping start from a standing position. Whether a cat is jumping down from a tree, jumping onto a window sill, or starting after fleeing prey, its basic starting position is the same. Initially the body weight

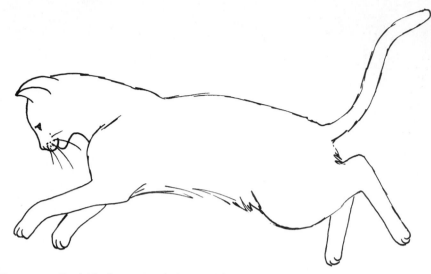

Figure 9-22 Caudal body rotation during air righting.

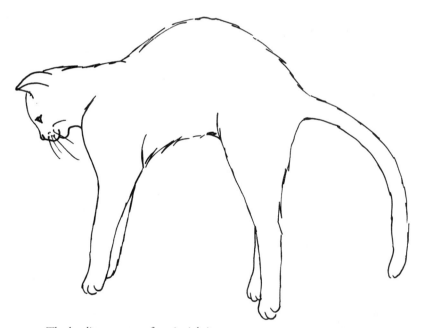

Figure 9-23 The landing posture after air righting.

is shifted over the hindlimbs, which are situated so that one is slightly in front of the other. Rapid extension of these limbs provides the propulsion for the cat's spring and is a modified form of the half-bound gallop gait (see Figure 9-17). The animal lands on its forelimbs, one at a time, with the second limb landing forward of the first. The amount of energy necessary for the initial propulsion is significantly greater than that

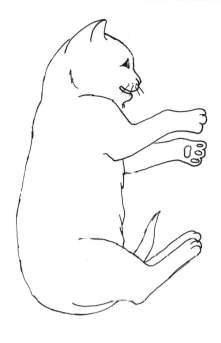

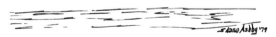

Figure 9-24 The air-righting reflex does not correct a position if the limbs are not in the same horizontal plane.

required for the other gaits, and the force of the support provided by each limb in turn is four to five times greater than that developed during walking.[39] This amount of power must be generated because the weight supported by each limb in turn is approximately four times body weight.[39]

The distances jumped by a cat are dependent on a number of factors, including the physical ability of the individual and the distance to the goal; however, if conditions are right, a maximal leap would cover approximately 170 cm (5.5 feet).[39]

Swimming

Like most mammals, cats are natural swimmers, although it is not usually a favored behavior. The Turkish cat is a breed exception to this dislike for swimming. The limb movements, which are used to provide slow forward progress, are commonly referred to as the *dog paddle,* the same combination of movements used in walking. This four-beat, symmetric pattern is also used by the dog, but the posture differs slightly in the cat because it keeps more of its back and tail out of the water.

Retrieving

Queens bring prey home for the young to use in practicing their hunting skills, and when the mouse escapes the young, the queen will catch it and bring it back for her offspring. This is the most common and natural form of retrieving exhibited by cats. For other individuals, live prey is repeatedly released only to be recaptured and dragged back. Members of the Kuiat breed, as well as a few other individuals, have an innate retrieving ability: They will catch a ball or other toy and bring it back for the owner to throw again.

Digging

The digging of soil by cats is well known as being part of the eliminative behavior pattern. Cats are capable of earth-raking only relatively loose dirt because their claws are retractable and not available to break the ground initially. The toes must do all the work of loosening and moving the dirt. This is the primary reason cats do not dig into rodent burrows after their prey, as other animals do. Digging behavior can be shown by moving one forepaw exclusively, using one paw for a while and then the other, and occasionally by alternating paws in a sequential fashion.

Paw Dominance

Felis catus shows a paw dominance similar to the right and left handedness observable in humans. Although reported paw dominance has varied by researcher, two studies report 49.5% to 51.5% of cats have a right-paw preference, 36.4% to 40.4% have a left preference, and 10.1% to 12.1% are ambidextrous.[126,129] These studies had more females than males. Other studies found that right-forepaw usage is preferred by 20% to 39% of the cats, and another 13.6% to 38.3% favor the left side for manipulatory tasks.[18,32,141] The remaining 41.7% to 47.7% are ambidextrous. The genders of the cats used in this later report were not given. Another study of adult male cats reported a strong left-paw preference in 80.7% of the trials.[80,81] Practice decreased left-paw usage to 71.4% and one cat even became a right-paw–exclusive user.[80] Results from my own study of a group with equal numbers of males and females show a slight left-paw bias (Figure 9-25 and 9-26). Preferences are determined by the sensorimotor cerebral cortex, influenced by testosterone, and can be modified only slightly by environmental factors, such as convenience for reaching something.[32,125,141,142]

Female cats are more right-paw dominant, with 44% strongly favoring the right paw and an additional 10% using their right paw the most.[126] This compares with 28% of male cats that are strongly right pawed, and 15% more right-paw tending. There is no difference in sex for those that are left-paw dominant.[126] Weight also seems to be associated with laterality. In right-pawed males, the trend toward being ambidextrous increases as body weight increases.[123] In left-pawed females, the use of the left paw increases with increased weight.[123] Various drugs such as lithium and imipramine affect the asymmetry of paw use, suggesting a biochemical asymmetry in the brain.[124] There may also be a hormonal influence. Testosterone is thought to suppress the left brain to induce ambilaterality.[125]

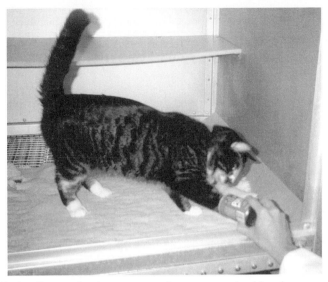

Figure 9-25 Testing for paw dominance means the cat can reach with only one paw at a time.

Accuracy and reaction times are affected by which paw is used. When a cat uses its preferred paw, it is considerably more accurate than when it uses the nondominant paw.[32] In addition, there is a much faster reaction time for the dominant paw.[32,81]

Limb Flicking

Cats respond to foreign material on their feet by lifting the paw and rapidly shaking it outward from the body. If more than one limb is involved, the cat will alternately shake each limb, repeating the cycle as often as necessary to rid the foot of the substance. Cats that have been dosed with *d*-lysergic acid diethylamide (LSD) will spontaneously exhibit limb-flicking behavior.[63]

Bipedal Standing

A cat is capable of standing on its hindlimbs for relatively long periods. This posture is often displayed when the cat is begging or searching for food (Figure 9-27). The cat is an exception with this behavior because the posture is considered uncommon for predatory animals; their long, slender limbs do not readily adapt to bipedal balance.[23]

Unusual Patterns of Locomotion

Occasionally, otherwise normal cats are observed to show episodes of slow-motion movement. The events described are of varying duration and may include a period of apparently normal sleep. Walking movements are less than half as fast as normal, as are eating and grooming motions. Even urination has been observed at this slow speed.

	Free Reach	Reach into Tube	Reach for Block
MALE CATS			
1	A	L	R
2	L	L	L
3	L	R	L
4	A	R	A
5	A	R	R
6	L	L	L
7	R	R	R
FEMALE CATS			
1	L	L	L
2	A	L	L
3	A	A	A
4	A	L	A
5	L	L	A
6	R	A	R

ALL MALES				TOTAL
Left paw	3	3	3	9
Right paw	1	4	3	8
Ambidextrous	3	0	1	4
ALL FEMALES				
Left paw	2	4	2	8
Right paw	1	0	1	2
Ambidextrous	3	2	3	8
ALL CATS				
Left paw	5	7	5	17
Right paw	2	4	4	10
Ambidextrous	6	2	4	12

*The cat had to use one paw at least 75% of the time in each trial to be labeled with a laterality. A, *Ambidextrous;* L, *left-paw dominant;* R, *right-paw dominant.*

Figure 9-26 Paw preferences on three trials of cats at Texas A&M University.*

Another unusual pattern observed in cats is a sudden aversion to a particular carpet, such that the cat will do almost anything to avoid walking on it. In seeking the reason for this behavior, several aversive causative situations must be considered. Chemicals used in rug cleaning may be physically irritating or leave an offensive odor. A traumatic event associated with laying a new carpet or even the odor of a new carpet are other factors for consideration. Sometimes an adequate history is difficult to obtain, and at other times the history may not provide any clues to the cause of the problem.

RESTING BEHAVIORS

The resting stage of cat activity varies from sitting to sleeping, with several associated postures in between. Owned cats kept indoors use an average of five locations.[49] During the day, preference is given to rest high up for 39.4% of cats, for 7 hours total time. Another 33.4% rest on a couch/sofa for 5 hours (Figure 9-28); 31.3% use a window sill/seat for 1 hour at a time. At night 52.4% rest on or in the bed for 5 hours. A blanket is the favorite spot for 28.1% of cats for 6 hours, equally divided between day and night. Fewer than 25% use material, chairs, cat baskets, carpet, wood, cat trees, or other smooth surfaces.[49]

Sitting

In a sitting posture, the thoracic limbs are positioned much like those of a normal standing cat, with the angulation of each joint remaining about the same. In contrast, the major joints of the pelvic limbs are flexed to lower the caudal portion of the body until the skin covering the ischiatic tuberosities contacts the ground. The tail may be directed caudally, especially when the sit is of short duration (Figure 9-29, *A*), or the tail may be wrapped around the paws during a less transient period (Figure 9-29, *B*). House cats spend approximately 16% of their day sitting.[4]

Lying Down

Resting is often equated with the lying positions, and although that usually is true, it does not necessarily have to be. Adult farm cats will rest between 2.8 and 7.8 hours a day.[101] In households with two cats, cats spend 3% of their time crouched, 30% lying with their head down, and 45% lying with their head up.[4]

To lie down the cat can lower either the sternum or the pelvis to the ground first, and to rise the cat can raise either end first or both ends at one time, as is most often done when springing after prey or stretching. If resting on a window sill, the cat may also slide head first off its perch to the ground.

There are four basic body postures associated with lying. Sternal recumbency is the first, and with it the forepaws may be pointed forward, usually with the tail directed caudally (Figure 9-30, *A*). Another more common version of sternal recumbency has the forepaws rotated and flexed so they are tucked back under the cat (Figure 9-30, *B*). In this situation the tail is generally curled around the cat's body and across its paws.

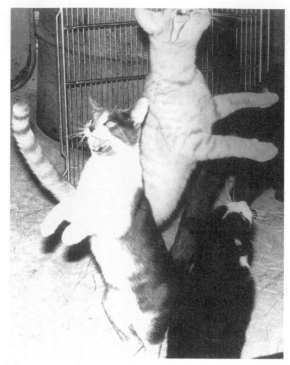

Figure 9-27 Bipedal posture used to request food.

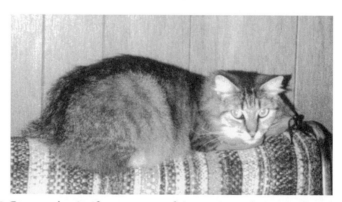

Figure 9-28 Cats spend a significant amount of time resting at locations relatively high off the ground, such as on the back of a sofa.

This posture should be considered when treating ear mites. Unless the cat's whole body is initially treated, the mites can survive on other body areas and return to the ears when the treatment has been discontinued. Transfer of this parasite to the tail while the cat is lying in this curled position is a common occurrence in individuals whose ears alone are treated.

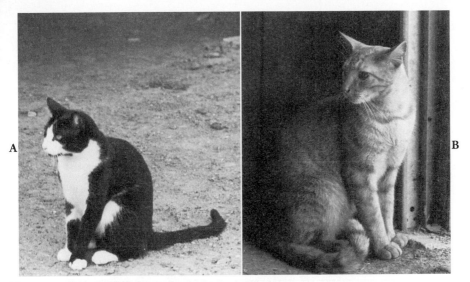

Figure 9-29 A and **B,** Common sitting postures of the cat.

The second lying posture is complete lateral recumbency (Figure 9-31). Either side may contact the ground, and the cat may be stretched out or curled into a ball with the paws folded around one another. In the former case the tail is also outstretched, and in the latter the tail is curved around the body. The cooler the environmental temperature, the more tightly curled is the posture, so that the cat's head and paws are tucked under its body and enclosed by its tail.[14] Both of these are the postures associated with true sleep.

The third of the general postures associated with lying is a combination of cranial sternal recumbency and caudal lateral recumbency (Figure 9-32). This position is commonly used by cats and is often associated with a "quiet alert" conscious phase.[144]

A few cats sleep on their back, a fourth posture (Figure 9-33). This posture is generally not used for long periods, and it is much less commonly used by thin individuals.

Preferences for sleeping places will change periodically, but they often involve areas that are warm, quiet, and elevated. When attempting to persuade a cat to accept a bed, it is best to encourage an area's use by providing warmth with a lamp or hot-water bottle.[13] An enclosed sleeping compartment may also be beneficial, especially for nervous or upset individuals.

Sleeping

The phenomenon known as sleep is not a state of absence of activity, as has been generally described, but is an active process. It begins with the neural initiation of a search for a place to sleep. Special posturing for sleep is also part of this appetitive portion.[31,96] Sleep and wake cannot be differentiated by electroencephalographic means before days 2 through 5.[114] Also, the two consummatory phases of sleep are behaviorally

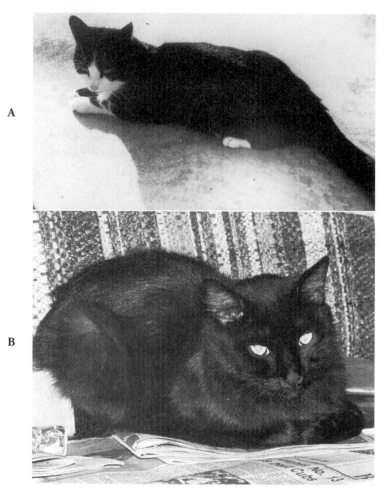

Figure 9-30 A and **B,** The sternally recumbent lying postures.

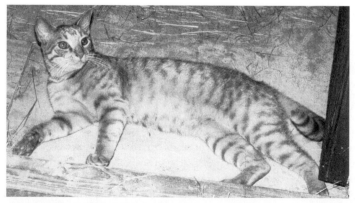

Figure 9-31 The laterally recumbent lying posture.

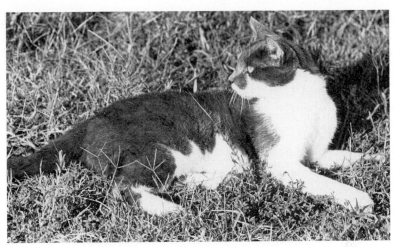

Figure 9-32 The combination of sternally and laterally recumbent lying postures.

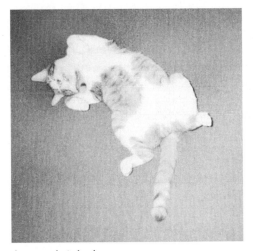

Figure 9-33 Some cats sleep on their back.

evident at birth but cannot be differentiated until the kitten is 2 or 3 weeks of age.[38] Until that time, approximately 50% of the kitten's day is spent sleeping, but only the deep phase is evident electronically.[2,46] Complete organization of electroencephalographic sleep and wake patterns may not be adultlike until near the end of the second month of life.[114] The amount of sleeping done by kittens is inversely proportional to the amount of play participation. Sleep takes up between 7.4 and 11.7 hours of an adult farm cat's day, but laboratory cats kept in controlled lighting sleep 10 to 15.6 hr/day[61,101] (Figure 9-34). The amount of deep sleep needed by a cat gradually decreases from three fourths of the sleep time to about one fourth for an adult.[56] Older cats have increased sleep bout fragmentation and show significantly less deep sleep.[10]

	Awake (min)	Drowsy (min)	Slow-Wave Sleep (min)	Paradoxical Sleep (min)
Normal cat fed once daily	484±36	257±15	566±50	112±23
Reduced external stimuli			453±20	
Continuous light		496±81		
Reduced food intake			388±19	
Three meals per day		147±14		
Overfeeding				185±49

Figure 9-34 Factors that significantly alter the sleep patterns for cats with 12-hour light-dark cycles.[112]

Slow-wave (light) sleep usually occurs when the cat is in either a sternally recumbent posture with its forepaws tucked under and its tail wrapped around its body or the curled-up form of lateral recumbency. For both positions, some muscle tone must be maintained for balance and head posture.[46,67] There is a low-voltage, synchronized, slow cortical activity[35,68] generated in the thymus.[54] Physiologic conditions also reflect this slowed state: Breathing and heart rates are decreased and steady; blood pressure is lowered; and the eyes exhibit myosis of the pupils, stillness of the extrinsic muscles, and protrusion of the third eyelid.[54,68] Most sleep states of the cat are slow wave in nature, taking up between 9 and 12 hours, about 40% to 50% of each day. However, because the nocturnal activity patterns of cats are not observed, the relative amount of slow-wave sleep may appear to be greater than it actually is. Afternoon naps are easily observed, but hunting in the dark of night is not. Sleep studies indicate that modern cats are phasic throughout the day and night and thus are not truly nocturnal. They have 62.6% of their active time during daylight hours, and 82.1% of their sleep occurs during dark hours.[101,131] There is also evidence to support the idea that when deprived of slow-wave sleep a cat can neurally compensate for this deficit during conscious minor activity.[33]

Within 10 to 30 minutes after falling asleep, a cat may progress into paradoxical sleep, a deeper stage.[67,68] Electroencephalographic recordings show desynchronization of the high-voltage cortical activity, some of which resembles normal wake patterns.[11,54,56,76,94] Although neck and general body muscle tone is lax because of active inhibition of spinal motor neurons,[94] superimposed bursts of excitatory volleys from as yet unknown sources resulting in periodic movement of various parts can be observed. Digital flexion, twitching of the ears, irregular breathing, movement of vibrissae, flicking of the tongue, twitching of the tail, and sudden pupillary dilation often occur. If the atonia is experimentally prevented, the cat leaps up and chases or pounces on invisible prey, but it remains oblivious to observers.[54] Rapid eye movements (REMs) of 8 to 30 at a time are responsible for the other name for paradoxical sleep, REM sleep.[67]

The sleep-wake cycle of a laboratory cat has a mean duration of 104 minutes.[83] The 26 minutes of wakefulness are followed by sleep that contains 2.6 REM sleep bouts.[83] Lasting 6 to 7 minutes, REM sleep usually alternates with 20 to 30 minutes of slow-wave sleep, but it takes up approximately 15% of a 24-hour period.* This represents approximately one fourth of the total sleep time.[56,57] The phase of paradoxical sleep is known to be the time when dreaming occurs in human sleep, and although it may never be known whether animals do in fact dream, there is no reason to assume that they do not.[46,47,56,93] The body movements that accompany REM sleep do not necessarily indicate the subject of the dream, however.[47]

Cats that are forced to remain awake for prolonged periods become increasingly irritable, even to the point of illness, but effects of sleeplessness on learning are not conclusively defined.[135] Apparently, deprivation of paradoxical sleep is the most significant aspect of this prolonged wakefulness, because when allowed to sleep, the cat increases the amount of the REM phase until its deficit has been made up.[67,76,82,102] Not until that time will the accelerated heart rate associated with sleep deprivation return to normal.[67] Drowsiness increases with continuous light and decreases when the meals are divided[112] (see Figure 9-34). Fasting, reduced food intake, antihistamines, and increased external stimulation all decrease sleep episodes, but the opposite is true for added food intake, glucose, and quiet.

Awakening

Cats usually awaken from a slow-wave phase of sleep because the arousal threshold for REM sleep is 300 times greater than that needed for slow-wave sleep.[68] A detailed comparison of the neurologic pattern of waking and of slow-wave sleep suggests that they are controlled by different neural mechanisms.[5] Cats that are sleeping on the lap of a person while being petted may awaken in a somewhat disoriented state and react to being "caught" by clawing. It is not until they have jumped free that full consciousness brings back the reality of the situation. When awaking naturally, most cats will exhibit stretching behavior, usually of the thoracic limbs first. In addition, scratching nearby objects may serve as an action that in itself is a form of stretching[43] (see Figures 3-14 and 3-15).

Reflexive Immobility

A young kitten is carried from place to place by the queen holding the dorsum of its neck (see Figure 6-10). It results in a partial flexor dominant position and passivity, which function to keep the kitten from struggling and to keep its tail out of the way so that the queen will not step on it. Humans can successfully use the same method to immobilize adult cats, although its effectiveness decreases with the age of the cat. This reflexive posture, which might also be responsible for passivity during the male's mating neck grip, may be initiated by a number of factors.[45] External stimuli, such as visual, auditory, and tactile factors, as well as internal stimuli, such as emotional, visceral, or proprioceptive factors, are known to bring about reflexive immobility.[72]

*References 46, 54, 55, 57, 67, 93, 112, 122, 132.

BRAIN AND LOCOMOTION

The cerebellum has long been recognized for functioning in motor coordination as a regulator, not an initiator. The functions of maintenance of equilibrium and body posture are also performed by this neural area. Degeneration or hypoplasia of the cerebellum generally does not become obvious until the kitten is at least 4 weeks of age, because normal ambulation will not stabilize until then. Malnutrition of kittens from the prenatal period to as late as 6 weeks after birth will significantly and permanently affect the cerebellum and thus motor coordination.[44,118,119] Ablation of the cerebellum does not produce any significant changes in the various sleep states, except relative to the amount of muscle activity and tone during REM sleep.[100]

Visually directed forelimb placement, although regulated by the cerebellum, is probably under fine control by the caudal sigmoid gyrus.[40] The frontal lobes are also known to affect motor abilities, particularly placing. Vertigo can be associated with motion sickness; labyrinthitis; cerebellar lesions; proprioception problems; and drug intoxication, including that from salicylates and streptomycin.[104,115,117]

The reticular activating system of the brainstem maintains consciousness and is opposed by other central areas collectively called the *forebrain inhibitory system*.[17] The amount of arousal, related to the neuromodulator adenosine, decreases as a function of duration of wakefulness.[105] The thalamus of the brain is associated with sleep because stimulation of that region produces this homeostatic response, possibly by way of the thalamocortical radiations.[64,96] Thalamic connections with the hypothalamus regulate the sleep-wake cycle, with destruction of the hypothalamus producing an abnormal amount of sleepiness. Conversely, stimulation of these areas results in hyperactivity and increased locomotion. The hypothalamic association with somatomotor responses, such as circling, rolling over, limb extension, claw extension, and head movements, can be demonstrated by stimulation soon after a kitten's birth.[73] Temperature reduction in the anterior hypothalamus occurs during sleep,[1] although the significance of that is not known. Damage to this area has been associated with a reduction in urine spraying but an increase in the startle response when awaking.[48] The hippocampus has been experimentally shown to facilitate REM sleep, and the rostral raphe nuclei provide the major control of slow-wave sleep and the capacity of the brain to shift to sleep patterns.[2,70,71]

During sleep, pontine activity stimulates the medullary inhibitory center, which then inhibits spinal cord motor neurons from initiating muscle contractions.[93,95] Stimulation of or damage to the forebrain system's pontine formations is also associated with disruptions in normal sleep-wake rhythms.[3,17,87] Mesencephalic brainstem lesions have shown the relationship of that area to normal behavior.[121] The result is a marked deficit in several of the senses and hyperexploratory activity. There is also a lack of responsiveness to pleasurable or noxious stimuli and an exaggeration of oral activities including overeating, holding excessively large objects, swallowing small objects, holding other animals by the back of the neck, and chewing their own hair or skin.[121] The brainstem also affects the equilibrium and level of locomotor activity and thus speed.[98]

Lesions in the caudate nuclei result in hyperactive behavior.[79] The importance of this area to active young or excessively hyper adult cats is not known. Furthermore, specific cerebral cortical areas regulate movement of certain body areas by the time kittens are 47 days old.[143]

Locomotion is motivated by homeostatic drives, which are associated with rest and sleep and elicited by internal stimuli, and by nonhomeostatic drives caused by external stimuli, such as movement to escape a dog's approach. A combination of homeostatic and nonhomeostatic drives can also be effective, such as the prey-catching behavior of a cat that is initiated by both hunger and the squeak of a mouse.[96]

The brain has been studied relative to paw dominance to some extent. Right-pawed males and females show a stronger tendency toward laterality with increasingly asymmetric brains in which the right side gets larger.[127,128] The left-side correlation is not the same, sometimes depending on a relationship with an increased left side of the brain and sometimes with a decreasing right side.[127,128] The differences found between males and females tend to support variations found in paw dominance between the sexes.

LOCOMOTIVE BEHAVIOR PROBLEMS

Most problems associated with locomotion are related to lameness, but because these problems are of minor significance in a feline practice, and because they are traditionally covered in other subjects of veterinary medicine, this chapter does not discuss lameness.

Narcolepsy

Narcolepsy is an uncommon neurologic condition in the cat that results in sudden, recurring episodes of sleep. It is usually emotional stimuli that cause the REM sleep cataplexy.[94] There has been speculation that the spinal motor inhibition normally associated with REM sleep may be inappropriately triggered by stimuli affecting the reticular activating system.[94] The condition can occur at any time and thus could be potentially dangerous to the animal. Treatment of narcolepsy with dextroamphetamine and other stimulants can be successful.[74]

Other Sleep Disorders

With the exception of narcolepsy, sleep disorders are not well understood in domestic animals. Only a few cats with spontaneous sleep disorders have been studied.[55] Seizurelike activity during REM sleep has been reported in an otherwise healthy cat.[57] Damage of the pons can release muscle inhibition during sleep, resulting in cats that sleep walk, attack, show exploratory behaviors, or reach and grasp.[94]

Reversal of day/night activities is fairly common in geriatric cats. It and increased vocalization are the two most common signs of feline cognitive dysfunction.[20] Melatonin is showing promise for treating this activity change, and selegiline is being evaluated for the feline version of cognitive dysfunction.

Stereotyped Behavior

A stereotypy is a repetitive behavior that is nonfunctional, noninjurious, predictable in its sequence of actions, and performed in a specific rhythmic manner.* It becomes more rigid

*References 6, 25, 26, 85, 86, 91, 148.

and ritualized in its pattern over time, and it appears to be purposeless in the context in which it occurs. This behavior probably develops as a coping mechanism to deal with stress, frustration, or conflict.* Physical evidence of stress is less in an animal that shows a stereotypy than in one in which a stereotypy is not allowed to be performed.[86] In addition, there is evidence to suggest that there may be a genetic predisposition for a particular stereotypy or at least a lower tolerance for some stressors.[86,91] Eventually these behaviors will be performed even though the initiating stressors are gone. The action patterns chosen become more fixed in their performance with repetition. The caged cat begins to randomly walk within its confined space. It is theorized that stress releases endorphins, which act on nigrostriatal dopaminergic neurons to increase motor activity and stimulate pleasure centers of the brain, subsequently reinforcing the behavior.[28] The hypothesis on coping suggests that the adaptive significance in chronic stress may be in the attenuation of the deleterious consequences of chronic stress.[153]

Animals that are in chronically frustrating situations, such as being confined in small cagelike environments or not getting enough exercise or environmental enrichment, commonly develop this behavioral vice. Although generally associated with zoo animals, stereotyped behavior patterns can also be developed by cats and are characteristic for each individual regardless of the cause. Two basic patterns have been described in cats. The first involves the movement of the head and neck in a continuous lateral to-and-fro motion.[36,138] The animal may have enough momentum to cause weight shifting over the appropriate forepaw at the same time. The second stereotyped behavior is that the cat stands at a particular location, usually near the cage door, and sniffs.[138] Certain drugs have been shown to potentiate these behaviors in cats known to have already acquired them.[138] Affected cats may also be increasingly irritable to environmental stimuli, striking out at minor changes, such as new people feeding them or cleaning their cages.

Neutering has been the most successful control because of its calming effect on the animal.[12] Narcotic antagonists have been helpful at reducing or eliminating the problem because they block the internal reward the animal gets from endorphin release. The tricyclic antidepressant and selected serotonin reuptake inhibitor (SSRI) drugs have also been used with some success. They probably reduce the overall anxiety state of the individual and address the problem as a possible obsessive-compulsive disorder. Progestins and tranquilizers have also been used successfully, but in all cases it is highly desirable to change the exercise plan for the cat. This can readily be accomplished by providing movable toys or another cat if space and social natures permit.

Obsessive-Compulsive Disorders

In humans, an obsession is a state of a single subject monopolizing the person's thought processes excessively, to the point that he or she feels compelled to act on that thought. This occurs repeatedly. Although all of the obsessive-compulsive disorders (OCDs) are repetitive, not all must be repeated according to a rigid motor pattern. Thus an OCD is different from a stereotyped behavior, but it could involve a stereotypy.

---

*References 6, 15, 27, 84, 86, 148.

Because we cannot ask cats what they are thinking, we can evaluate only their behavior. Approximately 12% of feline behavior cases relate to OCD.[99] By looking at the various repetitive behaviors that a cat may show, several have been identified as possible OCD candidates, including head shaking, pacing, roaming, and freezing (not moving for long periods).[24,29] This reluctance to move, along with circling, pica, and star gazing, have also been associated with polycythemia vera.[69]

The neurologic basis for OCD is not well described yet. Serotonin systems have been implicated in several behaviors including motor activity,[106] and dopa, dopamine, and dexamphetamine can experimentally induce signs.[19]

OCD is currently being treated with SSRI drugs. The success rate is low, with only 50% showing partial to complete reduction in symptoms. This rate is similar in human patients. Hopefully, advances in drug therapy will eventually allow us to understand OCD and more effectively treat these problems.

Overactivity

Overactivity as a problem for approximately 1.9% of cats,[49] and it can have a number of causes.[136] In young cats, play behaviors may involve a lot of running, especially in sporadic bouts. The channeling of this energy into a play bout before bedtime can allow owners a night without the kitten bouncing over them. Hyperthyroidism is a common clinical entity associated with increased activity and restlessness.[66] The result is a young-acting geriatric cat. Thus owners need to be warned that the animal's activity may decrease after treatment. Other clinical conditions must be considered as causes of excess activity, including pain, feline immunodeficiency viral infections, feline infectious peritonitis, and metabolic encephalopathies.[29,113] Valproic acid, used to treat the seizures of cerebral palsy in humans, has also been associated with excessive activity.[154]

Hyperactivity and hyperkinesia have been described in dogs[6,7] and probably exist in cats too. Clinically, both conditions are similar—short attention span, excessive awareness of surroundings, no habituation, and overactivity. It is the response to therapy that differentiates the two conditions. Hyperactivity is reduced to normal behavior by phenothiazine tranquilizers, and hyperkinesis requires a stimulant like methylphenidate.

The feline hyperesthesia syndrome is also manifested by overactivity and is discussed in Chapter 10.

Jumping on Counters/Tables

Cats frequent high places. They are particularly prone to jump onto kitchen counters and tables because they are often rewarded with some type of food. Prevention involves allowing the cat to have certain desirable high spots, but teaching them that others are unacceptable. From the beginning, it is easier to teach a cat to stay off of something where it has never had a strong positive experience. This means owners must be conscientious about keeping food out of the reach of the cat. The lesson of staying off a particular table or counter is then taught by using remote punishment.[97] Covering the surface with upside-down or two-sided sticky tape, cookie trays filled with water, bubble wrap, irregular objects like books or boxes, electric shock mats, covered or upside-down mousetrap, or upside-down vinyl carpet runners will make the surface undesirable.

Remote-controlled or motion sensor–controlled alarms or aimed hair dryers can startle the cat as it lands on the top of the counter. The possibilities of "booby traps" are limited only by one's imagination. The cat should not be able to see the items on the table from the floor so that it does not learn to visually determine whether it is safe to jump. Even more important than the specific method used is the concern that each occurrence receive the same negative treatment. Intermittent success must not serve as its own reward.

Because cats usually start from the floor, another technique can be paired with remote punishment. Drape a piece of paper, string, fly swatter, or some other object over the edge of the table so that it is easily seen from the ground. This can be used to mark any location where the remote punishment technique is being used, but only those locations. Over time the cat will come to learn that the visual signal means the area is not a good place on which it should attempt to jump. This visual signal can then be used occasionally on other areas for short periods when it is desirable to keep the cat off.

Escaping

Approximately 1.4% of cats exhibit problem escape or roaming behavior.[49] Some of these cats are outdoor cats confined indoors, but others are indoor ones that apparently like the challenge of getting out. Confining the cat to its own room for a few weeks works best, particularly if this has been an outdoor cat that is to now remain indoors.[60] Careful monitoring or double barriers will usually control the situation, although an occasional escape can still occur. Allowing controlled access to the outside by leash or screened area may be enough to keep the cat from attempting additional escapes.

REFERENCES

1. Adams T: Hypothalamic temperature in the cat during feeding and sleep, *Science* 139:609, 1963.
2. Adrien J: Lesion of the anterior raphe nuclei in the newborn kitten and the effects on sleep, *Brain Res* 103:579–583, Feb 27, 1976.
3. Bard P, Macht MB: The behavior of chronically decerebrate cats. In Wolstenholme GEW, O'Connor CM, editors: *Neurological basis of behavior,* Boston, 1952, Little, Brown and Company.
4. Barry K: Time-budgets and social behavior of the indoor domestic cat. Paper presented at American Veterinary Society Animal Behavior meeting, Pittsburgh, July 10, 1995.
5. Basar E, Durusan R, Gönder A, Ungan P: Combined dynamics of EEG and evoked potentials. II. Studies of simultaneously recorded EEG-programs in the auditory pathway, reticular formation, and hippocampus of the cat brain during sleep, *Biol Cybern* 34(1):21–30, 1979.
6. Beaver BV: *The veterinarian's encyclopedia of animal behavior,* Ames, 1994, Iowa State University Press.
7. Beaver BV: *Canine behavior: a guide for veterinarians,* Philadelphia, 1999, WB Saunders.
8. Berman M, Dunbar I: The social behaviour of free-ranging suburban dogs, *Appl Anim Ethol* 10(1–2):5–17, 1983.
9. Blaszczyk J, Loeb GE: Why cats pace on the treadmill, *Physiol Behav* 53(3):501–507, 1993.
10. Bowersox SS, Baker TL, Dement WC: Sleep-wakefulness patterns in the aged cat, *Electroencephalogr Clin Neurophysiol* 58:240–252, Sep 1984.

11. Brooks DC, Gershon MD: Eye movement potentials in the oculomotor and visual systems of the cat: a comparison of reserpine induced waves with those present during wakefulness and rapid eye movement sleep, *Brain Res* 27:223–239, April 2, 1971.

12. Brunner F: The application of behavior studies in small animal practice. In Fox MW, editor: *Abnormal behavior in animals,* Philadelphia, 1968, WB Saunders.

13. Bryant D: *The care and handling of cats,* New York, 1944, Ives Washburn.

14. Burton M: *The sixth sense of animals,* New York, 1973, Taplinger Publishing.

15. Cabib S, Puglisi-Allega S, Oliverio A: Chronic stress enhances apomorphine-induced stereotyped behavior in mice: involvement of endogenous opioids. *Brain Res* 298:138–140, 1984.

16. Carmichael L: The genetic development of the kitten's capacity to right itself in the air when falling, *J Genet Psychol* 44:453–458, 1934.

17. Clemente CD: Forebrain mechanisms related to internal inhibition and sleep, *Cond Reflex* 3(3):145–174, 1968.

18. Cloe J: Paw preference in cats related to hand preference in animals and man, *J Comp Physiol Psychol* 48:137–140, April 1955.

19. Cools AR, van Rossum JM: Caudal dopamine and stereotype behaviour of cats, *Arch Int Pharmacodyn* 187:163–173, 1970.

20. Cooper LL: Personal communication, July 23, 2000.

21. Coulmance M, Gahéry Y, Massion J, Swett JE: The placing reaction in the standing cat: a model for the study of posture and movement, *Exp Brain Res* 37(2):265–281, 1979.

22. Cruickshank RM: Animal infancy. In Carmichael L, editor: *Manual of child psychology,* New York, 1946, John Wiley and Sons.

23. Dagg AI: Gaits in mammals, *Mammal Rev* 3:135–154, 1973.

24. Dallaire A: Stress and behavior in domestic animals: temperament as a predisposing factor to stereotypies, *Ann N Y Acad Sci* 697:269–274, Oct 29, 1993.

25. Dantzer R: Behavioral, physiological and functional aspects of stereotyped behavior: a review and a reinterpretation, *J Anim Sci* 62:1776–1786, 1986.

26. Davis KL, Gurski JC, Scott JP: Interaction of separation distress with fear in infant dogs, *Dev Psychobiol* 10(3):203–212, 1977.

27. Dodman NH: Pharmacological treatment of behavioral problems in cats, *Vet Forum* pp 62–65, 71, April 1995.

28. Dodman NH, Shuster L: Pharmacologic approaches to managing behavior problems in small animals, *Vet Med* 89(10):960–969, 1994.

29. Dow SW, Dreitz MJ, Hoover EA: Exploring the link between feline immunodeficiency virus infection and neurologic disease in cats, *Vet Med* 87(12):1181–1184, 1992.

30. English AW: Interlimb coordination during stepping in the cat: an electromyographic analysis, *J Neurophysiol* 42:229–243, Jan 1979.

31. Ewer RF: *Ethology of mammals,* London, 1968, Paul Elek.

32. Fabre-Thorpe M, Fagot J, Lorincz E, et al: Laterality in cats: paw preference and performance in a visuomotor activity, *Cortex* 29(1):15–24, 1993.

33. Ferguson J, Dement W: The effect of variations in total sleep time on the occurrence of rapid eye movement sleep in cats, *Electroencephalogr Clin Neurophysiol* 22:2–10, Jan 1967.

34. Fish MW, Windle WF: The effect of rotatory stimulation on the movements of the head and eyes in newborn and young kittens, *J Comp Neurol* 54(1):103–107, 1932.

35. Foulkes D: Dream reports from different stages of sleep, *J Abnorm Soc Psychol* 65:14–25, July 1962.

36. Fox MW: New information on feline behavior, *Mod Vet Pract* 56(4):50–52, 1965.

37. Fox MW: *Understanding your cat,* New York, 1974, Coward, McCann & Geoghegan.

38. Fox MW: The behavior of cats. In Hafez ESE, editor: *The behavior of domestic animals,* ed 3, Baltimore, 1975, Williams & Wilkins.

39. Gambaryan PP: *How mammals run,* New York, 1974, John Wiley and Sons.
40. Glassman RB: Cutaneous discrimination and motor control following somatosensory cortical ablation, *Physiol Behav* 5(9):1009–1019, 1970.
41. Gottlieb G: Ontogenesis of sensory function in birds and mammals. In Tobach E, Aronson LR, Shaw E, editors: *The biopsychology of development,* New York, 1971, Academic Press.
42. Gray J: *Animal locomotion,* New York, 1968, WW Norton & Company.
43. Hart BL: Behavioral aspects of scratching in cats, *Feline Pract* 2(2):6–8,1972.
44. Hart BL: Behavior of the litter runt, *Feline Pract* 4(5):14–15,1974.
45. Hart BL: Handling and restraint of the cat, *Feline Pract* 5(2):10–11, 1975.
46. Hart BL: Sleeping behavior, *Feline Pract* 7(4):8–10, 1977.
47. Hart BL: The client asks you: a quiz on feline behavior, *Feline Pract* 8(2):10–13, 1978.
48. Hart BL, Voith VL: Changes in urine spraying, feeding and sleep behavior of cats following medial preoptic-anterior hypothalamic lesions, *Brain Res* 145:406–409, 1978.
49. Heidenberger E: Housing conditions and behavioural problems of indoor cats as assessed by their owners, *Appl Anim Behav Sci* 52(3,4):345–364, 1997.
50. Hein A: Prerequisite for development of visually guided reaching in the kitten, *Brain Res* 71:259–263, May 17, 1974.
51. Hein A, Diamond RM: Locomotory space as a prerequisite for acquiring visually guided reaching in kittens, *J Comp Physiol Psychol* 8:394–398, 1972.
52. Hein A, Held R: Dissociation of the visual placing response into elicited and guided components, *Science* 158:390–392, Oct 20, 1967.
53. Held R, Hein A: Movement-produced stimulation in the development of visually guided behavior, *J Comp Physiol Psychol* 56(5):872–876, 1963.
54. Hendricks JC: Abnormal sleep in pets, *Mod Vet Pract* 64(6):458–462, 1983.
55. Hendricks JC, Lager A, O'Brien D, Morrison AR: Movement disorders during sleep in cats and dogs, *J Am Vet Med Assoc* 194(5):686–689, 1989.
56. Hendricks JC, Morrison AR: Normal and abnormal sleep in mammals, *J Am Vet Med Assoc* 178(2):121–126, 1981.
57. Hendricks JC, Morrison AR, Farnbach GL, et al: A disorder of rapid eye movement sleep in a cat, *J Am Vet Med Assoc* 178(1):55–57, 1981.
58. Hildebrand M: How animals run, *Sci Am* 202:148–157, May 1960.
59. Hildebrand M: Analysis of tetrapod gaits: general considerations and symmetrical gaits. In: Herman RM, Grillner S, Stein PSG, Stuart DG, editors: *Neural control of locomotion,* New York, 1976, Plenum Publishing.
60. Houpt KA: Transforming an outdoor cat into an indoor cat, *Vet Med* 95(11):830, 2000.
61. Houpt KA, Wolski TR: *Domestic animal behavior for veterinarians and animal scientists,* Ames, 1982, Iowa State University Press.
62. Internal gyroscope helps cats land on their feet following falls, *DVM* 19(2):76, Feb 1988.
63. Jacobs BL, Trulson ME, Stern WC: An animal behavior model for studying the actions of LSD and related hallucinogens, *Science* 194:741–743, Nov 12, 1976.
64. Jenkins TW: *Functional mammalian neuroanatomy,* Philadelphia, 1972, Lea & Febiger.
65. Johnson LN: Design of the master hunter, *Cat Fancy* 16:23, 24, 26, 27, 59, Dec 1973.
66. Jones RJ: Hyperthyroidism in the cat, *Pulse* 22:14, Nov 1980.
67. Jouvet M: The states of sleep, *Sci Am* 216:62–72, Feb 1967.
68. Jouvet M: Neurophysiology of the states of sleep, *Physiol Rev* 47:117–177, April 1967.
69. Khanna C, Bienzle D: Polycythemia vera in a cat: bone marrow culture in erythropoietin-deficient medium, *J Am Anim Hosp Assoc* 30(1):45–49, 1994.
70. Kim C, Choi H, Kim CC, et al: Effect of hippocampectomy on sleep patterns in cats, *Electroencephalogr Clin Neurophysiol* 38(3):235–243, 1975.

71. Kim C, Choi H, Kim JK, et al: Sleep pattern of hippocampectomized cat, *Brain Res* 29(2):223–236, 1971.

72. Klemm WR: Neurophysiologic studies of the immobility reflex ("animal hypnosis"), *Neurosci Res* 4:165–212, 1971.

73. Kling A, Kovach JK, Tucker TJ: The behavior of cats. In Hafez ESE, editor: *The behavior of domestic animals,* ed 2, Baltimore, 1969, Williams & Wilkins.

74. Knecht CD, Oliver JE, Redding R, et al: Narcolepsy in a dog and a cat, *J Am Vet Med Assoc* 162(12):1052–1053, 1973.

75. Kolata RJ, Kraut NH, Johnston DE: Patterns of trauma in urban dogs and cats: a study of 1,000 cases, *J Am Vet Med Assoc* 164(5):499–502,1974.

76. Lancel M: Cortical and subcortical EEG in relation to sleep-wake behavior in mammalian species, *Neuropsychobiology* 28(3):154–159, 1993.

77. Langworthy OR: Histological development of cerebral motor areas in young kittens correlated with their physiological reaction to electrical stimulation, *Contrib Embryol* 19:177–207, 1927.

78. Langworthy OR: A correlated study of the development of reflex activity in fetal and young kittens and the myelinization of tracts in the nervous system, *Contrib Embryol* 20:127–172, 1929.

79. Levine MS, Hull CD, Buchwald NA, Villablanca JR: Effects of caudate nuclei or frontal cortical ablations in kittens: motor activity and visual discrimination performance in neonatal and juvenile kittens, *Exp Neurol* 62(3):555–569, 1978.

80. Lorincz E, Fabre-Thorpe M: Effect of practice on paw preference in a reaching task in cats, *C R Acad Sci III* 317(12):1081–1088, 1994.

81. Lorincz E, Fabre-Thorpe M: Shift of laterality and compared analysis of paw performances in cats during practice of a visuomotor task, *J Comp Psychol* 110(3):307–315, 1996.

82. Lucas EA: Effects of five to seven days of sleep deprivation produced by electrical stimulation of the midbrain reticular formation, *Exp Neurol* 49:554–568, Nov 1975.

83. Lucas EA, Sterman MB: The polycyclic sleep-wake cycle in the cat: effects produced by sensorimotor rhythm conditioning, *Exp Neurol* 42:347–368, 1974.

84. Luescher A: Compulsive behavior in companion animals. In Houpt KA, editor: Recent advances in companion animal behavior problems, International Veterinary Information Service. Available at www.ivis.org.

85. Luescher UA: Conflict, stereotypic and compulsive behavior. Paper presented at American Veterinary Medical Association meeting, San Francisco, July 9, 1994.

86. Luescher UA, McKeown DB, Halip J: Stereotypic or obsessive-compulsive disorders in dogs and cats, *Vet Clin North Am Small Anim Pract* 21(2):401–413, 1991.

87. Mancia M: Electrophysiological and behavioral changes owing to splitting of the brain-stem in cats, *Electroencephalogr Clin Neurophysiol* 27(5):487–502,1969.

88. Manter JT: The dynamics of quadrupedal walking, *J Exp Biol* 15:522–540, Oct 1938.

89. Martin P, Bateson P: Behavioural development in the cat. In Turner DC, Bateson PPG, editors: *The domestic cat: the biology of its behaviour,* Cambridge, 1988, Cambridge University Press.

90. McDonald D: How does a cat fall on its feet? *New Scientist* 7:1647–1649, June 30, 1960.

91. McKeown DB, Luescher UA, Halip J: Stereotypies in companion animals and obsessive-compulsive disorder, behavior problems in small animals, *Purina Specialty Review* pp 30–35, 1992.

92. Miller S, Van Der Burg J, Van Der Meche FGA: Locomotion in the cat: basic programmes of movement, *Brain Res* 91:239–253, 1975.

93. Morrison AR: A window on the sleeping brain, *Sci Am* 248:94–102, April 1983.

94. Morrison AR: Contributions of animal models to sleep disorders medicine, *Lab Anim* 25(2):22, 23, 26–28, 1996.
95. Morrison AR, Mann GL, Hendricks JC: The relationship of excessive exploratory behavior in wakefulness to paradoxical sleep without atonia, *Sleep* 4(3):247–257, 1981.
96. Moruzzi G: Sleep and instinctive behavior, *Arch Ital Biol* 107:175–216, July 1969.
97. Nothwanger C, Reisner I, Hunthausen W: Counter attack, *Vet Forum* 22, June 1994.
98. Orlovsky GN, Shik ML: Control of locomotion: a neurophysiological analysis of the cat locomotor system. In Porter R, editor: *International review of physiology*, vol 10, Baltimore, 1976, University Park Press.
99. Overall KL: Understanding repetitive, stereotypic behaviors: signs, history, diagnosis, and practical treatment. Paper presented at American Veterinary Medical Association meeting, July 8, 1995.
100. Palmer C: Interpositus and fastigial unit activity during sleep and waking in the cat, *Electroencephalogr Clin Neurophysiol* 46(4):357–370, 1979.
101. Panaman R: Behaviour and ecology of free-ranging female farm cats (*Felis catus* L.), *Z Tierpsychol* 56:59–73, 1981.
102. Parmeggiani PL, Cianci T, Calasso M, et al: Quantitative analysis of short term deprivation and recovery of desynchronized sleep in cats, *Electroencephalogr Clin Neurophysiol* 50:293–302, 1980.
103. Paul A: Glucocorticoid therapy in cats, *J Am Vet Med Assoc* 179(2):158, 1981.
104. Pierce JH: Disturbed equilibrium in small animals, *Mod Vet Pract* 49:32–35, Oct 1968.
105. Porkka-Heiskanen T, Strecker RE, Thakkar M, et al: Adenosine: a mediator of the sleep-inducing effects of prolonged wakefulness, *Science* 276:1265–1268, May 23, 1997.
106. Rapoport JL, Ryland DH, Kriete M: Drug treatment of canine acral lick: an animal model of obsessive-compulsive disorder, *Arch Gen Psychiatry* 49:517–521, July 1992.
107. Rheingold HL, Eckerman CO: Familiar social and nonsocial stimuli and the kitten's response to a strange environment, *Dev Psychobiol* 4:71–89, 1971.
108. Riesen AH, Aarons L: Visual movement and intensity discrimination in cats after early deprivation of pattern vision, *J Comp Physiol Psychol* 52(2):142–149, 1959.
109. Robinson GW: The high rise trauma syndrome in cats, *Feline Pract* 6(5):40–43, 1976.
110. Rosenblatt JS: Suckling and home orientation in the kitten: a comparative developmental study. In Tobach E, Aronson LR, Shaw E, editors: *The biopsychology of development*, New York, 1971 Academic Press.
111. Rosenblatt JS: Learning in newborn kittens, *Sci Am* 227:18–25, 1972.
112. Ruckebusch Y, Gaujoux M: Sleep patterns of the laboratory cat, *Electroencephalogr Clin Neurophysiol* 41:483–490, Nov 1976.
113. Sawyer DC: Pain control in small-animal patients, *Appl Anim Behav Sci* 59(1–3):135–146, 1998.
114. Scheibel M, Scheibel A: Some structural and functional substrates of development in young cats, *Progr Brain Res* 9:6–25, 1964.
115. Schmidt JP: Psychosomatics in veterinary medicine. In Fox MW, editor: *Abnormal behavior in animals*, Philadelphia, 1968, WB Saunders.
116. Schneirla TC, Rosenblatt JS, Tobach E: Maternal behavior in the cat. In Rheingold HL, editor: *Maternal behavior in mammals*, New York, 1963, John Wiley and Sons.
117. Shimazu H, Precht W: Tonic and kinetic responses of cat's vestibular neurons to horizontal angular acceleration, *J Neurophysiol* 28:991–1013, Nov 1965.
118. Smith BA, Jansen GR: Early undernutrition and subsequent behavior patterns in cat, *J Nutr* 103(7):29, 1973.
119. Smith BA, Jansen GR: Behavior and brain composition of offspring of underfed cats, *Fed Proc* 36:1108, 1977.

120. Smith RC: *The complete cat book*, New York, 1963, Walker & Co.
121. Sprague JM, Chambers WW, Stellar E: Attentive, affective, and adaptive behavior in the cat, *Science* 133(3447):165–173, 1961.
122. Sterman MB, Knauss T, Lehmann D, Clemente CD: Circadian sleep and waking patterns in the laboratory cat, *Electroencephalogr Clin Neurophysiol* 19:509–517, 1965.
123. Tan Ü: Inverse correlation between right-paw use and body weight in right-pawed male cats and left-pawed female cats, *Int J Neurosci* 67(1–4):119–123, 1992.
124. Tan Ü, Kara I, Tan S: Lithium and imipramine effects on paw preference in cats, *Int J Neurosci* 52(1–2):25–28, 1990.
125. Tan Ü, Kara IL, Kutlu N: The effects of testosterone on paw preference in adult cats, *Int J Neurosci* 56(1–4):187–191, 1991.
126. Tan Ü, Kutlu N: The distribution of paw preference in right-, left-, and mixed pawed male and female cats: the role of a female right-shift factor in handedness, *Int J Neurosci* 59(4):219–229, 1991.
127. Tan Ü, Kutlu N: The relationships between paw preference and the right- and left-brain weights in male and female adult cats: ipsilateral and contralateral motor control with regard to asymmetric postural and manipulative actions, *Int J Neurosci* 69(1–4):21–34, 1993.
128. Tan Ü, Kutlu N: The role of right- and left-brain weights in cerebral lateralization of right- and left-pawed male and female cats, *Int J Neurosci* 68(3–4):185–193, 1993.
129. Tan Ü, Yaprak M, Kutlu N: Paw preference in cats: distribution and sex differences, *Int J Neurosci* 50(3–4):195–208, 1990.
130. Tilney F, Casamajor L: Myelinogeny as applied to the study of behavior, *Arch Neurol Psychiatry* 12:1–66, July 1924.
131. Turner DC, Meister O: Hunting behaviour of the domestic cat. In Turner DC, Bateson P, editors: *The domestic cat: the biology of its behaviour*, Cambridge, 1988, Cambridge University Press.
132. Ulrsin R: Sleep stage relations within the sleep cycles of the cat, *Brain Res* 20:91–97, May 20, 1970.
133. van Hof-van Duin J: Development of visuomotor behavior in normal and dark reared cats, *Brain Res* 104:233–241, March 12, 1976.
134. Villablanca JR, Olmstead CE: Neurological development of kittens, *Dev Psychobiol* 12:101–127, 1979.
135. Vogel GW: A review of REM sleep deprivation, *Arch Gen Psychiatry* 32(6):749–761, 1975.
136. Voith VL, Marder AR: Feline behavioral disorders. In Morgan R, editor: *Handbook of small animal practice*, New York, 1988, Churchill Livingstone.
137. Walk RD: The study of visual depth and distance perception in animals. In Lehrman DS, Hinde RA, Shaw E, editors: *Advances in the study of behavior*, vol 1, New York, 1965, Academic Press.
138. Wallach MB, Gershon S: The induction and antagonism of central nervous system stimulant-induced stereotyped behavior in the cat, *Eur J Pharmacol* 18(1):22–26, 1972.
139. Wand P, Prochazka A, Sontag K-H: Neuromuscular responses to gait perturbations in freely moving cats, *Exp Brain Res* 38(1):109–114, 1980.
140. Warkentin J, Carmichael L: A study of the development of the air righting reflex in cats and rabbits, *J Genet Psychol* 55:67–80, 1939.
141. Warren JM, Abplanalp JM, Warren HB: The development of handedness in cats and rhesus monkeys. In Stevenson HW, Hess EH, Rheingold HL, editors: *Early behavior, comparative and developmental approaches*, New York, 1967, John Wiley and Sons.
142. Warren JM, Cornwell PR, Webster WG, Pubols BH: Unilateral cortical lesions and paw preferences in cats, *J Comp Physiol Psychol* 81:410–422, Dec 1972.

143. Weed LH, Lanworthy OR: Physiological study of cortical motor areas in young kittens and in adult cats, *Contrib Embryol* 17:89–106, 1926.

144. West M: Social play in the domestic cat, *Am Zool* 14:427–436, Winter 1974.

145. Wetzel MC: Independently controlled EMG responses in treadmill locomotion by cats, *Am J Phys Med* 60:292–310, 1981.

146. Wetzel MC: Operant control and cat locomotion, *Am J Phys Med* 61:11–25, Feb 1982.

147. Whitney WO, Mehlhaff CJ: High-rise syndrome in cats, *J Am Vet Med Assoc* 191(11):1399–1403, 1987.

148. Wiepkema PR: Developmental aspects of motivated behavior in domestic animals, *J Anim Sci* 65:1220–1227, 1987.

149. Windle WF, Fish MW: The development of the vestibular righting reflex in the cat, *J Comp Neurol* 54(1):85–96, 1932.

150. Windle WF, Griffin AM: Observations on embryonic and fetal movements of the cat, *J Comp Neurol* 52(1):149–188, 1931.

151. Windle WF, O'Donnell JE, Glasshagle EE: The early development of spontaneous and reflex behavior in cat embryos and fetuses, *Physiol Zool* 6:521–541, Oct 1932.

152. Wood GL: *Animal facts and feats,* Garden City, NJ, 1972, Doubleday.

153. Würbel H, Stauffacher M: Prevention of stereotypy in laboratory mice: effects on stress physiology and behaviour, *Physiol Behav* 59(6):1163–1170, 1996.

154. Zoran DL, Boeckh A, Boothe DM: Hyperactivity and alopecia associated with ingestion of valproic acid in a cat, *J Am Vet Med Assoc* 218(10):1587–1589, 2001.

ADDITIONAL READINGS

AAHA's fourth annual pet survey looks at human animal bond, *Trends* 11(2):30–31, 1995.

Abraham LD, Marks WB, Loeb GE: The distal hindlimb musculature of the cat: cutaneous reflexes during locomotion, *Exp Brain Res* 58(3):594–603, 1985.

Alstermark B, Wessberg J: Timing of postural adjustment in relation to forelimb target-reaching in cats, *Acta Physiol Scand* 125:337–340, Oct 1985.

Anand BK: Nervous regulation of food intake, *Physiol Rev* 41:677–708, Oct 1961.

Ángyán L: Sleep induced by hypothalamic self-stimulation in cat, *Physiol Behav* 12(4):697–701, 1974.

Baust W, Böhmke J, Blossfeld U: Somato-sympathetic reflexes during natural sleep and wakefulness in unrestrained cats, *Exp Brain Res* 12(4):361–369, 1971.

Beadle M: *The cat: history, biology, and behavior,* New York, 1977, Simon & Schuster.

Beaver BV: Reflex development in the kitten, *Appl Anim Ethol* 4(1):93, 1978.

Beyer C, Almanza J, De La Torre L, Guznan-Flores C: Brain stem multi-unit activity during "relaxation" behavior in the female cat, *Brain Res* 29(2):213–222, 1971.

Bogen JE, Suzuki M, Campbell B: Paw contact playing in the hypothalamic cat given caffeine, *J Neurobiol* 6(1):125–127, 1975.

Bradshaw JL: Animal asymmetry and human heredity: dextrality, tool use and language in evolution—10 years after Walker (1980), *Br J Psychol* 82(1):39–59, 1991.

Burgess JW, Villablanca JR: Recovery of function after neonatal or adult hemispherectomy in cats. II. Limb bias and development, paw usage, locomotion and rehabilitative effects of exercise, *Behav Brain Res* 20(1):1–17, 1986.

Camuti LJ: Cat ahoy! *Feline Pract* 4(3):50, 1974.

DeLahunta A: *Veterinary neuroanatomy and clinical neurology,* Philadelphia, 1977, WB Saunders.

Dowd PJ: Effects of congenital feline cerebellar hypoplasia on developmental behavior and the vestibular system, *J Psychol* 62:89–97, 1966.

English AWM: An electromyographic analysis of forelimb muscles during overground stepping in the cat, *J Exp Biol* 76:105–122, Oct 1978.

Ewer RF: *The carnivores,* Ithaca, NY, 1973, Cornell University Press.

Goslow GE Jr, Reinking RM, Stuart DG: The cat step cycle: hind limb joint angles and muscle lengths during unrestrained locomotion, *J Morphol* 141(1):1–41, 1973.

Halbertsma JM: The stride cycle of the cat: the modelling of locomotion by computerized analysis of automatic recordings, *Acta Physiol Scand* 521:1–75, 1983.

Hall VE, Pierce GN: Litter size, birth weight and growth to weaning in the cat, *Anat Rec* 60:111–124, 1934.

Hart BL: Behavioral aspects of selecting a new cat, *Feline Pract* 6(5):8, 10, 14, 1976.

Hart BL, Voith VL: Sexual behavior and breeding problems in cats, *Feline Pract* 7(1):9, 10, 12, 1977.

Hemmer H: Gestation period and postnatal development in felids. In Eaton RL, editor: *The world's cats,* ed 3, Seattle, 1976, Carnivore Research Institute.

Jalowiec JE, Panksepp J, Shabshelowitz H, et al: Suppression of feeding in cats following 2-deoxy-D-glucose, *Physiol Behav* 10(4):805–807, 1973.

Johnson DL: Venipuncture in unrestrained cats, *Lab Anim* 10(7):35–38, 1981.

Kemp IR, Kaada BR: The relation of hippocampal theta activity to arousal, attentive behavior and somato-motor movements in unrestrained cats, *Brain Res* 95(2–3):323–342, 1975.

Kilham L, Margolis G, Colby ED: Cerebellar ataxia and its congenital transmission in cats by feline panleukopenia virus, *J Am Vet Med Assoc* 158(6):888–900, 1971.

Koepke JE, Pribram KH: Effect of milk on the maintenance of sucking behavior in kittens from birth to six months, *J Comp Physiol Psychol* 75(3):363–377, 1971.

Konrad KW, Bagshaw M: Effect of novel stimuli on cats reared in a restricted environment, *J Comp Physiol Psychol* 70:157–164, Jan 1970.

Langworthy OR: Behavior disturbances related to the decomposition of reflex activity caused by cerebral injury: an experimental study of the cat, *J Neuropathol Exp Neurol* 3:87–100, 1944.

Lockard DE, Traher LM, Wetzel MC: Reinforcement influences upon topography of treadmill locomotion by cats, *Physiol Behav* 16(2):141–146, 1976.

Meier GW: Infantile handling and development in Siamese kittens, *J Comp Physiol Psychol* 54:284–286, June 1961.

Munk MHJ, Roelfsema PR, König P, et al: Role of reticular activation in the modification of intracortical synchronization, *Science* 272(5259):271–274, 1996.

Munson JB: Multi-unit activity with eye movements during fast-wave sleep in cats, *Exp Neurol* 37:446–450, Nov 1972.

Orem J, Lydic R: Upper airway function during sleep and wakefulness: experimental studies on normal and anesthetized cats, *Sleep* 1(1):49–68, 1978.

Podberscek AL, Blackshaw JK, Beattie AW: The behaviour of laboratory colony cats and their reactions to a familiar and unfamiliar person, *Appl Anim Behav Sci* 31(1–2):119–130, 1991.

Prinz PAN: Pharmacological alterations of patterns of sleep and wakefulness in the cat, *Diss Abstr Int* 30:3794B-3795B, 1969.

Scott PP: Diet and other factors affecting the development of young felids. In Eaton RL, editor: *The world's cats,* ed 3, Seattle, 1976, Carnivore Research Institute.

Skoglund S: On the postnatal development of postural mechanisms as revealed by electromyography and myography in decerebrate kittens, *Acta Physiol Scand* 49(4):299–317, 1960.

Steriade M: Arousal: revisiting the reticular activating system, *Science* 272(5259): 225–226, 1996.

Suzuki J, Cohen B: Integration of semicircular canal activity, *J Neurophysiol* 29(6):981–995, 1966.

Tan Ü, Kutlu N: Asymmetrical relationships between the right and left heights of the sylvian end points in right- and left-pawed male and female cats: similarities with planum temporale asymmetries in human brain, *Int J Neurosci* 67(1–4):81–91, 1992.

Troncone LRP, Tufik S: Effects of selective adrenoceptor agonists and antagonists on aggressive behavior elicited by apomorphine, DL-DOPA and fusaric acid in REM-sleep–deprived rats, *Physiol Behav* 50(1):173–178, 1991.

Udo M, Matsukawa K, Kamei H: Hyperflexion and changes in interlimb coordination of locomotion induced by cooling of the cerebellar intermediate cortex in normal cats, *Brain Res* 166(2):504–408, 1979.

Velluti R, Velluti JC, García-Austt E: Cerebellum PO_2 and the sleep-waking cycle in cats, *Physiol Behav* 18(1):19–23, 1977.

Wada N: Effects of lesions of nucleus raphe magnus on behavior of the cat, *Jpn J Vet Sci* 52(3):643–644, 1990.

Warkentin J, Smith KU: The development of visual acuity in the cat, *J Genet Psychol* 50:371–399, 1937.

Watt DGD: Effect of vertical linear acceleration on H-reflex in decerebrate cat. I. Transient stimuli, *J Neurophysiol* 45(4):644–655, 1981.

Weigel I: Small cats and clouded leopards. In Grzimek HCB, editor: *Grzimek's animal life encyclopedia,* vol 12, New York, 1975, Van Nostrand Reinhold.

Widdowson EM: Food, growth and development in the suckling period. In Graham-Jones O, editor: *Canine and feline nutritional requirements,* New York, 1965, Pergamon Press.

Wilson M, Warren JM, Abbott L: Infantile stimulation, activity and learning by cats, *Child Dev* 36:843–853, Dec 1965.

Winterkorn JMS, Meikle TH Jr: Lesions of the tectospinal tract of the cat do not produce compulsive circling, *Brain Res* 190(2):597–600, 1980.

Worden AN: Abnormal behavior in the dog and cat, *Vet Rec* 71:966–978, Dec 26, 1959.

Zajac FE, Zomlefer MR, Levine WS: Hindlimb muscular activity, kinetics and kinematics of cats jumping to their maximum achievable heights, *J Exp Biol* 91:73–86, April 1981.

Zielinski C: Carpet runners keep cats away, *Vet Med* 93(12):1047, 1998.

10

Feline Grooming Behavior

The various grooming behaviors are important to a normal healthy cat. The lack of these behaviors can indicate depression or ill health. Their absence may also signal the potential for ectoparasite infestation or secondary conditions.

GROOMING FUNCTIONS

Newborn kittens depend on the dam for grooming, especially during the first few days of life. Her licking not only conditions their coats but also stimulates urination and defecation until the young are physically able to move to a special area to eliminate. This reflex control of eliminations keeps both the nest and the kittens clean. As motor skills mature, the kittens begin self-grooming, but it is incomplete and awkward at first.

As the cat matures, grooming becomes increasingly significant, until up to 50% of the awake time, or 15% of a 24-hour period, is spent performing some type of this behavior.[18,22,32] Variations do exist, probably as a result of early experience, genetic factors, and hair coat, with long hair needing more attention.

Grooming serves several purposes, with the most important probably being maintenance of healthy skin. Body hygiene is apparently learned early, because kittens that are not well cared for develop into unkempt adults more often than those with normal histories. Although hair is shed by normal cats year-round, losses are heaviest in the spring, when the cat is ill, or when it is staying in dry indoor heat. The hair between the eye and ear is normally thinner than that on other parts of the body but during shedding may almost disappear. Siamese cats may appear to almost lose their mask.[10] Removal of loose hair is necessary to keep the coat unmatted and free from dander. Grooming is also important to minimize ectoparasite infestations. In a flea-infested environment, prevention of oral grooming will result in twice the number of fleas and a scratch grooming frequency seven times higher than in a control group.[17]

In hot weather, as much as one third of the cat's evaporative cooling losses can be achieved by licking the skin and hair.[22] Another function of grooming is that of an affiliative behavior between two cats. Last, it can relieve tension, as may occur after a reprimand from the owner, after an encounter with a very aggressive cat, or preceding a thunderstorm.[21] Some evidence suggests static electricity may build in the cat's fur, so licking would also tend to defuse the charge and the tension.

GROOMING PATTERNS

Each type of grooming has an appetitive and a consummatory phase. The former phase is made up of the orienting components that direct the animal's attention to the affected body surface. The consummatory phase completes the response and consists of the lick, bite, or scratch.[51] Normal tactile stimulation to the cat's body results in either grooming of the region, or more commonly, no response.[51]

Oral Grooming

The cat grooms much of its body with its tongue or teeth. Licking as a form of grooming usually appears near the beginning of the kitten's second week with attempts at licking the forepaw. Within a few days, the kitten is licking the rest of its body. The caudally directed, well-developed lingual papillae are particularly suited for this form of grooming.

Oral grooming most often occurs after periods of rest or sleep.[18] It also occurs after eating, when a cat spends considerable time grooming by licking, particularly around the oral area. Direct licking is useful from the caudal to the midcervical area of the body (Figure 10-1). To reach various areas, the cat can assume some very unusual positions (Figure 10-2). The anogenital area is groomed after mating and during normal grooming periods. Oral grooming will involve multiple body areas 91% of the time and typically progresses from cranial toward caudal.[18] If a cat is prohibited from grooming for 72 hours, a 67% increase in oral grooming will be seen during the next 12 hours.[18]

The incisors are useful for pulling burrs and tangles out of the hair coat and are often used to clean between the toes. As would be expected, this type of grooming is most effective for the body caudal to the neck (see Figure 10-1).

It has been suggested that feline oral grooming, particularly through licking, could be a useful tool in evaluating the environment.[34] The cat's metabolic concentrations of pollutants gathered by grooming serve as sentinels of public health.

Paw Grooming

Areas that cannot be groomed directly by the mouth are cared for using either forepaws or hindpaws (see Figure 10-1). Because the head and neck are so difficult to care for, problems are more numerous in these areas.[22] The common form of grooming that follows eating, which is second only to licking, is use of the forepaw as a washing tool. The paw is licked several times (Figure 10-3), and then its medial side is wiped across the neck, the back of the head and ears, and finally the face (Figure 10-4). Often the head and neck are moved to accommodate this action. After every few swipes the cat again licks its paw. The young kitten usually begins this forepaw-washing behavior before it is 4 weeks of age.

Scratching various parts of the body with a hindpaw begins about 18 days after birth (see Appendix D). As in paw washing, the areas most often scratched are those that

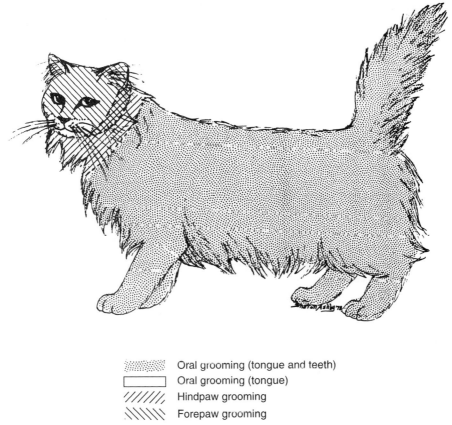

░░░░░	Oral grooming (tongue and teeth)
▭	Oral grooming (tongue)
//////	Hindpaw grooming
\\\\\	Forepaw grooming

Figure 10-1 Areas groomed in various manners by the cat.

cannot be licked, particularly the neck and auricular areas (see Figure 10-1). Scratch grooming is usually directed toward single regions and usually occupies only about 2% of the amount of time devoted to oral grooming.[18] If prevented from scratching itself for several days, a cat will show an increase of 200% in the amount of scratching during the first 12 hours it is permitted.[18]

The cat conditions its claws by scratching favorite objects, usually near its sleeping quarters, or by chewing off the frayed and worn parts (see Figure 3-16). Scratching usually grooms the thoracic claws, and claws on the pelvic limbs are primarily cared for by the teeth.

Mutual Grooming

Ancestors of the cat were not particularly social animals, so they did not have well-defined social behavior patterns. When two cats are together by mutual agreement, it is common for one to lick or rub against the other. Allogrooming involves one cat licking another. This type of mutual, or social, grooming usually involves the head and neck, the most difficult places for which to care (Figure 10-5). Females will groom other

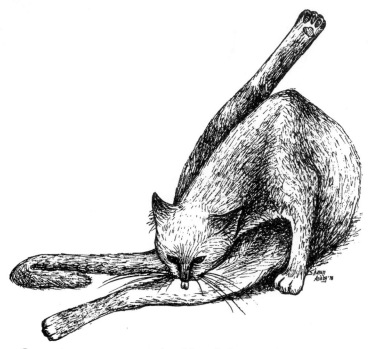

Figure 10-2 Cats can assume some unusual positions during grooming sessions.

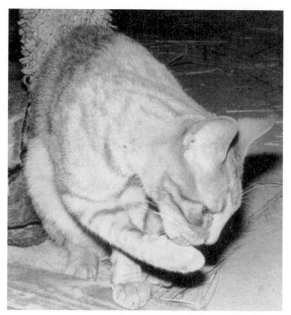

Figure 10-3 The licking of the forepaw before using it as a washing tool.

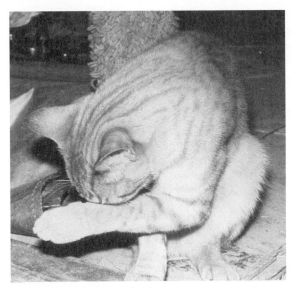

Figure 10-4 The forepaw is used to groom facial areas.

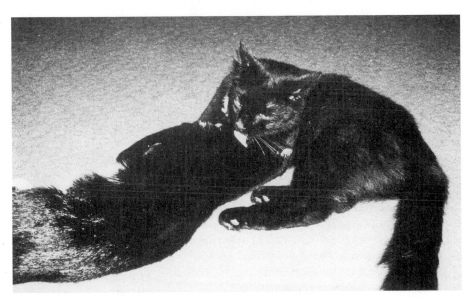

Figure 10-5 Mutual grooming of one cat by another.

females and males, whereas males will groom only females.[3] Cats, including queens grooming their kittens, have been known to chew off another's tactile hairs during a mutual grooming session.[10,19] Beginning at a few weeks of age, social behavior tends to reach a peak when the kitten is between 5 weeks and 4 months.[55] After that time, the frequency of the mutual grooming sessions decreases.

Allorubbing usually involves one cat rubbing its head against the head or body of another cat, although the entire body could be used, not just the head. Female cats will allorub males more than males show the behavior to females.[3] Females will also rub males more often than other females, to the point that in homes with only female cats, allorubbing is rarely to never observed.[3] It has also been noted that an individual cat may rub another disproportionately more or less than is expected at random.[12] It is theorized that mutual rubbing facilitates the regular exchange of body odors. This will familiarize cats with each other and gradually result in a group odor.[12]

Mutual grooming can be extended to humans by licking them and accepting their petting. Most cats patiently accept a prolonged session of caressing, probably because they have no built-in mechanism to limit it.[20] In nature, one cat spends only a limited amount of time grooming another cat, and the receiver becomes almost immobile. Humans often extend this grooming session well beyond the normal length of time, and the cat usually accommodates them by not moving.

Displacement Grooming

When a cat is in a conflict or stressful situation, it may appear ready to react but instead suddenly stops and performs an act that is out of context with the situation at hand, such as licking a paw and rubbing it across its face. Those are displacement activities. Presumably, this behavior reduces anxiety. A queen with kittens may increase her grooming of the young or of her own perineal and mammary regions during stress. If reprimanded for some behavior, a cat will often react by walking a distance away, then grooming. Cats that roll over and accidentally slide off a table or chair also respond with a grooming session, usually after glancing around the room.

NEUROENDOCRINE AND GROOMING RELATIONSHIPS

Central controls of grooming behavior are not completely understood but are related to the pontine area of the brain and may be the same as for locomotion.[14] When lesions are created in this location, a dissociation develops between the appetitive and consummatory phases of grooming.[37,47] This abnormality is exhibited as an immediate response to a tactile stimulus that is independent of the appetitive component. Thus although the response is appropriate, the orientation may be poorly directed. For example, touching the ear might produce midair scratching movements.[35,51] Similar abortive grooming has been observed with frontal neocortical lesions.[26,47–49] In both cases, tryptophan hydroxylase levels of the rostral colliculi decrease, indicating a relationship between this area of the mesencephalon and grooming behavior.[48,49]

Serotonin is the neurotransmitter currently receiving the most attention because it can be affected by several popular drugs. Serotonin has not been linked to normal grooming behavior.[25] It has been shown, however, that a cat's chewing or licking behavior can activate serotonin.[25]

Thyroid hormones and glucocorticoids play a role in central control of grooming behavior, although the exact mechanism is uncertain. Thyroidectomized cats show the reduced tryptophan levels in the rostral colliculi, but the relationship between these two situations is not understood.[51]

Hallucinogenic drugs can produce dissociated grooming. The body is positioned properly, but licking, biting, or scratching either does not occur or is poorly directed.[24]

Circadian rhythms are difficult to identify, but studies of fragmented grooming behaviors have provided evidence that such cycles exist in the cat. Body temperature, caloric intake, and abnormal grooming activity fluctuate in 3- to 4-month periods, peaking in October or November and in June, and ebbing between February and May and in August.[36,38,47,49–51]

Hormone levels affect hair coat. Castrated males show a significant tendency toward longer hair.[43] Queening, extended lactation, or both may result in hair loss, producing a thinner or shorter coat.

GROOMING BEHAVIOR PROBLEMS

Nongrooming Behavior

Stressful conditions that are emotionally upsetting to a cat can result in cessation of grooming behaviors[21,29] (see Figure 4-9). Certainly disease can be a causal factor, but so can such things as overcrowding or a new dog or child in the house. The security of a box or paper sack may be all that is needed. Older cats gradually develop an appearance suggesting they are not grooming as much. With age, salivary gland production decreases, so their tongues are less effective grooming tools. It is best to have owners brush these cats more often to assist in dead hair and dander removal.

Excessive Grooming Behavior

Nervousness, "boredom," desire for human contact, or other stresses can be expressed with forms of excessive grooming, particularly by Siamese and Abyssinian cats.[22,41] Licking is the most commonly used type of excessive grooming, and the caudal half of the body, particularly the medial thigh and ventral abdomen, is the most commonly targeted anatomic location. Groomed areas usually have well-defined borders, normal skin, and almost no hair within the area. In extreme cases, self-mutilation can result or queens may overgroom their kittens to the point of mutilation.[21] Tail chasing, flicking the tongue, shaking the head rapidly side to side, and excessive scratching of the head are other variations of this behavior.[16,53] When stress is a contributing factor, treatment involves removing or decreasing the significance of the cause.[56] This could include treating fleas, food allergies, or other causes of pruritus; minimizing visualization of stray cats; or decreasing environmental disturbances. The role of medical conditions relative to the excessive grooming must always be considered. In addition to the various causes of pruritic dermatoses to consider, a thorough physical examination would also look for impacted anal sacs and balanoposthitis.[41]

There are times when the excessive grooming continues even though the original stressor has been removed.[2] In these cats, the licking may have become a habitual, stereotypic, or even obsessive-compulsive problem.[*] In addition to environmental changes, some may need to be supplemented with anxiolytic medication—progestins, benzodiazepines,

---

[*]References 13, 16, 28, 30, 31, 41, 44.

tricyclic antidepressants, selective serotonin reuptake inhibitors, azaperone, or chlorpheniramine maleate.[31,39,54,55] Naltrexone has been used successfully in some cats that are excessively grooming.[16] This suggests that like lick granulomas in dogs, the condition might actually be complicated.[7] Most cases are probably short-term responses to a specific stressor, but a few become chronic. Some of those cats may show the behavior because of the stress relief from the endorphin release. Other individuals with chronic cases may show the behavior as a type of obsessive-compulsive disorder. The affection-craving individual should initially be given extra attention again,[8] but that attention should be made part of a strict routine that includes not rewarding the grooming behavior.

Excessive grooming may indicate involvement of the central nervous system, probably in a number of ways. Direct stimulation of the ventral hippocampus can produce reactions with emotional manifestations including restlessness, vocalizations, body postures of fear and retreat, and excessive perineal licking.[15] There is also a connection between grooming and several forms of epilepsy, an understanding of which is useful in combining several diagnoses and treatments into a more common grouping.[15] Feline leukemia apparently plays a role in the pathologic behavior of some of these cats because diagnostically positive individuals have a much lower success rate for treatment.[6,46]

A secondary problem in excessive grooming is the formation of hairballs. Because most of the hair that pulls loose during grooming sticks to the papillae of the tongue, it is eventually swallowed. If enough is ingested and not lost by normal vomiting or defecation, anorexia and generalized depression result.[22]

Feline Hyperesthesia Syndrome

The feline hyperesthesia syndrome (rolling skin syndrome, feline neurodermatitis) is another behavioral abnormality. It is exhibited by a cat suddenly rising with vertical tail and with the skin over the dorsum appearing to twitch or roll.[5,56] These have been characterized as paroxysmal agitation, focal spasms of the thoracolumbar epaxial muscles, biting at the caudal trunk and pelvic limbs, and exaggerated tail movements.[27] Then the cat howls and dashes away. Several drugs have been used in an attempt to control or cure the condition. Some include antiepileptics like phenobarbital, amitriptyline, carnitine, coenzyme-10, progestins, and steroids.* Affected cats have spontaneous electromyelographic activity from a number of sources and vacuoles in the epaxial musculature.[27] These findings are similar to those in humans diagnosed with inclusion body myositis/myopathy.[4,27] A similar startle reaction is seen with pontine and certain rostral hypothalamic lesions.[23]

Hair Loss

Generalized or localized hair loss and alopecia can occur in cats that are under severe emotional stress, especially nervous individuals and purebred animals.[11,28,40] The cat may be pulling out clumps of its own hair or the hair can fall out on its own. In contrast,

---

*References 1, 9, 27, 29, 33, 52.

localized hair loss caudal to the ears, possibly accompanied by ulceration, is a result of the vigorous scratching of this area by the hindfeet. This hair loss is generally indicative of an *Otodectes cynotis* infestation.

Skin Problems

In addition to dermatoses resulting from nongrooming, allergens, and bacteria, the cat can suffer from psychic eczema.[40] Affected individuals commonly lick excessively, producing skin trauma, until they are hospitalized, where new surroundings distract them. Lesions of cutaneous lymphedema or lymphadenic dermatitis are characteristic.

Feline-acquired skin fragility cases can be presented as cats that groom so excessively that they tear their own skin. Most of these cases have been associated with the excessive use of progestational compounds.[42]

The loss of its tongue presents many problems for the cat. Most can learn to eat soft food, but skin and coat care must be done for them.[45] Sebaceous gland secretions tend to accumulate and present the biggest challenge for the caregiver. Frequent baths become a necessity.

REFERENCES

1. Alterman HP, Hart BL, Mosier JE, Parker AJ: Use of primidone in cats questioned, *Feline Pract* 7(6):4, 6, 1977.
2. August J: Personal communication, Feb 14, 1992.
3. Barry KJ, Crowell-Davis SL: Gender differences in the social behavior of the neutered indoor-only domestic cat, *Appl Anim Behav Sci* 64(3):193–211, 1999.
4. Bartt R, Shannon KM: Autoimmune and inflammatory disorders. In Goetz CG, Pappert EJ, editors: *Textbook of clinical neurology,* Philadelphia, 1999, WB Saunders.
5. Beaver BV: Disorders of behavior. In Sherding RG, editor: *The cat: diseases and clinical management,* New York, 1989, Churchill Livingstone.
6. Beaver BV: Feline behavioral problems other than housesoiling, *J Am Anim Hosp Assoc* 25(4):465–469, 1989.
7. Beaver BV: *Canine behavior: a guide for veterinarians,* Philadelphia, 1999, WB Saunders.
8. Blackshaw JK: Management of orally based problems and aggression in cats, *Aust Vet Practit* 21(3):122–125, 1991.
9. Blum SR: Aggressive behavior, *Feline Pract* 9(2):9, 1979.
10. Bryant D: *The care and handling of cats,* New York, 1944, Ives Washburn.
11. Chertok L, Fontaine M: Psychosomatics in veterinary medicine, *J Psychosom Res* 7:229–235, 1963.
12. Crowell-Davis SL, Barry K, Wolfe R: Social behavior and aggressive problems of cats, *Vet Clin North Am Small Anim Pract* 27(3):549–568, 1997.
13. Dallaire A: Stress and behavior in domestic animals: temperament as a predisposing factor to stereotypies, *Ann N Y Acad Sci* 697:269–274, Oct 29, 1993.
14. Deliagina TG, Orlovsky GN, Perret C: Efferent activity during fictitious scratch reflex in the cat, *J Neurophysiol* 45(4):595–604, 1981.
15. Dhume RA, Gogate MG, deMascarenhas JF, Sharma KN: Functional dissociation within hippocampus: correlates of visceral and behavioral patterns induced on stimulation of ventral hippocampus in cats, *Indian J Med Res* 64(1):33–40, 1976.

16. Dodman NH: Pharmacological treatment of behavioral problems in cats, *Vet Forum* pp 62–65, 71, April 1995.
17. Eckstein R, Hart BL: Feline grooming: grooming controls fleas: fleas control grooming. Paper presented at American Veterinary Medical Association meeting, Reno, Nev, July 22, 1997.
18. Eckstein RA, Hart BL: The organization and control of grooming in cats, *Appl Anim Behav Sci* 68(2):131–140, 2000.
19. Ehrenlechner S, Unshelm J: Whisker trimming by mother cats, *Appl Anim Behav Sci* 52(3,4):381–385, 1997.
20. Ewer RF: *Ethology of mammals,* London, 1968, Paul Elek.
21. Fox MW: *Understanding your cat,* New York, 1974, Coward, McCann & Geoghegan.
22. Hart BL: The role of grooming activity, *Feline Pract* 6(4):14, 16, 1976.
23. Hart BL: Sleeping behavior, *Feline Pract* 7(4):8–10, 1977.
24. Jacobs BL, Trulson ME, Stern WC: An animal behavior model for studying the actions of LSD and related hallucinogens, *Science* 194:741–743, Nov 12, 1976.
25. Jerone R: A model of good grooming, *The Sciences* pp 5–6, Sep/Oct 1992.
26. Langworthy OR: Behavioral disturbances related to the decomposition of reflex activity caused by cerebral injury: an experimental study of the cat, *J Neuropathol Exp Neurol* 3:87–100, 1944.
27. March PA, Fischer JR, Potthoff A, et al: Electromyographic and histological abnormalities in epaxial muscles of cats with feline hyperesthesia syndrome, *Am Coll Vet Intern Med Abstracts* p 238, 1999.
28. McKeown DB, Luescher UA, Halip J: Stereotypies in companion animals and obsessive-compulsive disorder, *Behavior Problems in Small Animals, Purina Specialty Review* pp 30–35, 1992.
29. Mosier JE: Common medical and behavioral problems in cats, *Mod Vet Pract* 56(10):699–703, 1975.
30. Overall KL: Recognition, diagnosis, and management of obsessive-compulsive disorders. Part 1: A rational approach, *Can Pract* 17(2):40–44, 1992.
31. Overall KL: Rational behavior pharmacology, *The Friskies Symposium on Behavior* pp 18–28, 1996.
32. Panaman R: Behaviour and ecology of free-ranging female farm cats (*Felis catus* L.), *Z Tierpsychol* 56:59–73, 1981.
33. Parker A: Feline hyperesthesia syndrome, *Virg Vet Notes* 19:2–3, Jan/Feb 1986.
34. Priester WA: Cats are pollution sentinels, *J Am Vet Med Assoc* 160(3):341, 1972.
35. Randall W, Elbin J, Swenson RM: Biochemical changes involved in a lesion-induced behavior in the cat, *J Comp Physiol Psychol* 86(4):747–750, 1974.
36. Randall WL, Parsons V: The concomitancy in the rhythms of caloric intake and behavior in cats: a replication, *Psychom Sci* 15:35–36, 1969.
37. Randall WL, Parsons V: Thyroidectomy produces abnormal grooming behavior in cats, *Psychom Sci* 21:268–269, 1970.
38. Rogers W, Parsons V, Randall W: Consummatory grooming fragments: a model for periodic behaviors, *Psychom Sci* 23(5):375–376, 1971.
39. Sawyer LS, Moon-Fanelli AA, Dodman NH: Psychogenic alopecia in cats: 11 cases (1993–1996), *J Am Vet Med Assoc* 214(1):71–74, 1999.
40. Schmidt JP: Psychosomatics in veterinary medicine. In Fox MW, editor: *Abnormal behavior in animals,* Philadelphia, 1968, WB Saunders.
41. Schwartz S: Animal behavior case of the month, *J Am Vet Med Assoc* 208(11):1813–1814, 1996.
42. Scott DW, Miller WH Jr, Griffin CE: *Muller and Kirk's small animal dermatology,* ed 5, Philadelphia, 1995, WB Saunders.
43. Searle AG: Gene frequencies in London's cats, *J Genet* 49:214–220, Dec 1949.
44. Seksel K, Lindeman MJ: Use of clomipramine in the treatment of anxiety-related and obsessive-compulsive disorders in cats, *Aust Vet J* 76(5):317–321, 1998.

45. Stauffer VD: Loss of the tongue in a cat and the resulting skin problem, *Vet Med Small Anim Clin* 68(11):1266–1267, 1973.

46. Stein B: Personal communication, 1977.

47. Trulson ME: Biological bases for the integration of appetitive and consummatory grooming behaviors in the cat: a review, *Pharmacol Biochem Behav* 4(3):329–334, 1976.

48. Trulson ME: Role of superior colliculus serotonin in the grooming behavior of cats, *Neuropharmacology* 15(2):91–97, 1976.

49. Trulson ME, Nicolay J, Randall W: Abnormalities in grooming behavior and tryptophan hydroxylase activity in the superior colliculi in cats with pontile and frontal neocortical lesions, *Pharmacol Biochem Behav* 3(1):87–94, 1975.

50. Trulson ME, Randall W: 5-Hydroxytryptamine metabolism, superior colliculus, and grooming behavior in cats with pontile lesions, *J Comp Physiol Psychol* 85(1):1–10, 1973.

51. Trulson ME, Randall W: Similarities in the physiological bases of an abnormal grooming behavior in thyroidectomized cats and in cats with lesions of the central nervous system, *J Comp Physiol Psychol* 90(10):917–924, 1976.

52. Tuttle JL, Parker AJ: Diagnosing, treating feline hyperesthesia syndrome, *DVM* 11:72, Feb 1980.

53. van den Bos R: Post-conflict stress-response in confined group-living cats *(Felis silvestris catus)*, *Appl Anim Behav Sci* 59(4):323–330, 1998.

54. Voith VL, Marder AR: Feline behavioral disorders. In Morgan R, editor: *Handbook of small animal practice,* New York, 1988, Churchill Livingstone.

55. West M: Social play in the domestic cat, *Am Zool* 14:427–436, Winter 1974.

56. Young MS, Manning TO: Psychogenic dermatoses, *Dermatol Rep* 3:1–8, 1984.

ADDITIONAL READINGS

Beadle M: *The cat: history, biology, and behavior,* New York, 1977, Simon & Schuster.

Beaver BVG: Feline behavioral problems, *Vet Clin North Am* 6(3):333–340, 1976.

Blacklock GA: A cat's purr... on purpose? *Cat Fancy* 16:20–22, Aug 1973.

Boudreau JC, Tsuchitani C: *Sensory neurophysiology,* New York, 1973, Van Nostrand Reinhold.

Fox MW: New information on feline behavior, *Mod Vet Pract* 56(4):50–52, 1965.

Fox MW: Aggression: its adaptive and maladaptive significance in man and animals. In Fox MW, editor: *Abnormal behavior in animals,* Philadelphia, 1968, WB Saunders.

Hart BL: Behavioral aspects of scratching in cats, *Feline Pract* 2(2):6–8, 1972.

Hart BL: Social interactions between cats and their owners, *Feline Pract* 6(1): 6, 8, 1976.

Hart BL: Aggression in cats, *Feline Pract* 7(2): 22, 24, 28, 1977.

Kling A, Kovach JK, Tucker TJ: The behavior of cats. In Hafez ESE, editor: *The behavior of domestic animals,* ed 2, Baltimore, 1969, Williams & Wilkins.

Podberscek AL, Blackshaw JK, Beattie AW: The behaviour of laboratory colony cats and their reactions to a familiar and unfamiliar person, *Appl Anim Behav Sci* 31(1–2):119–130, 1991.

Randall W, Parsons V: Rhythmic dysfunctions in 11-hydroxycorticoid excretion after midbrain lesions and their relationship to an abnormal grooming behavior in cats, *J Interdiscipl Cycle Res* 3:3–24, March 1972.

Randall W, Trulson M, Parsons V: Role of thyroid hormones in an abnormal grooming behavior in thyroidectomized cats and cats with pontile lesions, *J Comp Physiol Psychol* 90(3):231–243, 1976.

Tilney F, Casamajor L: Myelinogeny as applied to the study of behavior, *Arch Neurol Psychiatry* 12:1–66, July 1924.

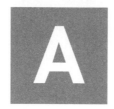

Phonetics of Feline Vocalization*

Murmur patterns
1. Grunt
2. Purr   ['hrn-rhn-'hrn-rhn...]
   a. Greeting (request)   ['mhrn]
3. Call   ['əmhrn]
4. Acknowledgement   ['mhrŋ]

Vowel patterns
1. Demand   ['mhrn-a':ou]
   a. Whisper   ['mhrn-ɛ̃']
   b. Begging demand   ['mhrn-a:ou]
2. Bewilderment   ['maou:?]
   a. Worry   ['mæ ou:?]
3. Complaint   ['mhŋ-a:ou]
4. Mating cry (mild form)   ['mhrn-a:ou]
5. Anger wail   [wa:ou:]

Strained intensity patterns
1. Growl   [grrr...]
2. Snarl   ['æ:o]
3. Hiss   ['sss...]
   a. Spit   [fft!]
4. Mating cry (intense form)   ['ø-ø':ə]
5. Scream   [æ!]
6. Refusal   ['æ^{v}'æ^{v}'æ]

Data from Moelk M: Am J Psychol 57:184–205, 1944.

KEY

[a] as in father, [æ] as in cat, [ɛ] as in get, [ə] as in momma, [o] as in go,
[ø] as in French eux, [u] as in pool, [f] as in fan, [g] as in gone, [h] as in hunt,
[m] as in mouse, [n] as in kitten, [ŋ] as in sung, [r] as in rat, [t] as in cat, [s] as in
see, [:] indicates prolongation, [~] indicates nasalization, ['] indicates stress-accent,
['] indicates inhalation, [?] indicates rising inflection, [ᶻ] indicates wavering or
discontinuity, [!] indicates abrupt, stress-accent ending.

Sensory Response Development

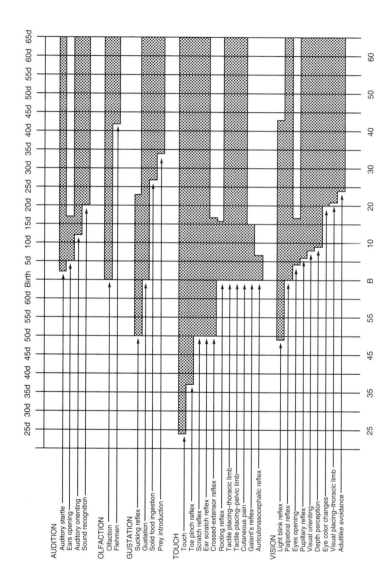

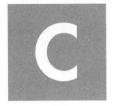

Motor Response Development

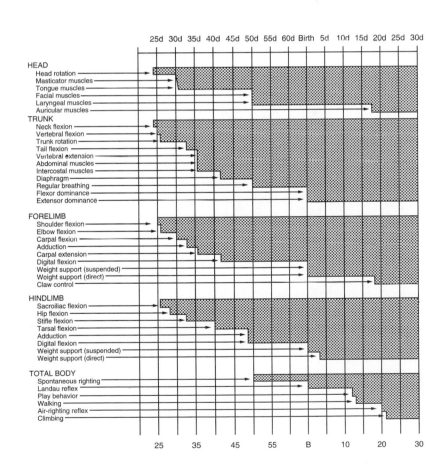

A P P E N D I X

Miscellaneous Response Development

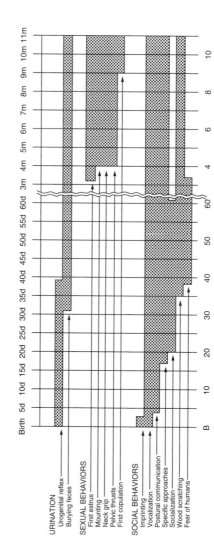

326

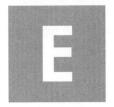

Psychopharmacologic Agents Used in Cats

(Please see Chapter 1 for Contraindications.)

Acepromazine maleate (Acepromazine)
Behavior Use: physical inhibition
Action: tranquilizer
Cat Dose: 0.5–2.0 mg/kg PO q8–36h[2]; 1–2 mg/kg PO q8h[4]; 1.1–2.2 mg/kg PO[11,17,18],
    IV, IM, SC[18]; 1–2 mg/kg PO[10]; 0.125–0.25 mg PO q12h[10]; 0.11–0.22 mg/kg IM,
    SC, IV[11,17]; 0.55–2.2 mg/kg PO[22]; 0.22–2.2 mg/kg IM, SC[22]

Alprazolam (Xanax)
Behavior Use: thunder phobias, panic attacks
Action: benzodiazepine
Cat Dose: 0.05–0.1 mg/kg PO q8h[4]; 0.1 mg/kg PO q8h or as needed[3]; 0.125–0.25 mg/kg
    PO q12h[11,16,17]

Amitriptyline HCl (Elavil, Etrafon, Limbitrol)
Behavior Use: excess grooming, separation anxiety, spraying, thunder phobias, excessive
    show-ring shyness
Action: tricyclic antidepressant (inhibits membrane pump mechanism responsible for
    uptake of norepinephrine and serotonin in adrenergic and serotonergic neurons)
Cat Dose: 0.5 mg/kg PO q12–24h[8]; 0.5–1.0 mg/kg PO q12–24h[15,21]; 0.5–2.0 mg/kg
    PO q12–24h[16]; 0.5–2.0 mg/kg PO q12–24h, start at 0.5 mg/kg PO q12h[17];
    5–10 mg PO q24h[9–12]; 5–10 mg PO q12–24h[12,20]; 2–4 mg/kg q12–24h[3]

Bethanechol Cl (Urecholine)
Behavior Use: excessive urination in females

Action: increases urinary bladder constriction (stimulates parasympathetic nervous system to increase tone on detrusor urinae muscle, resulting in initiation of micturition to empty the bladder; also increases gastric motility)

Cat Dose: 2.5–5.0 mg PO q8h[22]; 0.5–2.5 mg SC q12h[22]; 2.5–5.0 mg PO q8–12h[18]; 1.25–5.0 mg PO q8h[18]

Buspirone HCl (BuSpar)
Behavior Use: spraying, child aggression, barbering
Action: nonspecific anxiolytic, partial serotonin agonist (high affinity for serotonin receptors and moderate for D_2-dopamine brain receptors)

Cat Dose: 0.5–1.0 mg/kg PO q24h[21]; 0.5–1.0 mg/kg PO q8–12h[16,17]; 0.5–1.0 mg/kg PO q8–12–24h to 2.5–5.0 mg/cat PO q8–12–24h[15]; 0.5–2 mg/kg PO q8–12h[4]; 1 mg/kg PO q24h[12]; 2–4 mg/kg PO q12h[3]; 2.5–5.0 mg PO q8–12h[10,11]; 2.5–5.0 mg/cat PO q8–14h for 6–8 wk, some cats do well on q24h dosing[17]

Clomipramine HCl (Clomicalm, Anafranil)
Behavior Use: separation anxiety, excessive grooming, excessive compulsive behavior
Action: tricyclic antidepressant

Cat Dose: 0.4–0.7 mg/kg PO[20]; 0.5 mg/kg PO q24h[15,16,17,21]; 0.5–1.0 mg/kg PO q24h[4]; 1.0–1.5 mg/kg PO q24h[3]

Clorazepate dipotassium (Tranxene) (Schedule IV narcotic)
Behavior Use: thunder
Action: benzodiazepine

Cat Dose: 0.125–0.5 mg/kg PO q12–24h[2]; 0.2–0.4 mg/kg PO q12–24h[16,17]; 0.5–2.0 mg/kg PO prn for profound distress[16]; 0.5–2.2 mg/kg PO as needed for profound distress[17]; 0.55–2.2 mg/kg PO as needed[11]; 0.5–1.0 mg/kg q12–24h[11]

Cyproheptadine hydrochloride (Periactin)
Behavior Use: spraying cats
Action: antiserotonergic, anticholinergic, antihistaminic, sedative, also decreases serum testosterone levels

Cat Dose: 1–2 mg/cat PO q12–24h[19]

Diazepam (Valium)
Behavior Use: thunder, spraying
Action: benzodiazepine

Cat Dose: 0.05–1.0 mg/kg PO q12–24h[2]; 0.2–0.4 mg/kg PO q12–24h[16]; 0.2–0.4 mg/kg PO q12–24h, starting at 0.2 mg/kg PO q12h[17]; 0.25–1.0 mg/kg PO as needed[4]; 1–2 mg PO q12h[10,11,18]; 1–3 mg PO q12–24h[11]; 1–2 mg/kg PO q8–12h[3]; 2.5–5.0 mg PO, IV[22]

Diethylstilbestrol
Behavior Use: induction of estrus
Action: synthetic estrogen hormone

Cat Dose: 0.05–0.1 mg PO q24h or as needed[22]

Diphenhydramine (Benadryl, CJ-D, Hydramine)
Behavior Use: antianxiety
Action: sedative, antihistamine, antidepressant
Cat Dose: 4 mg/kg PO q12h[22]; 4 mg/kg PO q8h[18]; 2–4 mg/kg PO q8h[18]

Doxepin HCl (Adapin, Sinequan)
Behavior Use: excess grooming, has antipruritic action too
Action: tricyclic antidepressant
Cat Dose: 0.5–1.0 mg/kg PO q12–24h, starting low[17]

Fluoxetine (Prozac)
Behavior Use: excess grooming, compulsive behaviors, spraying
Action: selective serotonin reuptake inhibitor
Cat Dose: 0.5 mg/kg PO q24h[21]; 0.5–1.0 mg PO q24h[4,16,17]

Fluvoxamine
Behavior Use: compulsive behaviors
Action: selective serotonin reuptake inhibitor
Cat Dose: 0.25–0.5 mg/kg PO q24h[17]

Flurazepam
Behavior Use: appetite stimulant
Action: benzodiazepine
Cat Dose: 0.1–0.2 mg/kg PO q12–24h[17]

Haloperidol
Behavior Use: reduced defensive behaviors and aggression and cause sedation and muscle
    relaxation
Action: neuroleptic butyrophenones
Cat Dose: 0.25–0.5 mg/kg PO q24h[17]

Hydrocodone (Hycodan)
Behavior Use: excessive grooming
Action: phenanthrene-derivative opiate agonist structurally similar to narcotic antago-
    nists, antitussive
Cat Dose: 2.5–5.0 mg PO q12–24h[22]; 0.25–1.0 mg/kg PO q8–12h[16,17]

Imipramine HCl (Tofranil)
Behavior Use: antianxiety
Action: tricyclic antidepressant
Cat Dose: 0.5–1.0 mg/kg PO q12–24h, starting at 0.5 mg/kg PO q12h[17]

Lithium carbonate
Behavior Use: antidepressant
Cat Dose: 650–730 mg/m^2 PO[22]

Medroxyprogesterone acetate (Depo-Provera)
Behavior Use: antianxiety and antitestosterone

Action: progestin
Cat Dose: 5–10 mg/kg IM[4]; 10–20 mg/kg SC, IM[5,10,11,17]; 50 mg females, 100 mg males SC 3 times/yr[11,17]; 100 mg IM males q30d as needed[1]; 50 mg IM females q30d as needed[1]; 10–20 mg/kg SC as needed up to 3 times/yr[23]; 50–100 mg SC, repeat in 4–6 mo if needed[20]

Megestrol acetate (Ovaban, Megace)
Behavior Use: antianxiety, antitestosterone, postponement of estrus
Action: progestin
Cat Dose: 2–4 mg/kg PO q24h for 3–4 days, then q72h for 4–8 days, then twice weekly for 2–4 wk, then weekly[2]; 2.5–5.0 mg PO q24h for 7 days, then 2.5–5.0 mg/wk[10,11]; 2.5–5.0 mg PO q48h for 7–14 days, then 2.5–5.0 mg PO q7–14d[20]; 2.5–5.0 mg/cat q24h[17]; 2.5–5.0 mg/cat/wk[17]; 5–10 mg/cat PO q24h for 1 wk, then decrease to q2w to minimum effective dose[17]; 5 mg PO q24h for 7 days, then 5 mg q48h for 2 wk, then 5 mg once weekly, with 4–6 mo maximum[5]; 5–10 mg PO q24h for 1 wk, then decrease every 2 wk to minimum effective dose[11]; 2–5 mg/kg PO q24h for 1–2 wk, then reduce[4]; 2.5–5.0 mg PO q48h initially, then taper to lowest maintenance dose, weekly as needed[18]; 5 mg PO q24h for 5–7 days, then once weekly[18]; 2mg/kg PO q24h for 5 days, then 1 mg/kg q24h for 5 days, then 0.5 mg/kg q24h for 5 days[18]

Naltrexone (Trexan)
Behavior Use: stereotypies, compulsive behavior
Action: opiate antagonist
Cat Dose: 2.2 mg/kg PO q24h (up to 25–50 mg/cat)[16,17]; 25–50 mg PO q12–24h[14]; 25–50 mg PO q24h[11,13,20]

Oxazepam
Behavior Use: spraying
Action: benzodiazepine
Cat Dose: 0.2–0.5 mg/kg PO q12–24h[16,17]; 1.0–2.5 mg PO q12–24h[16,17]; 1–2 mg PO q12h[8]; 3 mg/kg PO as a bolus for appetite stimulation[17]

Paroxetine (Paxil)
Behavior Use: antidepressant, compulsive behavior, panic disorders
Action: selected serotonin reuptake inhibitor
Cat Dose: 0.5 mg/kg PO q24h[17]

Pentazocine and naloxone HCl (Talwin NX)
Behavior Use: stereotypies, compulsive behavior
Action: analgesic and partial opiate antagonist
Cat Dose: 1–3 mg/kg SC, IM, IV[22]; 2.2–3.3 mg/kg SC, IM, IV[18]

Phenobarbital
Behavior Use: tranquilizer, antiepileptic
Action: barbiturate
Cat Dose: 1 mg/kg PO q12h[18]; 2 mg/kg PO q8–12h[18]; 2–3 mg/kg IV, IM, PO as needed[11,17]; 2–4 mg/kg IV, IM, PO as needed[22]

Phenylpropanolamine HCl
Behavior Use: urination
Action: sympathomimetic amine that acts to tighten urinary bladder sphincter, antihis-
    taminic, bronchodilator
Cat Dose: 2 mg PO q12h[22]; 12.5 mg PO q8h[18]; 75 mg sustained-release capsule PO
    q24h[18]

Pindolol
Behavior Use: situational anxieties
Action: β-adrenergic receptor blocking agent
Cat Dose: 0.125–0.25 mg/kg PO q12h[4]

Promazine HCl
Behavior Use: tranquilizer
Action: propylamino phenothiazine
Cat Dose: 2–4 mg/kg PO, IM as needed[11,17]

Propranolol (Inderide, Inderal)
Behavior Use: mild thunder, fear aggression
Action: nonselective β-adrenergic receptor blocking agent
Cat Dose: 0.5–2.0 mg/kg PO q8h[4]; 2.5–5.0 mg PO q8h[22]

Selegiline (L-deprenyl) (Anipryl)
Behavior Use: cognitive dysfunction in geriatric animals
Action: irreversible monoamine oxidase inhibitor; two of three metabolites are
    L-amphetamine and L-methamphetamine; therapeutic effects thought to result in
    part from enhanced catecholaminergic nerve function and increased dopamine levels
Cat Dose: 0.5 mg/kg PO q24h in morning[6,7]; 0.25–0.5 mg/kg PO q12–24h, start low[17]

Sertraline (Zoloft)
Behavior Use: compulsive behaviors
Action: selected serotonin uptake inhibitor
Cat Dose: 0.5 mg/kg PO q24 h for 6–8 wk to start[17]

References

1. Beaver BV: Disorders of behavior. In Sherding RG, editor: *The cat: diseases and clinical management,* New York, 1989, Churchill Livingstone.
2. Burghardt WF Jr: Using drugs to control behavior problems in pets, *Vet Med* 86(11):1066, 1068–1071, 1074–1075, 1991.
3. Dodman NH: Pharmacological treatment of behavioral problems in cats, *Vet Forum* pp 62–65, 71, April 1995.
4. Dodman NH, Shuster L: Pharmacologic approaches to managing behavior problems in small animals, *Vet Med* 89(10):960, 1994.
5. Hart BL, Hart LA: *Canine and feline behavioral therapy,* Philadelphia, 1985, Lea & Febiger.
6. Landsberg G: Behavior problems in the geriatric dog and cat, *Friskies PetCare Symposium: Small Animal Behavior Proceedings* pp 37–42, Oct 4, 1998.

7. Landsberg GM: Behavior problems of older cats, *Proc Am Vet Med Assoc* pp 317–320, 1998.

8. Luescher AU: Compulsive behavior in dogs, *Friskies PetCare Symposium: Small Animal Behavior Proceedings* pp 9–18, Oct 4, 1998.

9. Mandelker L: Uncovering many new psychotherapeutic agents, *Vet Forum* p 28, Aug 1990.

10. Marder AR: Psychotropic drugs and behavioral therapy, *Vet Clin North Am Small Anim Pract* 21(2):329–342, 1991.

11. Overall KL: Practical pharmacological approaches to behavior problems, *Purina Specialty Review, Behavioral Problems in Small Animals,* St. Louis, 1992, Purina.

12. Overall KL: Recognition, diagnosis, and management of obsessive-compulsive disorders. Part 1: A rational approach, *Canine Pract* 17(2):40–44, March/April 1992.

13. Overall KL: Recognition, diagnosis, and management of obsessive-compulsive disorders. Part 2: A rational approach, *Canine Pract* 17(3):25–27, May/June 1992.

14. Overall KL: Recognition, diagnosis, and management of obsessive-compulsive disorders. Part 3: A rational approach, *Canine Pract* 17(4):39–43, July/Aug 1992.

15. Overall KL: Prescribing Prozac means taking thorough medical, behavioral history. *DVM* 27(11):2S, 24S, Nov 1996.

16. Overall KL: Pharmacologic treatments for behavior problems, *Vet Clin North Am Small Anim Pract* 27(3):637–665, May 1997.

17. Overall KL: Behavioral pharmacology, *Am Anim Hosp Assoc Proc* pp 65–75, April 2000.

18. Plumb DC: *Veterinary drug handbook,* pocket edition, White Bear Lake, Minn, 1991, PharmaVet Publishing.

19. Schwartz S: Use of cyproheptadine to control urine spraying and masturbation in a cat, *J Am Vet Med Assoc* 214(3):369–371, 1999.

20. Shanley K, Overall K: Psychogenic dermatoses. In Kirk RW, Bonagura JD, eds: *Current veterinary therapy,* ed 11, Philadelphia, 1992, WB Saunders.

21. Shanley K, Overall K: Rational selection of antidepressants for behavioral conditions, *Vet Forum* pp 30, 32–34, Nov 1995.

22. Texas A&M University: Formulary of the Texas A&M University Texas Veterinary Medical Center Veterinary Teaching Hospital. College Station, 1990, Texas A&M University.

23. Voith VL, Marder AR: Feline behavioral disorders. In Morgan RV, ed: *Handbook of small animal practice,* New York, 1988, Churchill Livingstone.

Index

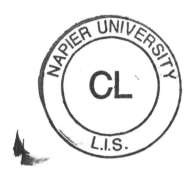

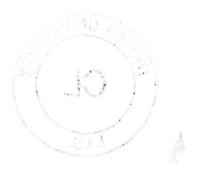